Mortimer

1989.

1989
YEAR BOOK OF
ANESTHESIA®

The 1989 Year Book® Series

Year Book of Anesthesia®: Drs. Miller, Kirby, Ostheimer, Roizen, and Stoelting

Year Book of Cardiology®: Drs. Schlant, Collins, Engle, Frye, Kaplan, and O'Rourke

Year Book of Critical Care Medicine®: Drs. Rogers and Parrillo

Year Book of Dentistry®: Drs. Rose, Hendler, Johnson, Jordan, Moyers, and Silverman

Year Book of Dermatology®: Drs. Sober and Fitzpatrick

Year Book of Diagnostic Radiology®: Drs. Bragg, Hendee, Keats, Kirkpatrick, Miller, Osborn, and Thompson

Year Book of Digestive Diseases®: Drs. Greenberger and Moody

Year Book of Drug Therapy®: Drs. Hollister and Lasagna

Year Book of Emergency Medicine®: Dr. Wagner

Year Book of Endocrinology®: Drs. Bagdade, Braverman, Halter, Horton, Korenman, Kornel, Metz, Molitch, Morley, Rogol, Ryan, Sherwin, and Vaitukaitis

Year Book of Family Practice®: Drs. Rakel, Avant, Driscoll, Prichard, and Smith

Year Book of Geriatrics and Gerontology: Drs. Beck, Abrass, Burton, Cummings, Makinodan, and Small

Year Book of Hand Surgery®: Drs. Dobyns, Chase, and Amadio

Year Book of Hematology®: Drs. Spivak, Bell, Ness, Quesenberry, and Wiernik

Year Book of Infectious Diseases®: Drs. Wolff, Barza, Keusch, Klempner, and Snydman

Year Book of Infertility®: Drs. Mishell, Lobo, and Paulsen

Year Book of Medicine®: Drs. Rogers, Des Prez, Cline, Braunwald, Greenberger, Wilson, Epstein, and Malawista

Year Book of Neurology and Neurosurgery®: Drs. DeJong, Currier, and Crowell

Year Book of Nuclear Medicine®: Drs. Hoffer, Gore, Gottschalk, Sostman, Zaret, and Zubal

Year Book of Obstetrics and Gynecology®: Drs. Mishell, Kirschbaum, and Morrow

Year Book of Oncology®: Drs. Young, Coleman, Longo, Ozols, Simone, and Steele

Year Book of Ophthalmology®: Dr. Laibson

Year Book of Orthopedics®: Dr. Sledge

Year Book of Otolaryngology—Head and Neck Surgery: Drs. Bailey and Paparella

Year Book of Pathology and Clinical Pathology®: Drs. Brinkhous, Dalldorf, Grisham, Langdell, and McLendon

Year Book of Pediatrics®: Drs. Oski and Stockman

Year Book of Perinatal/Neonatal Medicine: Drs. Klaus and Fanaroff

Year Book of Plastic, Reconstructive, and Aesthetic Surgery: Drs. Miller, Bennett, Haynes, Hoehn, McKinney, and Whitaker

Year Book of Podiatric Medicine and Surgery®: Dr. Jay

Year Book of Psychiatry and Applied Mental Health®: Drs. Talbott, Frances, Freedman, Meltzer, Schowalter, and Weiner

Year Book of Pulmonary Disease®: Drs. Green, Ball, Michael, Peters, Terry, Tockman, and Wise

Year Book of Rehabilitation®: Drs. Kaplan, Frank, Gordon, Lieberman, Magnuson, Molnar, Payton,and Sarno

Year Book of Sports Medicine®: Drs. Shephard, Sutton, and Torg, Col. Anderson, and Mr. George

Year Book of Surgery®: Drs. Schwartz, Jonasson, Peacock, Shires, Spencer, and Thompson

Year Book of Urology®: Drs. Gillenwater and Howards

Year Book of Vascular Surgery®: Drs. Bergan and Yao

1989
The Year Book of
ANESTHESIA®

Editor
Ronald D. Miller, M.D.
Professor and Chairman of Anesthesia and Professor of Pharmacology, Department of Anesthesia, University of California, San Francisco

Associate Editors
Robert R. Kirby, M.D.
Professor of Anesthesiology, University of Florida College of Medicine, Gainesville
Gerard W. Ostheimer, M.D.
Associate Professor of Anaesthesia, Harvard Medical School; Vice Chairman, Department of Anesthesia, Brigham and Women's Hospital, Boston
Michael F. Roizen, M.D.
Professor and Chairperson, Department of Anesthesia and Critical Care; Professor of Medicine, University of Chicago
Robert K. Stoelting, M.D.
Professor and Chairman, Department of Anesthesia, Indiana University School of Medicine, Indianapolis

Year Book Medical Publishers, Inc.
Chicago • London • Boca Raton

Printed in U.S.A.

International Standard Book Number: 0-8151-5935-8

International Standard Serial Number: 0084-3652

Editor-in-Chief, Year Book Publishing: Nancy Gorham
Sponsoring Editor: Gretchen Murphy
Manager, Medical Information Services: Laura J. Shedore
Assistant Director, Manuscript Services: Frances M. Perveiler
Assistant Managing Editor, Year Book Editing Services: Wayne Larsen
Production Coordinator: Max F. Perez
Proofroom Manager: Shirley E. Taylor

Table of Contents

The material covered in this volume represents literature reviewed through October 1988.

Journals Represented

Year Book Medical Publishers subscribes to and surveys more than 700 U.S. and foreign medical and allied health journals. From these journals, the Editors select the articles to be abstracted. Journals represented in this YEAR BOOK are listed below.

Acta Anaesthesiologica Scandinavica
Acta Chirurgica Scandinavica
Acta Obstetricia et Gynecologica Scandinavica
Age and Ageing
American Journal of Cardiology
American Journal of Medicine
American Journal of Obstetrics and Gynecology
American Journal of Perinatology
American Journal of Surgery
American Surgeon
Anaesthesist
Anesthesia
Anesthesia and Intensive Care
Anesthesia and Analgesia
Anesthesiology
Annales Chirurgiae et Gynaecologiae
Annals of Emergency Medicine
Annals of Internal Medicine
Annals of Otology, Rhinology and Laryngology
Annals of the Royal College of Surgeons of England
Annals of Surgery
Annals of Thoracic Surgery
Archives of Emergency Medicine
Archives of Internal Medicine
Archives of Neurology
Archives of Pathology and Laboratory Medicine
Archives of Surgery
Blood
British Journal of Anaesthesia
British Journal of Haematology
British Journal of Surgery
British Medical Journal
Canadian Journal of Anaesthesia
Canadian Medical Association Journal
Chest
Child Development
Circulation
Clinical Allergy
Clinical Orthopaedics and Related Research
Clinical Pediatrics
Clinical Pharmacology and Therapeutics
Convulsive Therapy
Critical Care Medicine
Developmental Medicine and Child Neurology
Diabetic Medicine
Diseases of the Colon and Rectum
European Journal of Anaesthesiology
Infections in Surgery

Intensive Care Medicine
International Surgery
Journal of Allergy and Clinical Immunology
Journal of the American Medical Association
Journal of Anesthesia
Journal of Cardiovascular Surgery
Journal of Clinical Anaesthesia
Journal of Clinical Epidemiology
Journal of Clinical Monitoring
Journal of Emergency Medicine
Journal of Laboratory and Clinical Medicine
Journal of Obstetrics and Gynaecology
Journal of Oral and Maxillofacial Surgery
Journal of Pediatric Orthopedics
Journal of Pediatric Surgery
Journal of Pediatrics
Journal of Thoracic and Cardiovascular Surgery
Journal of Trauma
Journal of Urology
Lancet
Life Sciences
Mayo Clinic Proceedings
Middle East Journal of Anesthesiology
Neurosurgery
New England Journal of Medicine
New York State Journal of Medicine
Obstetrics and Gynecology
Pain
Patient Education and Counseling
Pediatric Pathology
Postgraduate Medicine
Radiology
Regional Anesthesia
Science
Southern Medical Journal
Surgery
Surgery, Gynecology and Obstetrics
Thrombosis and Haemostasis

Introduction

The 1989 YEAR BOOK OF ANESTHESIA contains a wide spectrum of anesthesia-related articles from various specialties and journals worldwide. Overall, we have attempted to select those articles that may have the greatest importance in relation to the scientific and clinical basis of anesthesia practice. We also attempted to select those articles that are especially important to anesthesiologists even though they may not directly affect anesthesia practice. Although many of our articles were selected from anesthesia journals, we attempted to emphasize those journals that may not be widely read by anesthesiologists.

The 1989 YEAR BOOK OF ANESTHESIA has an emphasis different from that of the 1988 YEAR BOOK OF ANESTHESIA. This year, additional emphasis has been placed on the "outcome" type of studies; techniques are now being developed that will allow us to actually determine the short- and long-term effects of our anesthetic and surgical management. Because of the epidemic of acquired immunodeficiency syndrome (AIDS) there has been an increased awareness of health care worker protection, which is emphasized in this edition. Methods of providing analgesia in the postoperative period have been markedly improved during the last 5–10 years. This is reflected in the heavy emphasis in the 1989 YEAR BOOK on such techniques as epidural narcotics, patient-controlled analgesia, and transcutaneous electrical nerve stimulation. In the acid-base arena, the use of bicarbonate for cardiopulmonary resuscitation is constantly being evaluated. These represent only a few areas that have been discussed in the 1989 YEAR BOOK OF ANESTHESIA.

Several areas have received less emphasis this year; these include nutrition in critical care medicine, aspiration of gastric contents, and various subspecialties of anesthesia. We presume that our selections reflect a change in the overall emphasis of the literature. The reader should be reassured that we are constantly evaluating the many journals listed in the section "Journals Represented" to select those articles that we believe best cover the broad spectrum of clinical and scientific literature as it relates to anesthesia.

Ronald D. Miller, M.D.

1 The Informed Anesthesiologist

Outcome

Does Anesthesia Contribute to Operative Mortality?
Cohen MM, Duncan PG, Tate RB (Univ of Manitoba, Univ of Saskatchewan)
JAMA 260:2859–2863, Nov 18, 1988   1–1

Studies of surgical mortality have generally not included anesthesia as a possible risk factor for postoperative deaths. Recent studies of operative mortality from an anesthesia perspective did not control simultaneously for patient case-mix or surgical factors. The prospectively collected data from a large anesthesia follow-up study and vital statistics data were used to assess the role of anesthesia in operative deaths.

The study material consisted of data pertaining to 100,000 anesthetic administrations. Patient, surgical, anesthesia, and other factors were assessed using logistic regression analysis to determine which variables were predictive of death occurring within 7 days of the operative procedure.

The overall 7-day mortality rate was 71.40 per 10,000 anesthetics administered. Mortality increased with advanced age and showed a marked increase for patients older than age 80 years. Men had nearly twice the mortality of women. Physical status was a powerful predictor of postoperative mortality: mortality for normal, healthy patients was extremely low. Mortality for patients who were not expected to survive was 3,358 per 10,000 anesthetics. About one third of these patients died within 7 days of operation.

Other factors associated with increased mortality included major surgery, emergency procedures, procedures performed between 1975 and 1979, intraoperative complications, narcotic techniques, and having received only 1 or 2 anesthetic drugs. However, duration of anesthesia, experience of the anesthesiologist, and inhalation anesthesia techniques were not significantly associated with increased 7-day mortality.

Patient-related preoperative characteristics and surgery-related factors were more important in predicting mortality than were anesthesia-related factors. The low mortality found in this study reflects favorably on the effectiveness of modern anesthesia practices.

▶ Outcome studies are becoming increasingly important. This was an excellent study, which can serve as a model for what many other institutions should be doing.— R.D. Miller, M.D.

1

Evaluating Surgical Risk: The Importance of Technical Factors in Determining Outcome

Pettigrew RA, Burns HJG, Carter DC (Glasgow Royal Infirmary, Glasgow, Scotland)
J Surg 74:791–794, September 1987 1–2

Preoperative nutritional support seems to decrease postoperative morbidity and mortality. However, many surgeons remain skeptical of the place of prognostic formulas in clinical practice. Surgeons do recognize that many of the complications that occur after surgery are operator-dependent. Whether the technical aspects of surgery that contribute to a poor outcome can be quantified was studied.

One hundred thirteen patients undergoing elective alimentary resection were examined prospectively. The relationship of preoperative clinical and nutritional assessment to the development of major postoperative complications was evaluated. The operating surgeon also made a risk assessment on a linear analog scale before and immediately after surgery. Major complications developed in 25% of patients. Age, weight loss, and relative weight did not identify high-risk patients, but patients with a serum albumin level of less than 29 gm/L had significantly more complications than did those with higher levels. Clinical assessment identified some high-risk patients, but patients selected by the surgeon's preoperative assessment did not have significantly more complications than did those not selected. However, the surgeon's postoperative assessment was selective of patients at significantly increased risk. The surgeons changed their rankings postoperatively for 44 patients; in 36 cases, the reason given was the technical ease or difficulty of the procedure. Immediate postoperative assessment was better than any preoperative method of selecting high-risk patients.

Operative performance is the main factor in the development of postoperative complications. Operative performance should be assessed in future studies of outcome.

▶ It is clear that technically poor surgery can result in poor outcomes, and that's what this study shows. One wonders whether the postoperative assessment was surgeon-specific, and it's not clear how many different surgeons participated in this study. Clearly, when the surgeon changed his assessment of the patient's risk after surgery, that change was a very important factor in predicting outcome. The technical ease or difficulty of the procedure made the surgeon change his assessment of risk. Operating is a technical skill acquired during training and developed with experience, and most surgeons recognize that technical difficulties apparent at the time of operation have an important influence on outcome.

The major flaw in this study is that the roles of anesthesia and of the anesthetist are ignored. Perhaps the surgeons had uniformly good anesthesia, in which case one would only have to comment that great anesthesia can't save poor surgery, or perhaps there was a range of anesthesia quality (much like the range of surgical quality), and this confounding variable ended up causing the poor predictability that the surgeons experienced. One would only hope that future studies in this field would include assessment by the anesthesiologist, especially the anesthesiologist who knows which surgeon will operate and the surgical predictability in advance.—M.F. Roizen, M.D.

Pregnancy Outcome in Medically Complicated and Uncomplicated Patients Aged 40 Years or Older
Lehmann DK, Chism J (Tulane Univ)
Am J Obstet Gynecol 157:738–742, September 1987   1–3

Previous studies have had disparate findings as to the effects of increasing maternal age on the outcome of pregnancy. The hypothesis that increased complications in older mothers could be attributed to medical disorders antedating the pregnancy or to high parity rather than to advanced maternal age as such was examined in 183 women aged at least 40 years with a gestation of at least 20 weeks at the time of delivery. Sixteen patients were aged 45 years or more. Hospital records were evaluated and any readmission within 42 days was reviewed for the possibility of delayed complications. Patients were subgrouped on the basis of the presence or absence of medical disorders before pregnancy. A subgroup of patients of low parity comprised those who were para 2 or fewer at the time of delivery.

The average patient age was 41 years 7 months. At the time of admission for delivery, 150 patients were at least para 3. Preeclampsia, premature labor, precipitate labor, and malpresentation were significantly more common in the study group than in younger patients. Serious postpartum morbidity was relatively common, and the rate of vaginal delivery was significantly decreased. There was a significant increase in the incidence of stillbirth, abnormal birth weight, and perinatal mortality. Among the subgroups there were some differences in the type and frequency of complications, but all subgroups had higher complication rates than were found in the general obstetric population.

Women considering pregnancy after the age of 40 years should be advised of the increased risk of maternal and fetal complications. After age 40 the outcome is more likely to be unfavorable, even when the patient is of low parity and in good general health.

▶ This study complements a recent study that demontrated that there was increased maternal mortality among obstetric patients 35 years or older (Buehler et al: *JAMA* 255:53–57, 1986). The complication of deep venous thrombosis and pulmonary emboli was found in this study and was recently reported to be the major cause of maternal mortality over a 30-year period in the Commonwealth of Massachusetts. Your editor feels that the number of older women desiring pregnancy and therefore having the complications of pregnancy will in-

crease in the future as women delay having children for a variety of reasons.—
G.W. Ostheimer, M.D.

Regional Anaesthesia and Surgical Morbidity
Scott NB, Kehlet H (Hvidovre Univ Hosp, Hvidovre, Denmark)
Br J Surg 75:299–304, April 1988   1–4

A better understanding of postsurgical metabolic effects, together with rapid expansion of anesthetic knowledge and technique, have led to the concept of stress-free anesthesia. Proponents of this concept believe that the morbidity of surgery may not only result from imperfections in perioperative technique, but also from the body's metabolic stress response to the trauma of anesthesia and surgery. Regional anesthesia (RA) is currently considered the most effective way to reduce this stress response. The results of studies done to examine the influence of RA on surgical morbidity were reviewed. In this context, the use of RA does not imply operating on a conscious patient: in some studies patients were also given a light general anesthesia (GA) during surgery. Results of several studies have suggested that the moderating effect of RA on surgical morbidity is not affected by the addition of GA.

Because the mortality of modern elective surgery is low, large numbers of patients need to be studied before any benefit of a particular anesthesia regimen can be documented. Most published studies do not contain enough patients for a definite conclusion. To study the effect of anesthesia on mortality, the data of 12 existing controlled mortality studies that compared RA with GA in patients undergoing acute hip surgery were pooled for meta-analysis. For this body of pooled data, the early mortality in the RA group was 6.9%, and in the GA group, 10.3%. The difference was statistically significant.

Similarly, the data of other studies were pooled to compare the effects of RA and GA on the incidence of postoperative morbidity, including pulmonary infections, cardiac and gastrointestinal complications, immunocompetence, infective complications, blood loss, thromboembolism, cerebral function, duration of convalescence, and length of hospital stay.

Analysis of the various data bases constructed by pooling the data of existing controlled studies indicates that RA appears to reduce morbidity for operative procedures performed below the umbilicus. However, the evidence is not so clear for operations performed in the upper abdomen and thorax where it is coincidentally not possible to prevent the stress response.

By combining the data from different trials, the criteria to perform such a meta-analysis have not been fulfilled in all morbidity parameters considered in this study, with the exception of blood loss and mortality after hip surgery. Future studies of the stress-reducing effect of RA should therefore focus on specific operative procedures in well-defined patient populations.

▶ Bottom line: With the exception of a reduced morbidity for operative procedures performed below the umbilicus, the jury is still out on whether regional anesthesia is more efficacious in reducing the stress response in procedures above the umbilicus. Though we may never know the definitive answer, the efforts of surgeons and anesthesiologists to provide a stress-free or reduced-stress environment for the surgical procedure has tremendous merit. Only by a concentrated multidisciplinary approach will we be able to ascertain what is the best technique or techniques for the patient undergoing varying types of surgery.—G.W. Ostheimer, M.D.

Computer Records

The Computer-Stored Medical Record: For Whom?
Korpman RA, Lincoln TL (San Bernardino, Calif; Los Angeles)
JAMA 259:3454–3456, June 17, 1988   1–5

Computer automation facilitates the storage and retrieval of medical records. However, different branches of a medical institution have different information needs, and designing a computer-stored medical record (CSMR) data base that satisfies all end-users' needs for information is complex. Most development of CSMR data bases has evolved around the needs of hospitals; they generate the most data, have the sickest patients, and are associated with the most providers having a need for clinical data.

In today's cost-containing environment, many patients are cared for outside the hospital, in hospital-affiliated nursing homes, outpatient kidney dialysis centers, or other outpatient facilities. Any design of a CSMR data base should not only consider hospital-generated patient data but also allow for inclusion of and access to patient data generated by all the ancillary services.

However, each organized unit of care delivery protects its own unique requirements. Consequently, fragmented political interests have hampered the integrated approach to designing a unified data base structure for automated clinical record keeping. Until all involved parties realize that an integrated approach to automated clinical record keeping could significantly contribute to the quality of patient care while enhancing the effectiveness and efficiency of service, the design of a multipurpose information system will remain burdensome.

Computer-Stored Medical Records: Their Future Role in Medical Practice
McDonald CJ, Tierney WM (Indiana Univ)
JAMA 259:3433–3440, June 17, 1988   1–6

The increasing capabilities and lower cost of computers today, as well as third-party incentives to store medical information, will make computer storage of records more technically and economically feasible in the coming years. Many vendors of hospital data and billing systems are presently developing medical record modules. Hybrid systems of both computer and paper record keeping, which obtain data from existing ancillary service systems, soon will be widely available, and totally computerized record keeping will follow.

Computer-stored medical records solve many of the logistical problems involved in locating, organizing, and reporting patient information. Data are readily organized into special reports, flow sheets, or various types of specialized display. Reports may be tailored to a particular clinical context. Computerized systems can enhance physician decision making by performing difficult calculations and identifying clinical events requiring attention. These computer-based reminder systems have significantly benefited patient care. Finally, computerized systems are able to help guide future policies and practices by analyzing past clinical experience in a hospital or a physician's office.

Standards for exchanging clinical information between independent computers will elminate reentry or interfacing costs. Although storing all of the medical record is appealing, this may not be feasible for existing facilities. Hybrid systems can provide rapid access and useful organization of parts of the record, as well as retrieval, statistical analysis, and patient reminders. Eventually computers will directly transcribe the physician's voice messages into text, providing a more efficient system at lower cost.

▶ Most of us have bemoaned the day when we have had to repeat the history and physical on a patient who already had a history and physical and who was seen a long time before by another anesthesiologist. Wouldn't it be nice if we could call up that information and see that record of the previous anesthetic, see the previous history, get just an interval history from the patient to be able to evaluate him or her, and have all that done for us on a neatly printed computer sheet? Well, that's what the future holds, but there are many limitations to such a system at this time. The benefits are improved logistics and organization of the medical record to speed care and improve care giver's efficiency, automatic review of the medical record to limit errors and control costs, and systematic analysis to guide future practices and policies, as well as higher quality of care for the patient. What is driving the advent of the computer medical record is not these factors, though, but the wish for people to look at our individual quality of care and to assess outcome based on co-morbidity.

I believe it is in our best interest to take a lead role in instituting such a system so that the record will contain information that we as anesthesiologists believe is important to our patient's outcome and to assessment of us as anesthesiologists. Otherwise, it will be done and the assessment of us as anesthesiologists may not involve anything meaningful to the practice of anesthesia, I'm afraid.—M.F. Roizen, M.D.

Acquired Immunodeficiency Syndrome (AIDS): General and Blood Transfusion

Legal Limits of AIDS Confidentiality
Dickens BM (Univ of Toronto)
JAMA 259:3449–3451, June 17, 1988   1–7

Health care workers have a legitimate interest in knowing who is liable to transmit human immunodeficiency virus (HIV) infection. When they demand disclosure of those who have acquired immunodeficiency syndrome (AIDS), AIDS-related complex, or positive test results, hospital and public health officials come under pressure to disclose the information, even if it is necessary to compromise patients' rights to confidentiality. Some feel that, if disclosure is likely, those most in need of testing will not submit to it. There also is concern that persons tested during incubation of the AIDS virus will mistakenly be reported as negative.

The Supreme Court has confirmed that the protective privilege ends where public peril begins. If victims are identified, they have a right to be warned. And if they are not identifiable, warning of others, such as the police, may be legally necessary. In this circumstance, the police have the right to detain infected persons under quarantine provisions. Conscientious disclosure of test results is permissible even if the results prove to be falsely positive. However, disclosure should be restricted to those persons whose interests are threatened.

The law cannot be relied on to limit breaches of confidentiality, because so much in the law justifies and even compels disclosure of information. At the same time, members of risk groups, already subject to considerable discrimination, will not seek testing or help from public agencies unless reassured that they will not face hostile responses and a loss of liberty. This is more to the point than an exclusive concern about confidentiality. To contain the spread of AIDS, it will be necessary to reach and educate high-risk populations and make it possible for them to protect themselves and others.

▶ This is a very interesting article by a lawyer who cites case after case in which the legal responsibility to protect others is, in every case, decided to be higher than that of protecting confidentiality. In fact, as he cites from a major decision called *Tarasoff vs. Regents of the University of California,* the protective privilege (of AIDS confidentiality) ends where the public peril begins. Particularly if victims are identifiable, they are owed a duty by the physician to be warned. If the individuals are unidentifiable, warning to others, such as the police, is often legally required. It is of no consequence that the goal of the mandated protection of confidentiality, namely, to encourage recourse to professional care in the pubic interest, is thereby compromised. The author of this article goes on to say that, aware of their liability to suffer discrimination, members of these populations will not seek testing or help from public agencies unless reassured that they will not be further isolated by hostile responses and loss of liberties; more is likely to be gained by enacting and enforcing protection against discrimination in crucial areas for those affected persons whose identities are likely to become known.

This is the first time I've seen it spelled out that, for the protection of others, the physician has a responsibility to disclose HIV status, despite it being mandated in a specific law that you can't disclose HIV status. The article states that the courts have constantly held the responsibility to disclose for others' protection is a "higher" responsibility than the protective privilege of nondisclosure.— M.F. Roizen, M.D.

Documentation of an AIDS Virus Infection in the United States in 1968
Garry RF, Witte MH, Gottlieb AA, Elvin-Lewis M, Gottlieb MS, Witte CL, Alexander SS, Cole WR, Drake WL Jr (Tulane Univ; Univ of Arizona; Washington Univ; Biotech Research Labs, Inc, Rockville, Md; Univ of Missouri; et al)
JAMA 260:2085–2087, Oct 14, 1988   1–8

The acquired immunodeficiency syndrome (AIDS) has been recognized as a clinical entity in the United States since the early 1980s. Previous studies have suggested that the strain of the human immunodeficiency virus (HIV) responsible for the current epidemic was newly imported into the United States in the late 1970s from Central Africa, possibly via the Caribbean. However, the issue of when HIV was first introduced into at-risk populations in the United States remains unresolved.

In a previously published paper, a 15-year-old black adolescent male was described whose history bears on the origin of AIDS in the United States. This patient had been admitted in 1968 with extensive lymphedema of the genitalia and lower extremities. Chlamydial organisms were widely disseminated and isolated from numerous body fluids and organs. His condition deteriorated progressively over a 16-month period; at the time of death, the patient was severely wasted. Autopsy revealed the presence of Kaposi's sarcoma.

Later reexamination of preserved tissue sections indicated that the Kaposi's sarcoma was indistinguishable from the aggressive, disseminated type characteristic of that in contemporary AIDS patients. Because more sensitive and specific tests for the presence of antibodies specific for HIV and HIV antigens are now available, the serum and autopsy specimens of this patient, which had been frozen since his death in 1969, were reexamined.

Western blot and antigen capture assays revealed that the patient was infected with a virus that was either closely related or identical to HIV type 1. These findings add to other available clinical and immunologic evidence that an immunosuppressive retrovirus already existed in the United States before the late 1970s. It is suggested that, if a virus related to HIV has been present in the United States, Africa, or elsewhere for several decades, its failure to spread earlier may represent either a recent genetic change in the virus, a change in sociocultural factors involving sexual practices or numbers of sexual partners, or both.

▶ This article is useful for those individuals interested in the development of the AIDS problem in the United States.—R.D. Miller, M.D.

Risk of AIDS for Recipients of Blood Components From Donors Who Subsequently Developed AIDS
Perkins HA, Samson S, Garner J, Echenberg D, Allen JR, Cowan M, Levy JA (Irwin Mem Blood Bank, San Francisco; San Francisco Dept of Public Health; Ctrs for Disease Control, Atlanta; Univ of California, San Francisco)
Blood 70:1604–1610, November 1987   1–9

The risk of becoming infected with human immunodeficiency virus (HIV) and of contracting acquired immunodeficiency syndrome (AIDS) in recipients of blood components from donors who subsequently contracted AIDS was investigated. As of March 31, 1986, in San Francisco, 92 individuals who had donated blood subsequent to 1978 contracted AIDS. In all, 406 persons had received blood components from these individuals. Of the 336 recipients whose current status was known as of April 1, 1986, 223 had died as a result of the condition for which they were transfused; 7 had contracted AIDS, 5 of whom died, 2 before entry into the study and 3 subsequently. Of the 46 living recipients who did not have AIDS, 7 had AIDS-related complex (ARC), 19 had antibody to HIV but were otherwise healthy, and 19 had no detectable anti-HIV. Two had risk factors other than transfusion.

In general, recipients who contracted AIDS received more blood components than did those with ARC, anti-HIV only, or no evidence of infection, but the difference is not significant if a single atypical case is omitted. The frequency of infection of the recipient decreased as the time interval increased between transfusion and the diagnosis of AIDS in the donor.

These data indicate that recipients of blood components from donors who later contract AIDS are at relatively high risk of themselves contracting AIDS or of being infected with HIV. The shorter the interval between transfusion and onset of AIDS in the donor, the more likely it is that AIDS, as well as infection with HIV, will occur.

▶ This information speaks for itself. This is the famous "look back" study, which provides some very useful information regarding the epidemiology of transfusion-induced AIDS.—R.D. Miller, M.D.

Acquired Immunodeficiency Syndrome and Directed Blood Donations: A Dilemma for American Medicine
Kruskall MS, Umlas J (Beth Israel Hosp, Boston; Mount Auburn Hosp, Cambridge, Mass; Harvard Univ)
Arch Surg 123:23–25, January 1988   1–10

The incidence of transfusion-associated acquired immunodeficiency syndrome (TA-AIDS) is low, but the devastating nature of the disease has prompted action to reduce the risk even further. Although careful donor screening and antibody testing have substantially improved the safety of the blood supply, some physicians and patients favor a "directed-donor" approach, whereby the patient recruits a selected individual to be the donor. However, because the incidence of TA-AIDS is already so low, there is no evidence that recipient-selected donors would be less likely to carry the AIDS virus than nonselected donors. In addition, this proposal implies significant medical, ethical, and logistic problems.

For example, the directed donor would not be anonymous, and both the donor and the hospital might lose legal protection if the patient were to contract an illness or experience complications from the blood product. Further, donors would not be immune from coercion, and designated donors might be paid to donate. Other potential pitfalls include the question of who owns the rights to the blood should the hospital desire to use it for another patient in an emergency, the ethical question of a double standard in which blood from designated recipients is thought to be superior to blood from volunteer donors, the possibility that volunteer donations might dwindle, and the logistics of labeling and segregating recipient-designated blood. A directed-donor program might also be used by the collecting institution as a marketing device for its facility.

Directed-donor programs should not be permitted. Physicians would be better advised to make patients aware of the relative safety of the products already available and to use medically sound procedures for safer transfusion therapy.

▶ Although there is an inherent belief that directed or designated blood donations should be safer, they clearly have not proven to be so. This probably means that we do not know our friends and relatives as well as we think we do. Plus, there are many disadvantages of the designated blood program, which are nicely outlined in this article.—R.D. Miller, M.D.

Transmission of Human Immunodeficiency Virus (HIV) by Blood Transfusions Screened as Negative for HIV Antibody
Ward JW, Holmberg SD, Allen JR, Cohn DL, Critchley SE, Kleinman SH, Lenes BA, Ravenholt O, Davis JR, Quinn MG, Jaffe HW (Ctrs for Disease Control, Atlanta; Denver Disease Control Service; American Red Cross Blood Service, Atlanta, Los Angeles, Miami; Clark County Health District, Las Vegas; Central Blood Bank–South Bend Med Found, South Bend, Ind; et al)
N Engl J Med 318:473–478, Feb 25, 1988   1–11

Some persons at risk for human immunodeficiency virus (HIV) donate blood, and not all infected donors are detected through tests for HIV antibody. Reported instances of HIV transmission from screened antibody-negative donors were investigated to discover why these donors were not identified.

Thirteen persons seropositive for HIV had received transfusions from 7 donors screened as negative for HIV antibody. With the exception of the transfusions, 12 of the 13 recipients had no identifiable risk factors, but at follow-up, after 8–12 months, 3 had HIV-related illnesses and 1 had acquired immunodeficiency syndrome. All 7 donors were infected with HIV. Six reported a risk factor for HIV infection, and 5 had engaged in high-risk activities or had a previous illness indicative of an acute retroviral syndrome within 4 months of seronegative HIV testing.

These donors apparently had been infected recently before the time of screening and therefore tested negative on available antibody tests when blood was donated. Thus there is a small but identifiable risk of HIV infection for recipients of transfusions, even when blood is screened. Educational policies should emphasize the need for deferral in donors who engage in high-risk behavior. New tests that detect HIV infection earlier are desirable.

▶ Although this article indicates that the human immunodeficiency virus can be transmitted by blood transfusions that were originally screened as negative for the HIV antibody, the infectivity rate has decreased markedly. In the San Francisco Bay Area, the incidence of hepatitis has decreased to about 2% to 4% and the incidence of transfusion-induced AIDS has decreased dramatically. Now the estimate is that the risk of contracting AIDS from a blood transfusion is about 1:50,000. Therefore, the blood supply is probably safer than it has been in the last 20 years in regard to overall infectivity. The development of an antigen-based test should eliminate the so-called "window."—R.D. Miller, M.D.

Seroprevalence and Epidemiological Correlates of HTLV-I Infection in U.S. Blood Donors
Williams AE, Fang CT, Slamon DJ, Poiesz BJ, Sandler SG, Darr WF II, Shulman G, McGowan EI, Douglas DK, Bowman RJ, Peetoom F, Kleinman SH, Lenes B, Dodd RY (American Red Cross Jerome H Holland Lab, Rockville, Md; Univ of California, Los Angeles; State Univ of New York, Syracuse; American Red Cross Blood Services, Washington, DC, Atlanta; et al)
Science 240:643–646, Apr 29, 1988   1–12

After isolation of virus from patients with adult T-cell leukemia/lymphoma (ATL) and extensive cross-sectional serologic studies of ATL patients, human T-lymphotropic virus type I (HTLV-I) was conclusively identified as the causative agent of ATL. An association between HTLV-I antibodies and ATL was shown within distinct geographic clusters in southwestern Japan, Africa, and the Caribbean basin. Several other retrospective studies, conducted in Japan among donor-recipient pairs, suggested that HTLV-I can be transmitted from infected blood donors to recipients of cellular blood products. There is also evidence that HTLV-I infection is currently endemic in intravenous drug abusers residing in certain urban areas of the eastern United States.

Because of a concern that there could be asymptomatic HTLV-I carriers in the United States blood donor pool who could contribute to the introduction of HTLV-I into populations in which the infection is not endemic, the sera from 39,898 blood donors at 8 blood centers in geographically distinct areas were screened for the presence of HTLV-I antibodies.

Enzyme immunoassay identified 10 donors (0.025%) who had evidence of HTLV-I seropositivity, which was confirmed by protein immunoblot and radioimmunoprecipitation. Antibodies to HTLV-I were found predominantly in donors from the southeastern and southwestern United States. Seven of the 10 seropositive individuals, 5 women and 2 men, were interviewed; 4 reported intravenous drug abuse or sexual contact with an intravenous drug user. Sexual contact with native inhabitants of an HTLV-I endemic area was the only identified risk factor in 1 man.

These results suggest that testing for HTLV-I markers in blood donors may be necessary to prevent the spread of HTLV-I to transfusion recipients.

▶ Very soon all blood banks will be automatically testing for the presence of HTLV-I and eliminating positive-testing units of blood.— R.D. Miller, M.D.

Resident Training

Assessment of Surgical Residents' Competence Based on Postoperative Complications

Haddad M, Zelikovski A, Gutman H, Haddad E, Reiss R (Beilinson Med Ctr, Petah Tiqva; Tel Aviv Univ, Tel Aviv, Israel)
Int Surg 72:230–232, October–December 1987   1–13

Many methods have been developed for evaluating the competence of surgical residents. The surgical residents' operative skills were evaluated in a prospective study on the assumption that differences in training may have a significant effect on postoperative complications. Using a departmental microcomputer and a special noncommercial personally developed software program, 691 surgical procedures were monitored in a general surgery department having a vascular unit. Of these, 61% were performed by a senior surgeon; 37%, by a resident; and 2%, by an intern.

In the 207 minor operations performed by the junior staff, the complication rate was 6.3%; in the 170 performed by the senior staff, the complication rate was 8.8%; the difference was not significant. In matched operative groups, there was no significant clinical difference in the postoperative complication rate between those operated on by a senior staff member and those operated on by a resident. Close supervision by the senior staff may have influenced this outcome. Analysis of subgroups showed that, among the moderate to severely complicated procedures, the rate of postoperative complications was significantly higher for operations performed by the senior staff, possibly reflecting the inherently more complex operative problems dealt with by the senior staff and the preselection of poor-risk patients for treatment by these surgeons.

Because of the inherent practice of bias against the senior staff in case selection, assessment of surgical residents' competence based on postoperative complications is not a practical method of evaluating their surgical competence.

▶ Is this a reasonable approach with anesthesiologists both in training and in practice?—R.D. Miller, M.D.

The Effects of Acute Sleep Deprivation During Residency Training
Bartle EJ, Sun JH, Thompson L, Light AI, McCool C, Heaton S (Univ of Colorado Health Sciences Ctr, Denver)
Surgery 104:311–316, August 1988   1–14

Previous studies suggested that acute sleep deprivation can seriously affect the judgment and performance of interns and residents in training. However, those studies are now outdated, as internship and residency are even more difficult and stressful in the 1980s than they were in the past. To reevaluate the effects of sleep deprivation on house staff members, the performance of surgical residents who performed a battery of neuropsychologic tests when fatigued and when rested was studied.

All surgical residents were invited to take a battery of 8 tests that assessed verbal and symbol concentration, learning, problem solving, clear thinking, manual skills, and memory, and to complete a questionnaire on mood states. Tests and questionnaires were completed both when fatigued and when rested, with at least 7 days between tests. To eliminate the effects of learning from the first test series, the residents were randomized so that one half were first evaluated when rested and one half, when fatigued. Only the effects of acute sleep deprivation, defined as less than 4 hours of sleep, were evaluated because residents in general become used to chronic sleep deprivation.

Forty-two of the 50 residents who had been invited to participate in the study completed the tests. Analysis of the data showed that, although residents were less energetic and more fatigued, depressed, anxious, confused, and angry with less than 4 hours sleep than when in a rested state, their responses on all of the functional tests did not differ between states, and sleep deprivation, no matter what the amount, was not associated with impaired performance.

Although acute sleep deprivation alters mood state, it does not change performance in test situations in which concentration, clear thinking, and problem solving are important.

▶ The issue of resident working hours is complex and open to many distorted interpretations. There is no doubt, however, that inadequate sleep may impair physician judgment and ability. In anesthesia, the maintenance of vigilance seems particularly vulnerable to sleep deprivation, especially when the "stable" state of anesthesia is achieved. An airline pilot who had not slept for 24 hours would not be allowed to fly. It is increasingly difficult for physicians to justify working without sleep.—R.K. Stoelting, M.D.

2 Pharmacology

Inhaled Anesthetics

Attenuation of Endothelium-Mediated Vasodilation by Halothane

Muldoon SM, Hart JL, Bowen KA, Freas W (Uniformed Services Univ of the Health Sciences, Bethesda, Md; George Mason Univ)
Anesthesiology 68:31–37, January 1988
2–1

The vascular endothelium modulates vascular smooth muscle activity through several mechanisms. Because halothane reportedly causes vasodilation, the effects of halothane on endothelium-mediated vascular smooth muscle vasodilation were studied using isolated ring preparations of rabbit aorta and canine femoral and carotid arteries. Isometric tension was recorded in Krebs-Ringer bicarbonate solution at 37 C.

Acetylcholine and bradykinin relax norepinephrine-contracted arteries by an endothelium-dependent process. These relaxing effects were reversibly attenuated by 2% halothane, but halothane did not affect nitroglycerin-induced relaxation, an endothelium-independent phenomenon. During norepinephrine-induced contractions, halothane decreased tension in the canine carotid artery and rabbit aorta but increased tension in the femoral artery rings. These effects were unchanged after removal of the endothelium.

A direct action of halothane on vascular smooth muscle is suggested by these findings. Tension may increase or decrease, depending on the specific vessel. If halothane interferes with endothelium-derived relaxing factor-mediated relaxation of vascular smooth muscle, this may contribute to the vascular changes seen clinically during halothane administration. In vitro studies support in vivo indications of regional heterogeneity of vascular responses to halothane.

▶ Although this study does not provide any information that would be useful clinically, it does provide useful information regarding the mechanism of the vascular changes caused by halothane anesthesia.—R.D. Miller, M.D.

Comparison of the Effects of Subanaesthetic Concentrations of Isoflurane or Nitrous Oxide in Volunteers

McMenemin IM, Parbrook GD (Royal Infirmary, Glasgow, Scotland)
Br J Anaesth 60:56–63, 1988
2–2

Nitrous oxide is a useful sedative when used in subanesthetic concentrations, but its specific effects on vitamin B_{12} metabolism and amino acids can produce toxicity in patients after prolonged use. Isoflurane has a rapid uptake and excretion and undergoes minimal metabolism, and its long-term use is associated with few after-effects and lack of toxicity. Subanesthetic concentrations of isoflurane and nitrous oxide were compared in volunteers.

Twelve volunteers were given 25% nitrous oxide or 0.4% isoflurane, breathed for 20 minutes. Oxygen served as a control. Effects were observed for 35 minutes after the drugs were given. Choice reaction time, ability to tap 2 areas on a board, and ability to do mathematical problems were significantly impaired when inhaling nitrous oxide. With isoflurane, the effects were found to be significantly greater than with nitrous oxide. Isoflurane obtained its maximum effects after 15 minutes of inhalation, whereas the maximum effects of nitrous oxide were obtained after 5 minutes. After discontinuation of the test agent, levels returned promptly to base-line values. Subjective assessment of physical and mental sedation indicated that 0.4% isoflurane was more potent than 25% nitrous oxide. Significant effects were noted up to 15 minutes after the inhalation of the agent was stopped.

Isoflurane is an acceptable alternative to nitrous oxide. For clinical use, less than 0.4% should be sufficient. The problem of nausea and the specific analgesic effect of isoflurane require more study.

▶ It is not clear to me what this article means, other than that, at subanesthetic concentrations, impairment of psychomotor function in individuals can be detected. The doses of isoflurane and nitrous oxide were chosen to reach equivalent brain levels in 20 minutes. that is, using 0.4% isoflurane and 25% nitrous oxide, even though the equipotent concentrations at equilibrium would be 25% nitrous oxide and 0.3% isoflurane. Perhaps the reason that isoflurane impaired more and was more sedating was that these were not equivalent doses in the patients they used, and perhaps minimal alveolar concentration is not a linear measure of anesthetic potency. Nevertheless, this study does indicate that isoflurane may be useful as a dental analgesic as it appears to be more potent than nitrous oxide, but its safety and the safety of those in the dental operatory were not assessed in this study.—M.F. Roizen, M.D.

Plasma Glutathione S-Transferase Concentration as a Measure of Hepatocellular Integrity Following a Single General Anaesthetic With Halothane, Enflurane, or Isoflurane
Hussey AJ, Aldridge LM, Paul D, Ray DC, Beckett GJ, Allan LG (Univ of Edinburgh)
Br J Anaesth 60:130–135, February 1988   2–3

Some inhaled halogenated anesthetics may injure the liver. Plasma transaminase estimates are not very sensitive and may have poor organ specificity. An alternative is to measure plasma concentrations of the hepatic isoenzymes of glutathione S-transferase (GST) by radioimmunoassay. The course of plasma GST was followed in patients anesthetized with halothane, enflurane, or isoflurane. The patients were in American

Society of Anesthesiologists groups I and II, and underwent hernia repair or varicose vein surgery.

Concentrations of halothane were 1.0% to 1.5%, and those of isoflurane and enflurane were 1% to 3%. No significant changes in levels of bilirubin, alanine aminotransferase, or γ-glutamyltransferase accompanied anesthesia and surgery. However, the GST increased significantly after 3 hours of halothane or enflurane anesthesia. In the isoflurane group, GST levels remained stable. Changes in GST were not correlated with the total dose of anesthetic.

The increase in plasma GST accompanying halothane or enflurane anesthesia suggests impaired hepatocellular function. Isoflurane appears not to produce such impairment.

▶ Unrecognized hepatocyte hypoxia is often considered the likely explanation for transient liver dysfunction that follows surgery. This hypoxia may reflect mechanical disturbances produced by the surgery, hypovolemia, or anesthetic-induced reductions in hepatic blood flow despite relative maintenance of perfusion pressure. With respect to this latter mechanism, the present data support previous observations that hepatic blood flow is better maintained during administration of isoflurane than during administration of halothane.—R.K. Stoelting, M.D.

Prolonged Anaesthesia With Isoflurane and Halothane: Effects on Hepatic Function
Jantzen J-PAH, Kleemann PP, Witton PK, Mertzlufft F, Klein AM, Dick WF (Johannes Gutenburg Univ, Mainz, West Germany)
Anaesthesia 43:186–189, March 1988   2–4

The mechanisms that underlie hepatic injury induced by volatile anesthetics are unknown. The duration of anesthesia contributes to toxicity, and some studies suggest that isoflurane is the volatile agent of choice for prolonged anesthesia. To determine the effects of prolonged isoflurane and halothane anesthesia on biochemical and hematologic measurements of hepatic function, 40 healthy adults scheduled for prolonged maxillofacial surgery were randomly assigned to receive either isoflurane or halothane. Hepatic function was assessed preoperatively and on the first and sixth postoperative days.

There were no significant changes seen in hepatic enzyme activity (Fig 2–1) or bilirubin level in either the isoflurane or halothane group. One-stage prothrombin time and factor VII concentrations decreased significantly on the first postoperative day, with subsequent recovery to baseline values on day 6. The decrease was more pronounced in patients who received halothane and included values far below the physiologic range.

These results support the use of isoflurane rather than halothane for prolonged anesthesia. The decrease in factor VII and clotting activity

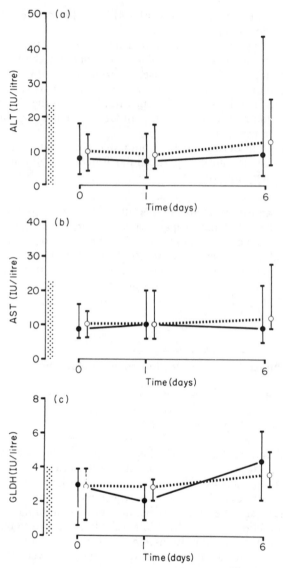

Fig 2–1.—**A,** alanine aminotransferase *(ALT)* changes; **B,** aspartate aminotransferase *(AST)* changes; and **C,** glutamate dehydrogenase *(GLDH)* changes after prolonged anesthesia with isoflurane *(black dot)* and halothane *(white dot)* (median, range). *Dotted column* indicates physiologic range. (Courtesy of Jantzen J-PAH, Kleeman PP, Witton PK, et al: *Anaesthesia* 41:186–189, March 1988.)

value in the halothane group reflects a decrease synthesizing activity of the liver, possibly as a result of reduced hepatic blood flow.

▶ Prolonged anesthesia and surgery may introduce the potential for a number of adverse events, which may or may not be related to the anesthetic. Better maintenance of hepatic blood flow, and thus hepatocyte oxygenation, is likely to be associated with isoflurane compared with halothane. This may be a logical, but not mandatory, reason to select isoflurane when hepatic effects of the anesthetic are most important.—R.K. Stoelting, M.D.

Single Breath Induction of Anaesthesia With Isoflurane
Lamberty JM, Wilson IH (Freedom Fields Hosp, Plymouth, England)
Br J Anaesth 59:1214–1218, October 1987   2–5

Two studies have shown that inducing anesthesia using a single breath of halothane and oxygen alone or halothane, nitrous oxide, and oxygen is effective and safe. However, concern has been expressed recently about the dangers associated with repeated halothane anesthesia. The suitability of isoflurane for use as an alternative to halothane in a single-breath induction technique was explored.

Seventy-two patients aged 11–65 years in American Society of Anesthesiologists classes I or II were divided randomly into a control group and a single-breath induction group. The patients were having minor outpatient surgery under general anesthesia. In the control group, anesthesia was induced through a Mapleson A breathing system with an initial mixture of 0.5% isoflurane and 66% nitrous oxide in oxygen. Isoflurane was increased by 0.5% after every fifth breath to a maximum concentration of 4%. The single-breath induction group inhaled a vital capacity breath of 2% isoflurane, with 66% nitrous oxide in oxygen. A modified Mapleson A breathing system, to which an extra 2-L reservoir bag had been added, was used in this group.

Single-breath induction was associated with fewer problems on induction, although it required more patient cooperation. In all, 94% of the patients were willing to repeat the single-breath induction technique, compared with 74% of the patients receiving conventional inhalation induction.

Isoflurane was concluded to be a viable alternative to halothane for use in a single vital capacity breath induction when halothane is not suitable. Also, single-breath induction is more acceptable to the patient.

▶ The same results can be accomplished in 1 circulation time with appropriate drugs administered intravenously. It is likely that the adult patients described in this study would have found the intravenous induction of anesthesia quite acceptable. In my opinion, the need for 2% isoflurane as utilized in this report introduces more potential risks than a conventional approach, be it a slow inhalation or rapid intravenous induction of anesthesia.—R.K. Stoelting, M.D.

The Enflurane-Sparing Effect of Alfentanil in Dogs
Hall RI, Szlam F, Hug CC Jr (Emory Univ)
Anesth Analg 66:1287–1291, December 1987   2–6

Some researchers believe that the dog is less sensitive than human beings to the anesthetic and analgesic actions of opioids. The alfentanil plasma concentration (ALF) vs. anesthetic effect relationship has been es-

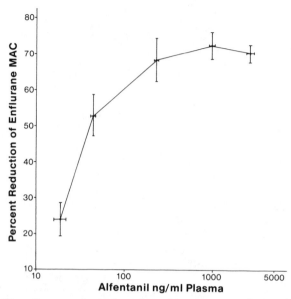

Fig 2–2.—Alfentanil concentration in plasma (log scale) vs. percentage reduction of enflurane MAC. Each point represents mean (±SEM) reduction in enflurane MAC produced by stable plasma concentration of alfentanil (ng/ml ± SEM) maintained by continuous infusion. (Courtesy of Hall RI, Szlam F, Hug CC Jr: *Anesth Analg* 66:1287–1291, December 1987.)

tablished for persons undergoing surgery. A study was done to determine the ALF vs. anesthetic relationship for alfentanil in enflurane-anesthetized dogs.

Ten mongrel dogs were anesthetized with enflurane. Enflurane minimal alveolar concentration (EMAC) was determined for each dog. Each then received at least 3 incremental infusions of alfentanil using infusion rates of 0.625, 1.6, 8, 32, or 80 μg/kg per minute. During each infusion rate, EMAC and ALF were determined. Incremental infusions of alfentanil produced a linear increase in ALF. Alfentanil administration produced a dose-dependent reduction of EMAC up to a maximum of 72.5% ± 3.7% at 32 μg/kg per minute; a ceiling effect was observed (Fig 2–2). The degree of EMAC reduction produced by the infusion rate of 8 μg/kg per minute was not significantly different from the EMAC reductions produced by infusion rates of 32 or 80 μg/kg per minute.

The relative potency of alfentanil was one seventh to one tenth that of fentanyl under identical conditions. The ALF-producing maximal EMAC reduction in enflurane-anesthetized dogs in response to a tail-clamp stimulus was similar to the ALF needed to provide adequate anesthesia of patients for skin incision in the presence of nitrous oxide.

Alfentanil, like other μ-receptor agonists, is capable of reducing EMAC by only 70% in dogs. The anesthetic efficacy of alfentanil in human beings and dogs appears to be similar.

▶ These data support the ability of opioid agonists to substantially reduce anesthetic requirements for volatile anesthetics. It is intriguing that high doses of these drugs combined with muscle relaxants are occasionally viewed as "complete" anesthetics in critically ill patients. Obviously, the amounts of opioid or inhaled anesthetic necessary to prevent skeletal muscle movement (MAC) and provide amnesia are not similar. In contrast to opioid agonists, the magnitude of agonist-antagonist-induced reductions in anesthetic requirements are probably insufficient to even produce amnesia.— R.K. Stoelting, M.D.

Awakening Concentrations of Isoflurane Are Not Affected by Analgesic Doses of Morphine
Gross JB, Alexander CM (Univ of Pennsylvania, Philadelphia VA Med Ctr)
Anesth Analg 67:27–30, January 1988   2–7

Ranges of MAC-awake—the alveolar concentration of an anesthetic at the time patients are first able to open their eyes in response to verbal command during recovery from anesthesia—have been established during recovery from halothane, fluroxene, and methoxyflurane. However, no MAC-awake data for isoflurane have been published, despite this agent's increasing popularity. A randomized, double-blind study was done to assess MAC-awake during recovery from isoflurane anesthesia and to determine whether an analgesic dose of morphine significantly affects MAC-awake.

Fourteen patients aged 21–59 in American Society of Anesthesiologists classifications I or II were studied. All were scheduled for general, orthopedic, or oral surgery. The effect of morphine, 0.1 mg/kg intravenously, or placebo given about 80 minutes before the end of surgery on recovery from isoflurane/oxygen anesthesia was determined. End-tidal isoflurane was constant at a mean of 1.1% in both treatment groups during surgery. No other anesthetics were given after administration of morphine or placebo. Duration of anesthesia was comparable in both groups.

Mean times from discontinuation of isoflurane until eye-opening at verbal command were 19 minutes in the morphine group and 22 minutes in the placebo group. At the time of eye opening, end-tidal isoflurane concentrations did not differ between the morphine and placebo groups. Those mean values were 0.2% and 0.18%, respectively.

The MAC-awake for isoflurane was 0.19% during emergence from surgical anesthesia under clinical conditions. This figure, as well as the time required for patients to awaken after isoflurane administration is discontinued, appeared to be independent of administration of analgesic doses of morphine 1 hour before the end of surgery.

▶ The goal is to provide patient comfort and safety in the early postoperative period. There is an implicit suggestion that a patient who can open his eyes on command would also possess protective laryngeal reflexes. The present data suggest that morphine, which would be presumed to enhance patient comfort, would not also contribute to delayed awakening. It is always important to recognize the importance of dose and timing when interpreting data derived from studies such as this one.— R.K. Stoelting, M.D.

Narcotics

Opioid Analgesia at Peripheral Sites: A Target for Opioids Released During Stress and Inflammation?
Joris JL, Dubner R, Hargreaves KM (Natl Inst of Dental Research, Bethesda, Md)
Anesth Analg 66:1277–1281, December 1987   2–8

Opioid receptors are present on afferent nerve fibers, but the role of these receptors in analgesia is unclear. Carrageenan was used to produce inflammation in the hind paws of rats. Groups of animals had fentanyl, ethylketocyclazocine, or saline injected into sites of inflammation and subcutaneously at the neck.

Both agonists reduced the paw withdrawal latency compared with saline. Doses that did not have systemic action were effective. Levorphanol, the same type of agonist as fentanyl, blocked carrageenan-induced hyperalgesia, but its isomer dextrorphan was inactive.

If opiates acted only in the central nervous system to produce analgesia, systemic effects would be expected. The peripheral effect observed probably involves primary afferent nerves or leukocytes, both of which have opioid receptors. Opioids may act directly on the nerve terminals by regulating nociceptive transmission, or indirectly through an anti-inflammatory effect. Peripheral injection of small doses of opiate might provide prolonged analgesia restricted to a delimited region. Quaternary opiates that did not cross the blood-brain barrier could be of use in the management of analgesia and anesthesia.

▶ In this study for which the rat paw injected with carrageenan was used as a model of inflammation, there appears to be a benefit of kappa and mu opioids injected locally into the tissue. This apparently is not systemic effect, as the local injection does not produce bilateral analgesia and, in fact, the doses were what we would call trivial. The mechanisms for this effect are speculated to be either peripheral terminals of primary afferents or leukocytes, both of which are known to possess opioid receptors. Other possible mechanisms are a direct effect on other peptides and amines locally released that increase pain sensation. I think this study has potential therapeutic implications in that perhaps it is possible to give opioids locally and not have undesirable CNS side effects such as respiratory depression. In addition, it means that perhaps we could develop quaternary analgesics that don't cross the blood/brain barrier and that could be used in treating postoperative pain with minimal side effects.

Perhaps we can find other drugs (that is, drugs other than narcotics) that will modify the action of nociceptive stimuli from the direct periphery and that can then be administered peripherally without having the central effects that narcotics have. The localization of narcotic effects is a fascinating subject. Is the nausea created by narcotics a central peripheral mechanism? We really don't know. It is thought that the area postrema is outside the blood/brain barrier, and thus we should be able to manipulate the narcotic molecule to just get central narcotic effect without the nausea or vice versa. This study implies that we should be able to get peripheral analgesic effect without any of the central side effects of narcotics, and it cites specific drug therapy, which I believe will be a major goal both for pharmaceutical firms and for anesthesia over the next decade.—M.F. Roizen, M.D.

Effects of Fentanyl and Sufentanil on Peripheral Mammalian Nerves
Gissen AJ, Gugino LD, Datta S, Miller J, Covino BG (Brigham and Women's Hosp, Boston; Harvard Univ)
Anesth Analg 66:1272–1276, December 1987   2–9

Fentanyl and sufentanil are widely used intravenously during balanced anesthetic techniques. Their analgesic action, when injected into the epidural space, is thought to be related to diffusion of the drugs into the subarachnoid space and to their interaction with opiate receptors in the spinal cord. Few data are available on the possible local anesthetic effect of these analgesics or on their possible neurotoxicity. The local anesthetic activity of fentanyl and sufentanil was evaluated in an isolated mammalian nerve preparation, and whether or not localized neural damage occurs was determined.

Albino rabbits, weighing 2 kg to 2.5 kg, were studied. The action potential amplitudes of A and C fibers were noted before and after a 30-minute exposure to 50 μg/ml and 100 μg/ml fentanyl and sufentanil. After 100 μg/ml of each drug, a reversible decrease in the action potential amplitude of A fibers in desheathed nerves was seen. The action potential amplitude of C fibers was also reduced, but not to the same extent. Pretreatment with naloxone did not block the reduction in action potential amplitude produced by the opiates. No evidence of irreversible conduction blockade indicating local neural toxicity was observed.

Fentanyl and sufentanil seem to have minimal effects on conduction in isolated sheathed rabbit vagus nerves. In desheathed nerve preparations, however, both drugs significantly decreased the action potential amplitude, particularly of A fibers. At high concentrations, both fentanyl and sufentanil may partially suppress conduction in peripheral nerves.

▶ It is comforting to know that these 2 highly lipid soluble opioids, fentanyl and sufentanil, have no neurotoxic effect. Extensive clinical experience with these agents supports the finding of these investigators.—G.W. Ostheimer, M.D.

Feeling No Pain: Alcohol as an Analgesic
Woodrow KM, Eltherington LG (Stanford Univ)
Pain 32:159–163, February 1988   2–10

Alcohol is widely perceived to have a blunting effect on sensation and emotion similar to that of the opiates. To document this effect, the analgesic potency and toxicity of alcohol were compared with the potency and toxicity of a narcotic analgesic during experimentally induced pain in 18 women, all volunteers. Ethyl alcohol (100%), mixed in a 1:1 ratio with tonic water, was administered orally in a dose of 2 mg/kg; morphine sulfate was given subcutaneously in a dose of 0.17 mg/kg. Both a pharmacologically active placebo (atropine) and a total inactive placebo (saline) were used. Pain was induced via mechanical pressure on the Achilles tendon using a device previously standardized in the clinical screening of more than 100,000 patients for pain awareness.

Ethyl alcohol in a dose equivalent to that in 2 cocktails produced pain tolerance comparable to that of 11.6 mg of subcutaneously administered morphine. Significantly, excellent analgesia occurred at blood alcohol concentrations of approximately 70 mg/100 ml, which is less than the legal level of intoxication in California. The pain threshold was not significantly altered by either alcohol or morphine.

These data indicate that alcohol, in nonintoxicating quantities, may be an effective adjunct to other analgesic modalities.

▶ An interesting study that could ultimately prove to be useful in the postoperative period. Should we be providing a martini to the postoperative patient?— R.D. Miller, M.D.

Delayed Respiratory Depression Following Fentanyl Anesthesia for Cardiac Surgery
Caspi J, Klausner JM, Safadi T, Amar R, Rozin RR, Merin G (Lady Davis Carmel Hosp, Haifa, Israel; Tel Aviv Univ, Tel Aviv, Israel)
Crit Care Med 16:238–240, March 1988   2–11

High-dose fentanyl anesthesia is widely used in cardiac surgery because of its very mild hemodynamic effects. Although its immediate side effects have been well studied, its late adverse effects, which include extreme truncal rigidity, decreased chest wall compliance, hypoventilation, respiratory acidosis, and hemodynamic instability, have received less attention.

During a 1-year study period, 380 patients underwent coronary bypass surgery under high-dose fentanyl anesthesia, 29 (7.6%) of whom suffered late adverse effects. All 29 patients (24 men and 5 women with a mean age of 58 years) had undergone aortocoronary bypass grafting, 23 because of unstable angina pectoris and 6 because of stable angina. None of the 29 patients suffered from congestive heart failure. Extreme thoracic and abdominal rigidity, which led to respiratory depression, developed 2–6 hours postoperatively in the 29 patients. A marked increase in peak inspiratory pressure 10–30 minutes before the onset of the complication was the first sign of an impending problem (table). Bradycardia at 50–65 beats/minute developed in 12 patients, and tachycardia at 120–150 beats/minute occurred in 8 patients. All patients appeared drowsy, with

Respiratory Variables in 29 Patients Who Suffered Late
Complications After Administration of Fentanyl Anesthesia
and in 351 Patients Who Did Not Suffer Complications

	351 Patients	29 Patients
PIP (cm H_2O)	24 ± 3.7	51 ± 5.5*
Paco$_2$ (torr)	32 ± 4.3	65.7 ± 2.8*
Pao$_2$ (torr)	96 ± 7.1	81.4 ± 11
pH	7.47 ± 0.07	7.21 ± 0.03*
Base excess (mEq/L)	1.8 ± 1.1	−2.7 ± 2.1

Note.—*PIP*, peak inspiratory pressure.
*P < .05 (unpaired *t* test) between groups.
(Courtesy of Caspi J, Klausner JM, Safadi T, et al: *Crit Care Med* 16:238–240,
March 1988.)

pinpoint pupils. None of the patients showed signs of bronchospasm, and chest x-ray films did not show any acute pathologic changes or endotracheal tube malposition. Fifteen patients had high plasma fentanyl levels, which correlated with their clinical status.

Treatment of the first 8 patients consisted of intravenous administration of pancuronium bromide and diazepam. Once the adverse reaction was recognized as a fentanyl-associated event, the next 21 patients with this type of complication were treated with naloxone, which is a fentanyl antagonist. Both regimens provided prompt resolution of muscular rigidity, stabilized the peak inspiratory pressure, and normalized hemodynamic values.

An awareness of the delayed, potentially life-threatening complications of high-dose fentanyl anesthesia in patients undergoing cardiac surgery is essential.

▶ This is a principle that has been well known and described for the past 10 years. That it also applies to cardiac surgery is interesting and should be taken into account by cardiac anesthetists.— R.D. Miller, M.D.

Mechanisms of Anesthesia

Partial Reversal of the Cerebral Effects of Isoflurane in the Dog by the Benzodiazepine Antagonist Flumazenil
Roald OK, Forsman M, Steen PA (Aker and Ullevål Hosp, Oslo; Univ of Oslo, Norway)
Acta Anaesthesiol Scand 32:209–212, 1988   2–12

Both coma caused by alcohol intoxication and shivering after inhalational anesthesia reportedly are reversed after administration of flumazenil, a benzodiazepine antagonist. To determine whether flumazenil could reverse some of the anesthetic action of inhalational anesthetics, 6 dogs initially anesthetized with isoflurane-N_2O–O_2 and maintained with 1% isoflurane-N_2–O_2 anesthesia were given 2-mg doses of flumazenil at an interval of 10 minutes. Cannulation of the sinus sagittalis was performed with the animals under anesthesia for direct measurement of cerebral blood flow (CBF). Cerebral and systemic variables were determined at 5 minutes and 10 minutes after the first dose and at 5, 10, and 15 minutes after the second dose.

Flumazenil significantly increased the cerebral metabolic rate for oxygen at all intervals, the increase in mean values varying from 9% to 14%. Flumazenil also converted the electroencephalogram from a sleep pattern to an awake pattern in 2 of 5 dogs, and caused no significant changes in CBF or mean arterial blood pressure. Brain biopsy specimens obtained at the end of the study showed a significant decrease in adenosine diphosphate and adenosine monophosphate, with no significant changes in the adenylate energy charge or lactate/pyruvate ratio, as compared with results in 5 dogs not given flumazenil.

These results indicate a partial reversal by flumazenil of the cerebral effects of isoflurane in dogs. It would be of interest to investigate the possible complete reversal of the cerebral effects of isoflurane by larger doses of flumazenil.

▶ Although this study has no direct clinical application, it does suggest that isoflurane acts in part by its action on a benzodiazepine receptor. This all assumes that flumazenil is a specific benzodiazepine antagonist with no other effects.—R.D. Miller, M.D.

The Imidazobenzodiazepine Ro 15-4513 Antagonizes Methoxyflurane Anesthesia
Moody EJ, Skolnick P (Natl Inst of Health, Bethesda, Md)
Life Sciences 43:1269–1276, Oct 17, 1988   2–13

Previous studies suggested that the anesthetic actions of barbiturates, steroids, and alcohols may be mediated through perturbation of the benzodiazepine/gamma-aminobutyric acid receptor chloride channel (supramolecular) complex. Although the mechanism of action for inhalation anesthetics differs from that of parenterally administered agents, inhalation anesthetics can also perturb the supramolecular complex. The imidazobenzodiazepine Ro 15-4513 is a high-affinity ligand for benzodiazepine receptors with inverse agonist properties. Whether Ro 15-4513 alone or in combination with other benzodiazepine receptor ligands could antagonize the anesthetic activity of methoxyflurane was investigated.

Groups of mice were exposed to 3.2% methoxyflurane in oxygen for 30 minutes. Immediately after removal from the anesthesia chamber, the animals were injected with vehicle or with 4 to 32 mg/kg of Ro 15-4513, given alone, or in combination with the benzodiazepine receptor antagonist flumazenil Ro 15-1788, the full inverse agonist 7-dimethoxy-4-ethyl-β-carboline-3-carboxylate (DMCM), or the partial inverse agonist N-methyl-β-carboline-3-carboxamide FG 7142. The animals were placed on their backs and observed until they awakened. Occurrence of the righting reflex was considered the point of awakening.

Methoxyflurane-exposed mice injected with vehicle only had a sustained loss of righting reflex with a sleep time of 47.5 minutes. Injection of Ro 15-4513 significantly decreased the methoxyflurane-induced sleep time, but only at doses of 8 mg/kg or higher. Coadministration of Ro 15-1788, FG 7142, or DMCM did not alter the methoxyflurane-induced sleep time, but all 3 agents blocked the Ro 15-4513-produced reduction in sleep time, suggesting that this reduction in sleep time is mediated via occupation of benzodiazepine receptors. However, because administration of other inverse agonists did not reduce the methoxyflurane-induced sleep time, the effect of Ro 15-4513 cannot be attributed solely to its inverse agonist properties, but rather suggests that this agent has unique pharmacologic properties which have not yet been elucidated.

The findings support those of recent studies reporting that inhalation anesthetics produce their depressant effects via perturbation of the supramolecular complex, and suggest that Ro 15-4513 may be useful as an antagonist to the depressant effects of inhalation anesthetics, such as methoxyflurane.

▶ This is another article that suggests that the inhaled anesthetics act in part on a benzodiazepine receptor.— R.D. Miller, M.D.

Nonnarcotic Intravenous Anesthetics

Haemodynamic Changes During Anaesthesia Induced and Maintained With Propofol
Claeys MA, Gepts E, Camu F (Flemish Free Univ of Brussels, Belgium)
Br J Anaesth 60:3–9, January 1988   2–14

Propofol is a strong hypnotic which might be suitable for anesthesia by continuous infusion. Ten patients, aged 50–75 years, who were to undergo total hip replacement were administered propofol, 2 mg/kg, followed by a continuous infusion of 6 mg/kg per hour. The patients received lorazepam, 1 mg, as premedication. One patient had a history of hypertension.

Heart rate, cardiac output, central venous pressure, and pulmonary artery pressures remained stable during anesthesia. Systemic arterial pressure decreased by about 25% during maintenance. Systemic vascular resistance also decreased significantly; pulmonary vascular resistance increased. Left ventricular stroke work decreased 30% during the infusion. Respiratory exchange was moderately impaired. The patients remained unconscious during the 1-hour infusion.

Propofol lowers systemic arterial pressure mainly by decreasing afterload. Resetting of the baroreflex may lead to a slower heart rate and inadequate peripheral perfusion. Ventilatory impairment may restrict the use of propofol in spontaneously breathing patients.

▶ The principal value of propofol to clinicians will be its onset and recovery characteristics and not its cardiopulmonary effects. As with thiopental, the rapid intravenous administration of propofol in the presence of hypovolemia seems potentially hazardous. Likewise, hypoventilation or apnea may be an expected response. In the vast majority of patients, however, these effects of propofol on blood pressure and breathing will be of minimal significance and will not detract from the frequent use of this drug.—R.K. Stoelting, M.D.

Sedative Doses of Midazolam Depress Hypoxic Ventilatory Responses in Humans
Alexander CM, Gross JB (Univ of Pennsylvania; Philadelphia VA Med Ctr)
Anesth Analg 67:377–382, 1988   2–15

Midazolam is often used as a sedative during regional anesthesia and in procedures such as endoscopy of the gastrointestinal tract and bronchoscopy. Whether sedative doses of the drug decrease ventilation was investigated, as were the effects of physostigmine, which reportedly reverses the action of midazolam.

A group of 8 volunteers entered the study. Blood pressure, heart rate, and levels of consciousness were recorded before and after midazolam injection to determine the hypoxic ventilatory response.

This response was significantly reduced by midazolam, 0.1 mg/kg, in hypercarbic volunteers. Patients with normal lung and respiratory function may become hypoxic after receiving midazolam, and those with depressed ventilation may be at a significantly greater risk for hypoxia after midazolam treatment.

A double-blind, crossover study analyzed the effects of physostigmine and a placebo on levels of consciousness and hypoxic ventilatory response. Physostigmine increased awareness but had no other significant effects. It did cause side effects, however, and should be used with midazolam only cautiously.

Hypoxia caused by midazolam may not be easily detected. It is associated with cyanosis and confusion, but not necessarily with tachycardia. Careful monitoring of arterial oxygen saturation is recommended for patients receiving midazolam.

▶ Midazolam has been under critical review nationally because of the many deaths associated with it during various diagnostic endoscopic procedures. This study validates that it not only is a classic respiratory depressant but also can be dangerous in that it depresses the hypoxic ventilatory response in humans.

Relation of Sedation and Amnesia to Plasma Concentrations of Midazolam in Surgical Patients
Persson MP, Nilsson A, Hartvig P (Univ Hosp, Lund, Sweden; Univ of Uppsala, Sweden)
Clin Pharmacol Ther 43:324–331, March 1988   2–16

The pharmacokinetics and pharmacodynamics of midazolam were investigated in 20 female patients undergoing lower abdominal surgery.

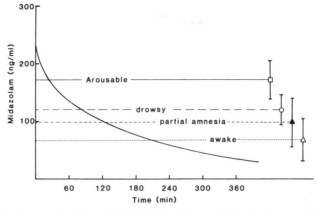

Fig 2–3.—Concentration-time profile of midazolam after extubation, showing mean (±SD) concentrations associated with various pharmacodynamic end points. (Courtesy of Persson MP, Nilsson A, Hartvig P: *Clin Pharmacol Ther* 43:324–331, March 1988.)

The relation between the plasma concentration of midazolam and postoperative sedation and amnesia was studied. Midazolam was infused intravenously in 10 patients given an epidural anesthetic. The other 10 patients were anesthetized with totally intravenous administration of midazolam and alfentanil.

There was no significant difference in the pharmacokinetics of midazolam between groups. There was a good correlation between the plasma levels of midazolam and pharmacodynamic response. A plasma midazolam concentration of 150–200 ng/ml corresponded with verbal responsiveness; 100–150 ng/ml, postoperative drowsiness; below 75 ng/ml, sedation (Fig 2–3). Amnesia was total at concentrations greater than 100 ng/ml. The relation between the quantal response data and the plasma midazolam concentration was represented by an S-shaped concentration-effect curve. Postoperative drowsiness was more pronounced in the group who received totally intravenous anesthesia. The concomitant administration of alfentanil shifted the concentration-effect curve regarding sedation to the left.

The results show that a midazolam concentration greater than 250–300 ng/ml is necessary to maintain a satisfactory hypnotic effect during surgery. The plasma midazolam concentration should be less than 100 ng/ml before the patient is considered sufficiently awake to be sent to the ward.

▶ These results are not surprising. This is an especially well performed study that should be read by all clinicians who use midazolam extensively.—R.D. Miller, M.D.

Comparison of the Recovery Characteristics of Diazepam and Midazolam
Galletly D, Forrest P, Purdie G (Wellington Clinical School of Medicine, Wellington, New Zealand)
Br J Anaesth 60:520–524, 1988   2–17

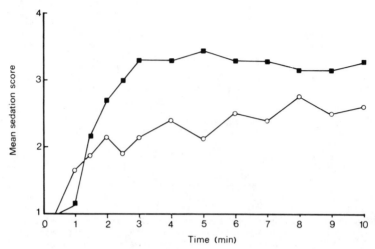

Fig 2–4.—Mean sedation score for 10 minutes following drug injection. ○, diazepam; ■, midazolam. (Courtesy of Galletly D, Forrest P, Purdie G: *Br J Anaesth* 60:520–524, 1988.)

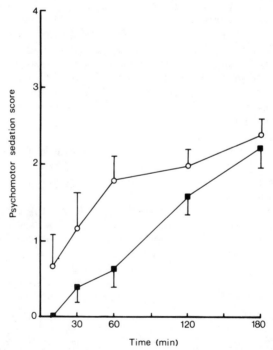

Fig 2–5.—Psychomotor/sedation test score. Mean number of tests returning to preinjection baseline score. ○, diazepam; ■, midazolam. (Courtesy of Galletly D, Forrest P, Purdie G: *Br J Anaesth* 60:520–524, 1988.)

Compared with diazepam in propylene glycol, water-soluble midazolam produces a lower incidence of pain on injection and of thrombophlebitis, and has advantageous physicochemical and pharmacokinetic properties. Although it has the shortest elimination half-life of all benzodiazepines commercially available, the recovery from equipotent doses of midazolam and diazepam seems similar. The efficacy and recovery characteristics of midazolam and diazepam after administration of equipotent doses of each drug were compared.

Eight volunteers, aged 22 to 28 years, were studied. The subjects received intravenously either 10 mg diazepam in propylene glycol or 5 mg midazolam. Mean times to onset of drug effect did not significantly differ. In the first 10 minutes, the observed degree of sedation was found to be significantly higher with midazolam (Fig 2–4). Recovery was better in the diazepam group at 10, 30, and 60 minutes. At 180 minutes, the midazolam group performed slightly better than the diazepam group (Fig 2–5). Amnesia for picture recall was significantly greater in the midazolam group.

Midazolam was found to be significantly more potent than diazepam and was associated with a delay in recovery. The doses used in this study, therefore, were believed not to be equipotent; the relative potency of the 2 drugs is significantly greater than 2 to 1, perhaps closer to 3 to 1. This would help explain the findings of other studies that showed that midazolam has a similar recovery and more intense amnesia than diazepam. If the newer formulations of diazepam—those mixed with micelle or lipid emulsion—were compared with midazolam, the discrepancy between their relative potencies would likely be even greater.

▶ This article clearly shows that, at the commonly used potency ratio, it takes the same time to recover from midazolam or diazepam. But the authors also conclude, as others have done, notably Drs. Lichtor and Korttila, that the potency is closer to 5 to 1 than 2 to 1. It is too bad that this study didn't include a dose-response curve so that they could examine recovery at equipotent doses.—M.F. Roizen, M.D.

Neuromuscular Blocking Drugs

Does Injection of Non-Depolarizing Neuromuscular Blockers Before Thiopentone Affect Their Speed of Onset? A Study of Tubocurarine and Vecuronium
Levack ID, Spence AA (Royal Infirmary, Edinburgh)
Br J Anaesth 59:1451–1453, November 1987   2–18

It is not known whether the order of administration of a neuromuscular blocker can affect its pharmacodynamic profile. The rate of onset of neuromuscular blockade using tubocurarine or vecuronium was measured in an open sequential pharmacodynamic study involving 40 patients. Four groups of 10 patients received either thiopentone followed by a blocker or a reverse sequence in which the blocker was injected before thiopentone. Isometric twitch tension was measured after nerve stimula-

Onset Times of Neuromuscular Blockade After
Administration of Vecuronium and Tubocurarine*

Depression of T1	Group 1 (T–V)	Group 2 (V–T)	Group 3 (T–Tc)	Group 4 (Tc–T)
50%	74 ± 19	73 ± 23	77 ± 24	68 ± 29
90%	109 ± 27	103 ± 46	210 ± 46	223 ± 41

*Values are expressed as mean ± SD. *T1*, first twitch of train-of-4 pattern; *T*, 2.5% thiopentone; *V*, vecuronium; *Tc*, tubocurarine. Group 1 received thiopentone followed by vecuronium; group 2, vecuronium followed by thiopentone; group 3, thiopentone followed by tubocurarine; group 4, tubocurarine followed by thiopentone.
(Courtesy of Levack ID, Spence AA: *Br J Anaesth* 59:1451–1453, November 1987.)

tion delivered with 0.2-msec impulses in a train-of-four pattern. The indices sought were 50% and 90% depression of the control twitch height in T1 and T4/T1 at 30%, 50%, and 70% depression of control height in T1.

There was a small difference between groups, amounting to a few seconds in rate of onset of block, but this was not suggestive of a systematic effect of the drug sequence. The mean times to 50% depression with vecuronium agreed to within 1 second regardless of whether thiopentone was given first or second (table). The mean time to the same level of depression after tubocurarine was 9 seconds faster when tubocurarine was given first. The time to 90% depression with tubocurarine was twice as long as that with vecuronium. The relationship between T1 depression and train-of-four ratio after either blocker was not affected by reversing the sequence with thiopentone.

There is neither advantage nor disadvantage in the reverse-sequence regimen for administration of either tubocurarine or vecuronium.

▶ I have always wondered whether this approach would work. Logically it seems as if it should, although this study does not confirm this reviewer's logic.—R.D. Miller, M.D.

Priming With Nondepolarizing Relaxants for Rapid Tracheal Intubation: A Double-Blind Evaluation
Baumgarten RK, Carter CE, Reynolds WJ, Brown JL, DeVera HV (Landstuhl Army Regional Med Ctr, Landstuhl, West Germany; Brooke Army Med Ctr, Fort Sam Houston, Tex)
Can J Anaesth 35:5–11, 1988   2–19

Succinylcholine is commonly used to facilitate muscle relaxation in patients who require rapid tracheal intubation; however, undesirable complications may ensue. Using the priming principle, excellent intubating conditions can be produced with nondepolarizing relaxants alone. A randomized, double-blind study investigated this premise.

In phase I of the study 2 groups of patients received a priming sequence with either atracurium or vecuronium. A control group received succinylcholine. In phase II the priming sequences were curare-vecuronium or vecuronium with a larger intubating dose. The control group received placebo. Researchers used vecuronium at 4-minute priming intervals in phase III. One control group received no prime and the other received succinylcholine.

In both phases I and III, succinylcholine provided uniformly excellent intubating conditions. All patients in both priming groups in phase I were successfully intubated, but intubating conditions were not equal to those with succinylcholine. The group that received no relaxant in phase II had significantly worse intubating conditions than the priming groups. In phase III priming significantly improved intubating conditions in comparison with an equivalent bolus dose of relaxant. Overall, the intubating conditions were good using the 4-minute priming interval, but in 7% of the patients, they were not equal to those with succinylcholine. When large priming doses were used, significant side effects developed; halving the doses mitigated the symptoms.

Priming produces significantly better intubating conditions than a single bolus does, and the 4-minute interval is as effective as a 7-minute interval. Intubating conditions are optimum, however, when succinylcholine is used. Because the results differ from those of other reports, further study is needed.

▶ Studies evaluating the ability of a muscle relaxant to produce adequate intubating conditions are fraught with difficulties, including investigator bias. Having tracheal intubating conditions evaluated in a double-blind fashion is one way to minimize these biases; in that respect the authors are to be congratulated. Otherwise they have shown results that are entirely predictable. First, even with priming, nondepolarizing muscle relaxants cannot produce adequate intubating conditions as rapidly as succinylcholine. Second, the time between the priming dose and intubating dose appears to be 4 minutes: this has been demonstrated by other investigators.—R.D. Miller, M.D.

Differential Effects of Neuromuscular Blocking Agents on Suxamethonium-Induced Fasciculations and Myalgia
O'Sullivan EP, Williams NE, Calvey TN (Whiston Hosp, Prescot, England)
Br J Anaesth 60:367–371, 1988   2–20

The side effects of suxamethonium, which include myalgia, hyperkalemia, and muscle twitching, can be pretreated with various nondepolarizing neuromuscular blockers. The effects of pretreatment agents (gallamine, pancuronium, and suxamethonium itself) were evaluated in a double-blind clinical trial.

Doses of the 3 drugs and of saline were given randomly to a group of 60 female surgical patients aged 18–66 years. Premedication, anesthesia, and the various tests administered were identical in all 60. Blood was analyzed for plasma potassium concentrations, both before and 5 minutes after the start of anesthesia, with the variations compared.

There was no correlation between muscle pain and contractions. Suxamethonium pretreatment did not significantly affect either score. Gallamine significantly reduced fasciculation as, to a lesser extent, did pancuronium. The latter was also most effective in reducing myalgia. None of the pretreatments had a significant effect on plasma potassium concentrations.

The results show that gallamine and pancuronium do not act identically, perhaps because of their differential activity at the neuromuscular junction. Blocking drugs with selective presynaptic and postsynaptic actions on neuromuscular transmission might be successful as pretreatment agents to prevent both postoperative myalgia and muscle fasciculations.

▶ The reader might ask why we have accepted another of the many studies regarding succinylcholine-induced fasciculations and myalgia. The personal bias of this reviewer, confirmed by this study, is that gallamine may be more effective in attenuating succinylcholine-induced fasciculations. I have had this bias for a long time and it was reassuring to see it confirmed by an objectively designed study.— R.D. Miller, M.D.

Muscle Relaxation With Succinylcholine or Vecuronium Does Not Alter the Rate of CSF Production or Resistance to Reabsorption of CSF in Dogs
Artru AA (Univ of Washington)
Anesthesiology 68:392–396, March 1988   2–21

Treatments that alter cerebrospinal fluid (CSF) pressure or the activity of adrenergic and cholinergic neurons can produce significant changes in the rate of CSF formation (Vf) and resistance to reabsorption of CSF (Ra). Although succinylcholine is reported to do so, vecuronium is reported to produce only minimal changes in CSF pressure or adrenergic and cholinergic nerve activity. Using the open ventriculocisternal perfusion method, Vf and Ra were studied in 6 halothane anesthetized dogs with and without continuous intravenous infusions of succinylcholine and 6 with and without vecuronium infusions. In addition, the effects of infusion of succinylcholine or vecuronium on CSF pressure and, in the case of succinylcholine, the magnitude of fasciculations, were recorded.

Both Vf and Ra during succinylcholine or vecuronium at both normal or elevated CSF pressures were not different from Vf and Ra values when no muscle relaxant was used. Succinylcholine caused transient muscle fasciculations and increases of CSF pressure, whereas vecuronium did not. When muscle relaxants were not used, the effects of cardiovascular and respiratory activity on the CSF pressure waveform were difficult to distinguish, and the coefficient of variability for determination of cisternal outflow rates was increased, making Ra values less reliable. In contrast, when muscle relaxants were used, the influences of cardiovascular activity and mechanical ventilation on CSF pressure were clearly evident. The coefficients of variability for volumes of cisternal outflow were significantly lower when either relaxant was used, thus improving the reliability of Vf and Ra.

Continuous infusion of succinylcholine or vecuronium does not affect Vf or Ra, suggesting that either muscle relaxant does not alter CSF volume to raise or lower CSF pressure. Immobilization of respiratory muscles is desirable during ventriculocisternal perfusion to improve both the reliability of Ra values and the usefulness of the CSF pressure waveform. Continuous infusion of either succinylcholine or vecuronium is suitable for studies on CSF dynamics because neither one significantly alters Vf or Ra.

▶ Anesthesiologists are accustomed to considering the role of increased cerebral blood flow (induced by volatile anesthetics or hypoventilation of the lungs) on intracranial pressure, especially in patients with space-occupying intracranial lesions. Drug-induced changes in rate of formation or resistance to reabsorption of cerebrospinal fluid and the subsequent impact on intracranial pressure are not often considered. In this regard, it is reassuring to learn that vecuronium or succinylcholine are not likely to alter dynamics of cerebrospinal fluid production or reabsorption.— R.K. Stoelting, M.D.

Mechanisms of Succinylcholine-Induced Arrhythmias in Hypoxic or Hypoxic:Hypercarbic Dogs

Leiman BC, Katz J, Butler BD (Univ of Texas, Houston)
Anesth Analg 66:1292–1297, December 1987   2–22

Succinylcholine is useful before tracheal intubation because it provides rapid onset of profound muscle relaxation. In cases of difficult intubation, patients may be hypoxic as well as hypercarbic and acidotic. The safety of succinylcholine in such cases may be questioned because of the potential development of cardiac arrhythmias that may be exacerbated by hypoxia and acidosis. A dog model was used to determine the effects of succinylcholine on cardiac rhythm and serum levels of potassium and catecholamines.

Dogs with hypoxia alone and with hypoxia and hypercarbia were studied during anesthesia with halothane or enflurane. After succinylcholine, 0.3 mg/kg, was injected, cardiac arrhythmias occurred in all halothane:hypoxia dogs and in 70% of dogs given halothane during hypoxia:hypercarbia. None of the dogs given enflurane anesthesia became arrhythmic. Serum potassium levels increased significantly 3 and 5 minutes after succinylcholine injection in all dogs. Serum epinephrine levels increased in the halothane-hypoxia:hypercarbia and enflurane:hypoxia groups.

After succinylcholine injection, epinephrine levels increased further in dogs in the halothane:control, halothane:hypoxia, halothane-hypoxia:hypercarbia, enflurane:hypoxia, and enflurane-hypoxia:hypercarbia groups. Norepinephrine levels rose with enflurane-hypoxia:hypercarbia and after succinylcholine injection in the halothane:hypoxia, halothane-hypoxia:hypercarbia, and enflurane-hypoxia:hypercarbia groups.

Succinylcholine induces arrhythmias by sympathetic stimulation. Halothane sensitizes the myocardium to arrhythmias at the same levels of serum catecholamines and potassium in the presence of hypoxia or hypoxia:hypercarbia more than enflurane.

▶ Hopefully, succinylcholine will rarely be administered to patients who are hypoxic, hypercarbic, or both. The exception may be patients with cyanotic congenital heart disease or those experiencing sustained laryngospasm. In the latter circumstance, the potential benefits of succinylcholine far outweigh its risks.—R.K. Stoelting, M.D.

Pharmacokinetics and Pharmacodynamics of Vecuronium Administered by Bolus and Infusion During Halothane or Balanced Anesthesia
Shanks CA, Avram MJ, Fragen RJ, O'Hara DA (Northwestern Univ, Chicago)
Clin Pharmacol Ther 42:459–464, October 1987   2–23

The pharmacokinetics and pharmacodynamics of vecuronium were studied in 2 groups of patients whose anesthesia was maintained with either halothane-nitrous oxide or fentanyl-barbiturate-tranquilizer-nitrous oxide. Vecuronium was administered in a single intravenous dose, 60 μg/kg, combined with an infusion, 1 μg/kg/hour, to 20 adults undergoing elective surgery.

At the end of infusion, the mean plasma vecuronium concentrations were 0.34 μg/ml in the halothane-treated group and 0.32 μg/ml in the fentanyl-treated group. These concentrations were associated with 93% and 88% depression of the twitch response, respectively. The difference between groups was not significant. Vecuronium plasma concentration-time data were combined with the simultaneous intensities of neuromuscular blockade to model the kinetic-dynamic values for each patient. There were no significant differences in the steady-state volume, clearance, or elimination half-life of vecuronium in either anesthetic group. Plasma vecuronium concentrations associated with 50% blockade averaged 0.2 μg/ml in both groups.

It appears that neither the pharmacokinetics nor the pharmacodynamics of vecuronium in man is affected during halothane or balanced anesthesia.

▶ This is probably the most sophisticated kinetics study demonstrating the usefulness of infusions of vecuronium. It is surprising that the pharmacodynamics of vecuronium were not different in halothane or balanced anesthesia because it is contrary to all of the other studies that have been performed. On the other hand, the choice of anesthetic agent seems to affect atracurium and vecuronium less than the long-acting neuromuscular blocking drugs.—R.D. Miller, M.D.

The Effect of Pancuronium Bromide on Polymorphonuclear Neutrophil Adherence In Vitro
Krumholz W, Käbisch S, Biscoping J, Wiedemann M, Hempelmann G
(Justus-Liebig-Universität Gieszen, West Germany)
Anaesthesist 37:246–248, 1988
2–24

Postoperative infection in surgical patients remains a significant problem. Polymorphonuclear neutrophil (PMN) granulocytes play a vital role in the body's defense against invading bacteria, but anesthetic agents may interfere with PMN function. An in vitro study was done to assess the influence of the muscle relaxant pancuronium bromide on PMN adherence.

Heparinized venous blood samples were collected from 18 healthy men aged 23–43 years. Half of each sample (5 ml) was used to measure the adherence of untreated PMN granulocytes. Pancuronium bromide was added to 9 samples in a concentration of 1.3 µg per ml of blood and to 9 samples in a concentration of 0.5 µg per ml of blood. Adherence was measured with the MacGregor assay method.

Both concentrations of pancuronium bromide caused inhibition of PMN adherence when compared with values obtained for the control samples. However, the difference was significant only for the higher pancuronium concentration.

Because the pancuronium concentration of 1.3 µg per ml of blood used in this in vitro study was similar to that attained 5 minutes after administration of 8 mg of pancuronium bromide during operation, it is possible that the risk of bacterial infection is increased by administration of this anesthetic agent.

▶ Whether this article has any useful clinical application is certainly questionable. Also, do muscle relaxants other than pancuronium produce this effect? It is an interesting article that proposes that the risk of infection might be increased by the administration of pancuronium. The authors will be hard-pressed to prove this.—R.D. Miller, M.D.

The Use of Intravenous Pancuronium Bromide to Produce Fetal Paralysis During Intravascular Transfusion
Copel JA, Grannum PA, Harrison D, Hobbins JC (Yale Univ)
Am J Obstet Gynecol 158:170–171, January 1988
2–25

Ultrasound-guided percutaneous umbilical blood sampling is increasingly being used as a prenatal diagnostic procedure. Most procedures are relatively brief once vascular access is obtained because the required amount of blood can be removed quickly. However, intravascular exchange transfusion takes considerably longer than simple fetal phlebotomy and may be complicated by difficulty in maintaining vascular access because of fetal movements.

Intravenously administered sedatives are often ineffective in significantly reducing fetal movements. Treatment with intramuscular pancuronium bromide has been proposed as a means of arresting fetal movements, but this form of treatment requires a separate puncture for injection. Experience with intravenous fetal injection of pancuronium bromide that avoids the need for a second puncture, was reviewed.

Four fetuses underwent 5 intravascular exchange transfusions under intravenously administered pancuronium paralysis. Ultrasound biometry was used to estimate fetal weight and calculate the pancuronium dosage. None of the fetuses was hydropic before the transfusion. A tuberculin syringe was used to draw up the appropriate volume of diluted pancuronium solution. After vascular access in the fetal umbilical vein was obtained, enough blood was drawn to measure the hematocrit level, the diluted pancuronium solution was infused into the umbilical vein, and the transfusion was started. Paralysis was rapidly induced and lasted from 25 to 75 minutes. No complications, such as fetal heart rate deceleration or maternal symptoms, occurred.

Fetal paralysis by intravenously administered pancuronium bromide is a safe and effective procedure that avoids the need for a second puncture.

▶ This is an interesting approach to an in utero problem. I wonder whether the fetus feels discomfort upon the intramuscular injection of the pancuronium?— G.W. Ostheimer, M.D.

Colonic Anastomotic Disruption in Myasthenia Gravis: Report of Two Cases
Herz BL (Coney Island Hosp; Maimonides Med Ctr, Brooklyn, NY)
Dis Colon Rectum 30:809–811, October 1987   2–26

Neostigmine is an anticholinesterase drug that is used in the treatment of myasthenia gravis. Neostigmine is also used intraoperatively for the reversal of the activity of neuromuscular blocking agents used during general anesthesia. Several investigators have reported that neostigmine can cause anastomotic disruption after colon surgery. In 2 patients with myasthenia gravis, fatal anastomotic disruption occurred after colon surgery during which neostigmine was used to reverse the neuromuscular blocking activity of anesthetic agents.

Case 1.—Man, 83, with confirmed myasthenia gravis was admitted because he was passing bright red blood from the rectum. Rectal examination revealed prolapsed nonbleeding hemorrhoids and colonoscopy revealed left-sided colonic bleeding. Because his hematocrit continued to drop despite transfusion with 10 units of packed red blood cells and 2 units of fresh frozen plasma, he underwent left hemicolectomy with primary anastomosis under halothane anesthesia. The patient also received neostigmine before, during, and after operation. During the early recovery phase he became bradycardic and required insertion of a temporary pacemaker. On the fourth postoperative day, the patient became hypotensive and was returned to the operating room where complete anastomotic disruption was discovered. He underwent colostomy, but did poorly postoperatively and remained respirator dependent. He died of multiple organ failure 43 days after the original operation.

Case 2.—Man, 44, with a 14-year history of myasthenia gravis, underwent elective closure of a colostomy during which he was given neostigmine perioperatively. Five days after colostomy take-down and reanastomosis, the patient had to be returned to the operating room because of septic shock; anastomotic breakdown with necrosis of the bowel ends was discovered. The patient died 41 days postoperatively of overwhelming sepsis.

These 2 case reports further confirm that the use of muscle relaxants during general anesthesia is highly questionable. Anticholinesterase therapy should be initiated with extreme caution in patients with myasthenia gravis because of their sensitivity to these drugs. Glucagon, which has been used to slow intestinal motility, may be a safe alternative to neostigmine in these patients.

▶ This is an unbelievable conclusion by this author. Furthermore, it is written in a journal that is unlikely to be read by anesthesiologists. It was published because of its unbelievable conclusions and because anesthesiologists should be aware of it.—R.D. Miller, M.D.

Anti-Curare Effect of Plasma From Patients With Thermal Injury
Storella RJ, Martyn JAJ, Bierkamper GG (Hahnemann Univ, Philadelphia; Harvard Univ; Univ of Nevada at Reno)
Life Sci 43:35–40, 1988   2–27

Burned patients are resistant to various neuromuscular blockers including d-tubocurarine (dTC) and pancuronium. The causes of this resistance are not fully understood. The hypothesis that the lowered potency of muscle relaxants in burned patients results from circulating substances in plasma was tested.

Blood samples were taken from burn victims and from healthy volunteers. The mean age for both groups was 28 years. Plasma preparations with either dTC or pancuronium were infused into rats, and the degree of muscular blockage was measured.

The dTC dosage dissolved in plasma from burned patients caused a significantly lower mean neuromuscular block than did the same amount of dTC in plasma from healthy volunteers (table). Similarly, pancuronium's effects were significantly decreased in plasma samples from burned patients.

The varied effects of dTC and pancuronium in patients' blood may be attributed to differences in the extent of the burns and the time after the burn. Because the rats had only plasma from burned patients, not burn-affected neuromuscular tissue, the anticurare effects must come from changes in plasma constituents brought about by the burn injury.

Percent Depression of Contractile Tension (0.2 Hz Nerve
Stimulation) in Rat Phrenic Nerve-Hemidiaphragm

2 μ M dTC in Plasma

CONTROL PLASMA		BURN PLASMA	
Subject	% Depression	Subject	% Depression
A	100	G	87
B	100	H	30
C	61	I	24
D	61	J	16
E	50	K	11
F	39	L	0
Mean	69	Mean	28*
SEM	10	SEM	1

dTC, d-tubocurarine.
*P < .05.
(Courtesy of Storella RJ, Martyn JAJ, Bierkamper GG: *Life Sci* 43:35–40, 1988.)

Clinical resistance to muscle relaxants is greater than the resistance noted in the rat model, however, indicating that other factors must be involved.

▶ This fascinating article suggests that the classic explanation of an increased number of receptors is not the cause when patients with thermal injuries are resistant to nondepolarizing muscle relaxants.—R.D. Miller, M.D.

Metocurine Kinetics in Patients Undergoing Operations Requiring Cardiopulmonary Bypass

Avram MJ, Shanks CA, Henthorn TK, Ronai AK, Kinzer J, Wilkinson CJ (Northwestern Univ, Chicago)
Clin Pharmacol Ther 42:576–581, November 1987   2–28

Metocurine is a nondepolarizing neuromuscular blocking agent that causes little or no cardioselective atropine-like action, autonomic blockade, sympathomimetic activity, or histamine release. Metocurine kinetics during cardiopulmonary bypass (CPB) were determined in 10 patients undergoing operations necessitating hypothermic CPB and were compared with those of 9 age-matched patients undergoing hip replacement operations, which do not necessitate CPB. Metocurine was administered as a bolus of 0.3 mg/kg, given concomitantly with the commencement of an infusion at a rate of 0.04 mg/kg/hour, a pharmacokinetic regimen designed to produce 95% depression of the twitch response. In the CPB group, anesthesia was induced with fentanyl and maintained with halothane; in the hip replacement group, anesthesia was induced with thiopental and maintained with enflurane.

Except for a small difference in elimination clearance, no differences in pharmacokinetic variables were observed between groups (table). However, there was a marked, but temporary, decrease in plasma metocurine concentration at the start of hypothermic CPB, which was often associ-

Metocurine Kinetics

Surgical group	Compartmental volumes (L/kg)				Clearances (ml/min/kg)			$t_{1/2}$ (hr)
	V_C	V_F	V_S	V_{SS}*	CL_F	CL_S	CL_E	
Hip replacement	0.06 ± 0.03	0.11 ± 0.02	0.19 ± 0.05	0.35 ± 0.06	7.9 ± 1.6	1.4 ± 0.4	1.3 ± 0.2	4.0 ± 0.8
CPB	0.05 ± 0.02†	0.09 ± 0.02	0.20 ± 0.04	0.34 ± 0.05	9.4 ± 3.6	1.9 ± 0.6	1.1 ± 0.1‡	4.4 ± 0.9

Note.—Values are expressed as mean ± SD. V_F, fast compartment volume; V_S, slow compartment volume; CL_F, fast intercompartmental clearance; CL_S, slow intercompartmental clearance; CL_E, elimination clearance.
*V_{SS} is sum of V_C, V_F, and V_S.
†Does not include pump prime.
‡$P < .05$ vs. hip replacement.
(Courtesy of Avram MJ, Shanks CA, Henthorn TK, et al: *Clin Pharmacol Ther* 42:576–581, November 1987.)

ated with the return of spontaneous diaphragmatic movements necessitating additional narcotic supplementation. The intensity of neuromuscular blockade decreased from 88% ± 11% after the start of CPB and maintained approximately 70% depression during hypothermia. With rewarming, blockade intensity returned to pre-CPB values without a change in plasma metocurine concentrations.

These data demonstrate that metocurine kinetics are affected minimally in patients undergoing operations necessitating hypothermic CPB. These results are in agreement with those reported by others for normal patients to whom metocurine was administered rapidly in a single intravenous dose. The changes in neuromuscular blockade with the onset of CPB and the return to original blockade intensities with rewarming suggest a decreased sensitivity to the effects of metocurine at lower temperatures.

▶ This is a well-done study of the pharmacokinetics of a nondepolarizing muscle relaxant during cardiopulmonary bypass. It also provides additional information to suggest that the sensitivity to d-tubocurarine and metocurine is decreased while it is increased to a steroidal muscle relaxant such as pancuronium. Why?—R.D. Miller, M.D.

Vecuronium in Alcoholic Liver Disease: A Pharmacokinetic and Pharmacodynamic Analysis
Arden JR, Lynam DP, Castagnoli KP, Canfell PC, Cannon JC, Miller RD (Univ of California, San Francisco: San Francisco Gen Hosp)
Anesthesiology 68:771–776, May 1988
2–29

Vecuronium is a nondepolarizing, pancuronium-type muscle relaxant, which is used in anesthetized surgical patients to facilitate tracheal intubation. Some investigators have found that vecuronium has a prolonged duration of action and decreased plasma clearance when a relatively large dose is administered to patients with hepatic cirrhosis, but other studies have not confirmed these findings. This study was done to further investigate whether the pharmacokinetics and pharmacodynamics of vecuronium are affected by alcoholic liver disease.

Ten surgical patients with alcoholic liver disease and 10 healthy surgical patients were anesthetized with nitrous oxide and isoflurane and were given vecuronium, 0.1 mg/kg intravenously for the induction of neuromuscular blockade. The force of thumb adduction in response to supramaximal ulnar nerve stimulation was recorded continuously throughout the study period. Plasma concentrations of vecuronium and its metabolite were measured by capillary gas chromatographic assay.

Only the mean time to attain 100% twitch depression at onset was prolonged in patients with liver disease compared with control patients. The mean time required to begin recovery of control twitch tension was 32.7 minutes for the patients with liver disease and 36.8 minutes for the control patients. The mean time to 50% recovery was 59.8 minutes for the patients with liver disease and 66.1 minutes for the control patients. These differences were not statistically significant. Vecuronium clearance, steady-state volume of distribution, and elimination half-time were also unaffected by alcoholic liver disease.

Alcoholic liver disease does not alter the pharmacokinetics or duration of action of vecuronium when given in an intravenous dose of 0.1 mg/kg.

▶ This study documents that patients with severe alcoholic liver disease do not have an altered response to vecuronium if doses less than 0.1 mg/kg are given.—R.D. Miller, M.D.

Effect of Biliary Obstruction on Muscle Relaxation With Vecuronium
Orko R, Alila A, Rosenberg PH (Helsinki Univ Central Hosp)
Eur J Anaesthesiol 5:9–14, 1988   2–30

Vecuronium, a muscle relaxant, is eliminated through the hepatobiliary route. The time required for elimination may be influenced by various factors including age and the presence of liver disease. Researchers compared vecuronium's neuromuscular blocking effects in 2 categories of patients: those with and those without biliary obstruction.

The 30 patients were undergoing elective biliary surgery. Ten were elderly, 10 were young or middle aged, and 10 (mean age, 66 years) had biliary obstruction. The dosage of vecuronium was started at 0.1 mg/kg and continued at 2 mg whenever the 20% level of control response was obtained.

The total intake of vecuronium was significantly lower in patients with biliary obstruction. No age-related differences were found, and no significant differences were noted in distribution half-lives or in distribution volumes of vecuronium among the 3 groups. All groups recorded a reduced mean heart rate and a moderate decrease in mean arterial pressure 20 minutes after induction.

Neuromuscular block is prolonged in patients with biliary obstruction, possibly because an increased concentration of bile salts in plasma prevents hepatic uptake of vecuronium. But the increased length of time is not clinically significant, and vecuronium can be given safely to patients with biliary obstruction.

▶ Whereas the influence of biliary obstruction and liver disease on vecuronium pharmacokinetics and pharmacodynamics is controversial, there can be no doubt that smaller doses should probably be given with monitoring via a peripheral nerve stimulator. The main contribution of this article is the demonstration that patients can have muscle pain even when no muscle relaxant is given.— R.D. Miller, M.D.

The Use of Fetal Neuromuscular Blockade During Intrauterine Procedures
Moise KJ Jr, Carpenter RJ Jr, Deter RL, Kirshon B, Diaz SF (Baylor College of Medicine, Houston)
Am J Obstet Gynecol 157:874–879, October 1987   2–31

A number of invasive therapeutic techniques are now attempted on the fetus. Fetal movement makes these procedures difficult and increases the risk of fetal injury. The authors examined the sedative effects of intramuscular *d*-tubocurarine, 3 or 1.5 mg/kg, or pancuronium bromide, 0.3 mg/kg, injected into the fetal gluteal region under ultrasound guidance before 70 invasive in utero procedures.

Short-term fetal paralysis was achieved in all cases. In 10 cases a second injection was required. All fetuses recovered. Among 31 fetuses 23 infants were born alive with no evidence of ill effects, 3 remain undelivered, 2 were aborted, and 3 infants died of causes that were unrelated to the sedation.

Fetal neuromuscular blockade appears to be a valuable adjunct to invasive in utero procedures. However, the long-term effects of this procedure require study. Prospective follow-up of the infants described in this study is being carried out.

▶ Fascinating!—R.D. Miller, M.D.

A Comparison of Computer-Controlled Versus Manual Administration of Vecuronium in Humans
Jaklitsch RR, Westenskow DR, Pace NL, Streisand JB, East KA (Univ of Utah)
J Clin Monit 3:269–276, October 1987   2–32

Because vecuronium has a short elimination half-life, it may be administered more efficiently by continuous infusion than by bolus injection. Manual administration was compared with computer-controlled administration of vecuronium after onset of anesthesia in 22 patients. A single-bolus injection of vecuronium was given to produce 100% twitch depression for tracheal intubation. Relaxation was maintained at 90% twitch depression by repetitive bolus injections in group 1, by manually controlled continuous infusion in group 2, and by computer-controlled continuous infusion in group 3.

Variability of relaxation differed significantly among the 3 groups: in group 1, it was 10.5%; in group 2, 12.4%; and in group 3, 7.1%. Twitch remained more nearly constant with computer control than with the other 2 methods. Differences in drug requirements were not statistically significant. The electromyogram produced less variability than did the mechanomyogram.

Computer-controlled infusion may be valuable when the anesthesiologist desires a stable level of patient relaxation during use of short-acting, nondepolarizing muscle relaxants. With this method, long periods of complete relaxation and overdosing can be avoided.

▶ Certainly a computer-controlled infusion may be successful for avoiding excessive neuromuscular blockade. However, this reviewer is concerned that anesthetists place greater emphasis on the degree of twitch depression rather than simply looking at the surgical field to see whether the surgeon is struggling because of tight musculature. Certainly there can be no doubt that in a deeply anesthetized patient, twitch depression does not need to be as extensive as with a lightly anesthetized patient. In my opinion the condition of the surgical field should rank as the number one criterion, whereas the response to peripheral nerve stimulation should be a secondary, although important, criterion.—R.D. Miller, M.D.

Neostigmine, Pyridostigmine, and Edrophonium as Antagonists of Deep Pancuronium Blockade

Donati F, Lahoud J, McCready D, Bevan DR (Royal Victoria Hosp, Montreal; McGill Univ)
Can J Anaesth 34:589–593, November 1987   2–33

Neuromuscular function affected by nondepolarizing muscle relaxants is usually restored by neostigmine, pyridostigmine, or edrophonium; however, the efficacy of these agents is altered by the intensity of blockade at the time of administration. Equipotent doses for the reversal agents at 90% and 99% pancuronium blockade were determined.

After anesthesia 60 patients were given pancuronium intravenously to achieve 100% blockade, after which tracheal intubation was accomplished. Patients were allowed to recover to 10% of first twitch height, and were then randomly selected to receive either neostigmine, pyridostigmine, or edrophonium. Researchers determined equipotent doses for the 3 agents. An equal number of patients were allowed only 1% recovery before administration of the reversal agents.

When administered at 10% spontaneous recovery, neostigmine, pyridostigmine, and edrophonium were equally effective; all produced recovery of first twitch height to 80% after 10 minutes. However, when given at 1% spontaneous recovery, edrophonium was rapid in onset, whereas pyridostigmine was slow (Fig 2–6). After 10 minutes neostig-

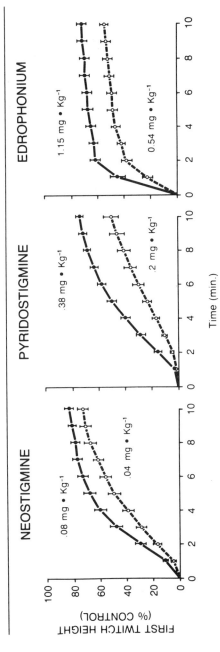

Fig 2–6.— First twitch height vs. time after administration of reversal agents, which were injected at 1% spontaneous recovery. (Courtesy of Donati F, Lahoud J, McCready D, et al: *Can J Anaesth* 34:589–593, November 1987.)

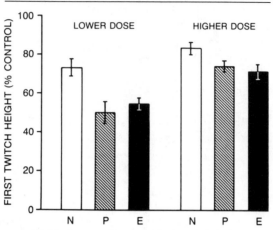

Fig 2–7.—First twitch height (percent of control) 10 minutes after administration of neostigmine (N), 0.04 mg/kg, or pyridostigmine (P), 0.2 mg/kg, or edrophonium (E), 0.54 mg/kg (lower dose), or 0.08 mg/kg, 0.38 mg/kg, or 1.15 mg/kg, respectively (higher dose). Bars, SEM. (Courtesy of Donati F, Lahoud J, McCready D, et al: Can J Anaesth 34:589–593, November 1987.)

mine produced a better recovery than the other 2 agents, especially at higher doses (Fig 2–7).

Neostigmine is more effective than either pyridostigmine or edrophonium in reversing the effects of deep pancuronium blockade. Because adequate neuromuscular recovery cannot be achieved with the usual doses of any of these agents sooner than 10 minutes after administration, it is preferable to avoid profound neuromuscular blockade entirely if possible.

▶ This is one of many articles indicating that the standard doses of edrophonium (0.5 mg/kg) are not effective in reversing an intense neuromuscular blockade (i.e., 95% or greater). There seems to be some controversy as to whether 1 mg/kg of edrophonium is effective in reversing these intense blocks. There seems to be little doubt that neostigmine, while slower in onset, is a more consistent antagonist of an intense neuromuscular blockade. Although it is of interest to compare the pharmacology of the antagonists, these authors correctly emphasize the need to avoid profound neuromuscular blockades in the first place.—R.D. Miller, M.D.

Relationship Between Posttetanic Count and Response to Carinal Stimulation During Vecuronium-Induced Neuromuscular Blockade
Fernando PUE, Viby-Mogensen J, Bonsu AK, Tamilarasan A, Muchhal KK, Lambourne A (King Khalid Univ Hosp, Riyadh; King Saud Univ, Riyadh, Saudi Arabia; Herlev Hosp, Herlev, Denmark)
Acta Anaesth Scand 31:593–596, October 1987   2–34

Sensitivity to muscle relaxants varies among muscle groups; therefore, the mechanical response to peripheral nerve stimulation does not necessarily reflect the degree of diaphragmatic paralysis. The number of re-

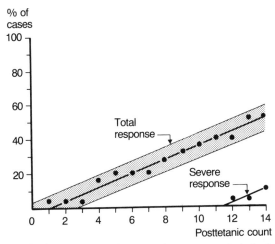

Fig 2–8.—Relationship between posttetanic count and response to carinal stimulation in 25 patients anesthetized with thiopental, N₂O, and halothane. (Courtesy of Fernando PUE, Viby-Mogensen J, Bonsu AK, et al: *Acta Anaesth Scand* 31:593–596, October 1987.)

sponses to posttetanic single-twitch stimulation can be correlated with the degree of peripheral neuromuscular blockade. The posttetanic count (PTC) recorded peripherally at the thumb was correlated with the degree of diaphragmatic paralysis induced by vecuronium in 50 patients randomly assigned to 1 of 2 equal groups.

One group was anesthetized with thiopental, nitrous oxide, and halothane; the other received thiopental, nitrous oxide, and fentanyl. The degree of peripheral blockade was determined by train-of-four (TOF) and

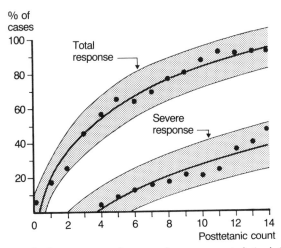

Fig 2–9.—Relationship between posttetanic count and response to carinal stimulation in 25 patients anesthetized with thiopental, N₂O, and fentanyl. (Courtesy of Fernando PUE, Viby-Mogensen J, Bonsu AK, et al: *Acta Anaesth Scand* 31:593–596, October 1987.)

PTC stimulation of the ulnar nerve. Diaphragmatic paralysis was evaluated by stimulating the carina. Muscular response was classified as severe, mild, or absent.

During halothane anesthesia at first response to PTC stimulation, 2% of patients had a mild response to carinal stimulation; at first response to TOF stimulation, 48% of patients had a mild response to carinal stimulation (Fig 2–8). When fentanyl was used, 20% of the patients reacted mildly when PTC was 1; however, at the first TOF response, 92% reacted to carinal stimulation, 24% so severely that intervention was required (Fig 2–9).

Peripheral elicitation of the TOF response is a late sign of neuromuscular recovery of the diaphragm. Evaluating early recovery of this muscle is better accomplished with the PTC method. Neuromuscular blockade should be so intense that no response to PTC can be obtained.

▶ Dr. Viby-Mogensen continues to ask interesting clinical questions; this is no exception. In essence, can one tell by examining the results to peripheral nerve stimulation whether a patient will cough when the carina is stimulated by an endotracheal tube? Clearly they have found that there should be no posttetanic count in order to assure that there will be no response to carinal stimulation. For example, if one is relying upon paralysis, rather than adequate anesthesia, to ensure that a patient will not cough during ophthalmologic surgery, then complete anesthesia (no response to peripheral nerve stimulation) is needed. Of course this reviewer's bias is that adequate anesthesia is preferable to a profound neuromuscular blockade.—R.D. Miller, M.D.

Monitoring Neuromuscular Blockade With Calf Stimulators
Beemer GH (Royal Melbourne Hosp, Melbourne)
Anaesth Intens Care 15:375–378, November 1987   2–35

Peripheral nerve stimulators used to monitor neuromuscular blockade are not widely used in Australia. As an alternative, anesthetists use the change in response to calf stimulation as an indication of the level of neuromuscular blockade. The efficacy of monitoring neuromuscular blockade during surgery using calf stimulators was determined in 25 patients. Stimulation of the ulnar nerve with a peripheral nerve stimulator also was performed. The calf stimulators were applied to the medial aspect of the calf and adjusted to produce a brisk ankle jerk. After an initial bolus dose of atracurium, 0.5 mg/kg, further incremental doses of 0.2 mg/kg were administered when the response to calf stimulation was small and obvious. The magnitude of the ankle jerk in response to calf stimulation was assessed visually and graded from 0 to 4.

Neuromuscular blockade was judged adequate throughout the surgical procedures in all patients, with an average of 5 incremental doses of atracurium administered. The response to calf stimulation was often greater and more often persisted than after stimulation of the ulnar nerve by a peripheral nerve stimulator. The mean spontaneous recovery time after the last incremental dose of atracurium was 42 minutes. The mean recovery time after administration of reversal agents for residual neuromuscular block was 5.5 minutes.

Calf stimulation has only limited accuracy in assessing neuromuscular blockade. It should not be considered as an alternative to a peripheral nerve stimulator when accurate monitoring is required. The difficulty in visually quantifying large responses limits the usefulness of calf stimulators, as well as the different sensitivities of the muscles being stimulated (both fast and slow muscles as against only fast muscle in peripheral nerve stimulation) to neuromuscular blocking agents. It may useful, however, in helping to avoid the wide fluctuations in blockade that are prone to occur with competitive neuromuscular blocking agents of intermediate duration.

▶ Although this may not have any practical use clinically, it is another way to monitor neuromuscular function.—R.D. Miller, M.D.

Prehospital Use of Neuromuscular Blocking Agents in a Helicopter Ambulance Program
Syverud SA, Borron SW, Storer DL, Hedges JR, Dronen SC, Braunstein LT, Hubbard BJ (Univ of Cincinnati)
Ann Emerg Med 17:236–242, March 1988   2–36

Airway interventions may be difficult during transport in a helicopter. The use of succinylcholine chloride and pancuronium bromide as an adjunct to airway management by the physician/nurse flight team of a hospital-based helicopter ambulance service (University Air Care) was evaluated in a prospective study. Data on 39 patients who received these agents at the scene of an accident (prehospital group) were compared with data on 35 patients who were paralyzed by the flight team in the emergency department of the transferring hospitals (control). According to protocol, succinylcholine was used primarily for endotracheal intubation and pancuronium bromide was used for prolonged paralysis after endotracheal intubation. The recommended dose of succinylcholine was 1.5 mg/kg, and of pancuronium, 0.06–0.1 mg/kg in an intravenous push.

The 74 patients received 1 or both neuromuscular blocking agents. Intubation attempts had failed previously in 54% of these patients; also, 12% were having seizures and 82% had significant intracranial pathology. Endotracheal intubation was the primary indication for paralysis in most patients, although intracranial pressure control, ventilation, agitation control, and seizure control were frequent secondary indications. After paralysis, 68 (96%) patients were successfully intubated. The 3 intubation failures resulted from an infiltrated intravenous line, poor visualization of the larynx, and upper airway hemorrhage after craniofacial trauma. Serious complications (i.e., dysrhythmias requiring drug therapy) occurred in 3 patients but resolved with appropriate therapy.

Minor complications (e.g., dysrhythmias not requiring therapy, histamine flush, or infiltrated intravenous line) occurred in 18 patients. There was no significant difference in successful intubation or complication rate between the prehospital group and controls. Furthermore, the flight team believed that, in most cases, safe helicopter transport could not have been accomplished without the use of neuromuscular blockade.

Neuromuscular blocking agents can be used safely and effectively at accident scenes by a physician/nurse team. Paralysis allows airway stabilization in a significant number of critically ill patients who could not otherwise be intubated endotracheally.

▶ Despite the success of this approach, this reviewer believes that the use of neuromuscular blocking drugs in a helicopter ambulance program is probably unwise. The ease of endotracheal intubation with the use of neuromuscular blocking drugs will encourage less experienced individuals to use them more frequently, which will provide the opportunity for disasters to occur.—R.D. Miller, M.D.

The Clinical Neuromuscular Pharmacology of Mivacurium Chloride (BW B1090U): A Short-Acting Nondepolarizing Ester Neuromuscular Blocking Drug
Savarese JJ, Ali HH, Basta SJ, Embree PB, Scott RPF, Sunder N, Weakly JN, Wastila WB, El-Sayad HA (Harvard Univ; Burroughs Wellcome Co, Research Triangle Park, NC)
Anesthesiology 68:723–732, May 1988   2–37

Mivacurium chloride (BW B1090U) is a newly developed, short-acting, nondepolarizing neuromuscular blocking agent intended for use during anesthesia. This study was done to define the neuromuscular blocking properties of mivacurium in human beings by determining its potency, dose-response for onset, duration of action, and ability to antagonize residual block by neostigmine.

The study population consisted of 72 American Society of Anesthesiologists Physical Status I or II patients, aged 18–49 years, who were undergoing nitrous oxide/oxygen-narcotic-thiopental anesthesia. The neuromuscular blocking effect of mivacurium was measured after administration of bolus doses of 0.03–0.30 mg/kg, as well as during and after continuous mivacurium infusions lasting 35–324 minutes. The force of thumb adduction in response to stimulation of the ulnar nerve at 0.15 Hz was measured at predetermined intervals.

The calculated ED95 for inhibition of thumb twitch was 0.08 mg/kg. At 0.1 mg/kg, 96% block developed, the mean time from onset to maximal neuromuscular blockage was 3.8 minutes, and recovery to 95% twitch height occurred 24.5 minutes after injection. At 0.25 mg/kg, the mean time to onset of maximal block was 2.3 minutes, and 95% recovery occurred within 30.4 minutes. Thus, an increase in duration of action of only 24% was observed with a 150% higher dose. Recovery indices did not differ significantly among all dosage groups from 0.1 to 0.3 mg/kg. Similarly, patients who received continuous mivacurium infusion also showed rapid recovery of neuromuscular blockade. Antagonism of residual block was seldom necessary.

It is thought that the rapid hydrolysis of mivacurium is caused by the catalytic activity of plasma cholinesterase. Even with increased doses, there was a surprisingly small increase in the duration of the blocking effect. Although the pharmacokinetic studies of mivacurium have not yet been fully completed, the findings to date suggest a short elimination half-life and a comparatively rapid clearance of mivacurium.

Mivacurium may be useful in short surgical procedures, such as are done in ambulatory care surgery, because it affords fast, spontaneous recovery.

▶ This is an excellent survey-type of study that described the neuromuscular blocking properties of a new nondepolarizing muscle relaxant. The main virtue of this relaxant is that it has a shorter duration of action than atracurium or vecuronium.— R.D. Miller, M.D.

Mivacurium Chloride (BW B1090U)-Induced Neuromuscular Blockade During Nitrous Oxide–Isoflurane and Nitrous Oxide–Narcotic Anesthesia in Adult Surgical Patients
Weber S, Brandom BW, Powers DM, Sarner JB, Woelfel SK, Cook DR, Foster VJ, McNulty BF, Weakly JN (Univ of Pittsburgh; Allegheny Gen Hosp, Pittsburgh; Burroughs Wellcome Co, Research Triangle Park, NC)
Anesth Analg 67:495–499, 1988   2–38

Mivacurium (BW B1090U) is a nondepolarizing, short-acting neuromuscular blocking agent that is metabolized by human plasma cholinesterase. Previous clinical trials have found it to be safe and effective. Evaluation was made of the dose-response relation for mivacurium, time of onset, and duration of neuromuscular blockade during nitrous oxide-oxygen-isoflurane (ISO) anesthesia and nitrous oxide-thiopental-fentanyl (BAL) anesthesia.

The study population consisted of 90 patients aged 18–67 years who were undergoing elective surgical procedures of low to moderate risk and requiring tracheal intubation. Anesthesia was induced with thiopental and fentanyl and maintained in 45 patients with ISO and in the other 45 patients with BAL. Neuromuscular blockade was measured using electromyographic activity of the adductor pollicis muscle after supramaximal stimulation of the ulnar nerve. Three subgroups of 9 patients each in the ISO group received mivacurium in doses of 0.025, 0.03, and 0.04 mg/kg, and 3 subgroups of 9 patients each in the BAL group were given mivacurium in doses of 0.03, 0.04, and 0.05 mg/kg.

The estimated ED_{50} in the ISO group was 0.029 mg/kg, and in the BAL group, 0.041 mg/kg. The estimated ED_{95} in the ISO group was 0.045 mg/kg, and in the BAL group, 0.058 mg/kg. The BAL group had a shorter recovery index than was found in the ISO group. Increasing the dose of mivacurium did not significantly prolong the neuromuscular blocking activity, as the difference in average time to any end-point of neuromuscular recovery between doses was about 2.0 minutes. The addition of isoflurane to nitrous-oxide-narcotic anesthesia, however, amplified the degree of neuromuscular blockade from a given dose of mivacurium and prolonged the recovery index. None of the patients experienced any significant changes in heart rate or blood pressure.

These findings confirm that mivacurium is safe and effective and has an extremely short half-life.

▶ This is a useful screen article with a new, nondepolarizing, neuromuscular blocking drug, which should be advantageous in the ambulatory surgery setting.—R.D. Miller, M.D.

Clinical Pharmacology of Doxacurium Chloride (BW A938U) in Children
Sarner JB, Brandom BW, Cook DR, Dong M-L, Horn MC, Woelfel SK, Davis PJ, Rudd GD, Foster VJ, McNulty BF (Children's Hosp of Pittsburgh; Univ of Pittsburgh; Burroughs Wellcome Co, Research Triangle Park, NC)
Anesth Analg 67:303–306, 1988   2–39

Neuromuscular blockade with doxacurium chloride was tested to determine its pharmacologic effects in children. A group of 26 children undergoing elective surgery that required tracheal intubation were enrolled in the study. The children, aged 2–12 years, received halothane-nitrous oxide-oxygen anesthesia.

Nine patients (group A) were given an initial dose of doxacurium, with additional doses after stabilization to achieve a minimum of 75% neuromuscular blockade. Another 9 patients (group B) received the calculated ED_{95} of doxacurium, 27.5 μg/kg, intravenously. Eight patients (group C) were given doxacurium, 50 μg/kg ($1.8 \times ED_{95}$).

During the monitoring period, no significant changes in blood pressure, mean arterial pressure, or cardiac rhythm appeared in the 3 groups of children. Nor were other adverse effects attributed to doxacurium. All 3 groups reported a similar recovery index. Neuromuscular transmission returned spontaneously in 14 patients.

In children, maximum blockade and recovery from blockade are achieved more quickly than in adults, thus children may need larger doses of doxacurium and higher plasma concentrations than adults do to receive the same degree of blockade. Although this study was limited to children receiving a single type of anesthesia and did not make use of a control group, the findings show doxacurium to be a muscle relaxant having no adverse effects on healthy children.

▶ This is a well-performed study, providing an overall survey of the use of this new, long-acting neuromuscular blocking drug in children.—R.D. Miller, M.D.

Clinical Pharmacology of Doxacurium Chloride: A New Long-Acting Non-depolarizing Muscle Relaxant
Basta SJ, Savarese JJ, Ali HH, Embree PB, Schwartz AF, Rudd GD, Wastila WB (Harvard Med School at Massachusetts Gen Hosp, Boston; Burroughs Wellcome Co, Research Triangle Park, NC)
Anesthesiology 69:478–486, October 1988   2–40

Doxacurium chloride is a long-acting, nondepolarizing, noncumulative muscle relaxant that is readily antagonized by neostigmine and edrophonium, has no autonomic effects, and has no histamine release (Fig 2–10). The compound's effects were assessed in 89 healthy American Society of Anesthesiologists physical status I and II patients, 74 males and 15 females, aged 18 to 59 years, who were undergoing low-risk elective surgical procedures.

Before anesthesia induction, each patient was pretreated with orally administered diazepam and morphine. General anesthesia was induced with thiopental and fentanyl and was maintained with nitrous oxide and oxygen. Doxacurium was given as a bolus injection in doses ranging from 10 to 80 µg/kg. The effects of doxacurium were compared with those in 8 control patients who received 100 µg/kg of pancuronium with an identical anesthesia. Neuromuscular function was monitored using the evoked mechanomyographic response of the ulnar nerve-adductor pollicis system. A mixture of neostigmine and atropine was used to antagonize any residual doxacurium-induced blockade.

The time between injection and maximum blockade was directly dose-related. Sixty-seven of the 81 doxacurium-treated patients and 8 of the 9 pancuronium-treated patients required varying doses of neostigmine and atropine to antagonize residual neuromuscular blockade, which was effectively antagonized in all patients. Doxacurium in doses up to and including 2.7 times the ED_{95} did not have any dose-related effects on the heart rate or mean arterial blood pressure, and it did not cause any elevation in plasma histamine concentrations.

Doxacurium is a long-acting nondepolarizing muscle relaxant with readily reversible neuromuscular blocking activity. It appears to have

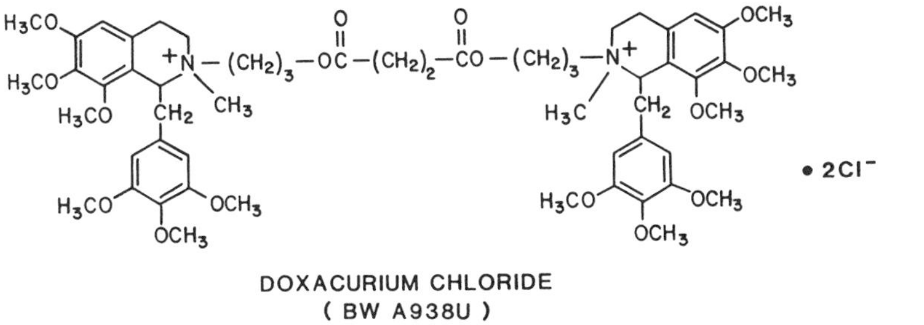

DOXACURIUM CHLORIDE
(BW A938U)

Fig 2–10.—Chemical formula of doxacurium chloride (BW A938U). (Courtesy of Basta SJ, Savarese JJ, Ali HH, et al: *Anesthesiology* 69:478–486, October 1988.)

clinical advantages over currently available long-acting neuromuscular blocking agents, which warrants its further testing in larger clinical trials.

▶ This is an excellent survey-type of study of a new, long-acting, nondepolarizing muscle relaxant.— R.D. Miller, M.D.

Allergy and Anaphylaxis

Atopy and Anaphylactic Reactions to Suxamethonium
Charpin D, Benzarti M, Hémon Y, Senft M, Alazia M, Arnaud A, Vervloet D, Charpin J (Hôpital Sainte-Marguerite; Hôpital de la Timone, Marseille, France)
J Allergy Clin Immunol 82:356–360, September 1988   2–41

The incidence of anaphylactic reactions (ARs) during general anesthesia appears to be increasing. Anaphylactic reactions to muscle relaxants are responsible for half of all adverse reactions during general anesthesia. To study the role of atopy as a potential risk factor for developing an immunoglobulin E (IgE)-dependent AR to muscle relaxants, a case-control study was done to assess the distribution of clinical and biologic signs of atopy among patients with a history of ARs to suxamethonium and among matched controls.

During a 6-year study period, each of 32 patients had an AR during general anesthesia with muscle relaxants, and 29 of them went into cardiac arrest. All patients had confirmed specific IgE and a positive leukocyte histamine release with suxamethonium. The matched control group consisted of 128 persons who had a negative skin test result for suxamethonium. All patients and controls were asked to complete questionnaires regarding prior personal history of hay fever, asthma, childhood dermatitis, and family history of atopic diseases. All patients and controls underwent skin testing to common aeroallergens and measurement of total serum IgE antibody levels.

Twenty-one (66%) of the 32 patients and 92 (72%) of the 128 controls had positive skin tests to common aeroallergens. Two (6.2%) patients and 6 (4.6%) controls had a history of hay fever. Fourteen (44%) patients and 47 (37%) controls had a family history of atopy. Thus, the distribution of symptoms suggestive of atopy and of skin tests and specific IgE to common aeroallergens was similar in both groups. However, total serum IgE levels were much higher among patients, suggesting the presence of specific IgE against suxamethonium or other drugs.

Atopy is not a risk factor for the occurrence of ARs to muscle relaxants.

▶ This is an interesting article that further elucidates the allergic or anaphylactic potential of muscle relaxants. Its only problem is that it intermingles nondepolarizing and depolarizing neuromuscular blocking drugs as if they are the same class of drugs, which is clearly not the case.— R.D. Miller, M.D.

Allergy to Suxamethonium: Persisting Abnormalities in Skin Tests, Specific IgE Antibodies and Leucocyte Histamine Release

Didier A, Benzarti M, Senft M, Charpin D, Lagier F, Charpin J, Vervloet D (Hôpital Ste-Marguerite, Unité INSERM, Marseille, France)
Clin Allergy 17:385–392, September 1987　　　　　　　　　　2–42

There have been a number of reports of anaphylactic reactions after general anesthesia with muscle relaxants, in particular with suxamethonium. Recent evidence indicates that these reactions are mediated by immunoglobulin E (IgE) antibodies against muscle relaxants. Various diagnostic tests are available to determine sensitivity. The reproducibility of several tests were assessed, the longevity of hypersensitivity to suxamethonium was investigated, and tests for use in retrospective diagnosis were evaluated.

Skin tests were performed in 21 patients approximately 2 months after anaphylactic reactions to suxamethonium and again 1–4 years later. In addition to suxamethonium, patients were tested for sensitivity to gallamine, pancuronium, and alcuronium. Sera from 19 patients were tested for choline-specific IgE antibodies, and leukocyte histamine release was measured in 17 patients.

All patients had positive skin tests to suxamethonium at the time of initial evaluation; 15 patients were positive for gallamine; 8, for alcuronium; and 5, for pancuronium. On retesting 1–4 years later, 96% of patients still had positive test results for suxamethonium; positivity had declined slightly for the other muscle relaxants. Twenty-six percent of patients had modification of anticholine IgE over the study period. On retesting, 1 patient had a reduction in leukocyte histamine release.

These findings indicate that skin tests, leukocyte histamine release, and detection of anticholine IgE are reliable methods of diagnosing allergic reaction to suxamethonium, even when testing occurs a long time after the initial anaphylactic reaction. It is possible that sensitivity to muscle relaxants may be maintained by exposure to its major antigenic determinants, quaternary ammonium compounds, which are found in cosmetics, antiseptics, and detergents.

▶ It is a common teaching that quaternary ammonium portions present in all muscle relaxants are the antigenic stimulus for production of immunoglobulin E antibodies. Acceptance of this concept allows one to recognize the predictable cross-sensitivity between all muscle relaxants and the likely continued antigenic stimulation from soaps and cosmetics that contain quaternary ammonium components. It seems the best clinical dictum is "once allergic, always allergic."—R.K. Stoelting, M.D.

Anaphylaxis to Intravenous Furosemide

Hansbrough JR, Wedner HJ, Chaplin DD (Washington Univ)
J Allergy Clin Immunol 80:538–541, October 1987　　　　　2–43

True systemic allergic reactions to furosemide, a potent loop diuretic and a sulfa compound, occurred in a patient who had an anaphylactic reaction to the drug.

Man, 41, with long-standing hypertension, experienced urticaria, periorbital edema, and significant hypotension within 5 minutes after the intravenous administration of furosemide for treatment of severe hypertension. Immediate hypersensitivity was documented by positive skin tests to furosemide and other related sulfonamide-based drugs. No adverse reaction was noted when the patient was challenged with nifedipine, the only other drug administered at the time of his reaction.

Although clinical experience with furosemide indicates that it is a safe drug free from life-threatening side effects under normal conditions, a hypersensitivity reaction to furosemide may occur. The possibility of such an adverse reaction should be considered in patients who are sensitive to other sulfonamide-containing drugs.

▶ This is perhaps not surprising when one considers the relationship of furosemide to sulfonamide drugs. A history of allergy to "sulfur" should now translate to concern should diuretics with a sulfonamide component (furosemide, chlorothiazide, and bumetanide, but not ethracrynic acid) be considered for intravenous administration.—R.K. Stoelting, M.D.

3 Preoperative

Medication

Do Patients Fasting Before and After Operation Receive Their Prescribed Drug Treatment?
Wyld R, Nimmo WS (Univ of Sheffield, England)
Br Med J 296:744, Mar 12, 1988   3–1

Periods of fasting perioperatively make normal drug treatment difficult to maintain. In one series, only 71% of patients had their normal drugs before surgery, and only 41% received them on the day of their operation. The sudden withdrawal of such drugs may be harmful. A study was done to determine whether patients fasting before and after their operations in 1 hospital received their prescribed drugs.

One hundred seventy patients admitted consecutively for surgery, excluding cardiac, neurosurgical, and orthopedic procedures, were studied. Seventy-two were taking drugs unrelated to their surgery or anesthesia. On the day of surgery and the day after surgery, 1,746 single prescriptions were recorded as to be given, but 256 (15%) were not given (table). All prescriptions of analgesics and premedicants were given. When these were excluded, the proportion of prescriptions that were not administered rose to 29%. Prescriptions omitted included 38 of 95 for drugs for cardiovascular disease, 34 of 103 for drugs for respiratory disease, and 10 of 61 for drugs for endocrine disorders. The omission of drugs was not known to the medical staff.

In this study, 15% of all prescriptions were omitted for fasting patients

Number of Prescriptions Intended to be Given and Number Not
Given Over 2 Days to 170 Patients Taking Operations,
by Drug Group

	No of prescriptions (% of total) (n=1746)	No (%) omitted (n=256)
Drugs affecting*:		
Gastrointestinal system	40 (2)	31 (78)
Cardiovascular system	95 (5)	38 (40)
Respiratory system	103 (6)	34 (33)
Central nervous system	73 (4)	36 (49)
Infections	255 (15)	32 (13)
Endocrine system	61 (4)	10 (16)
Urinary tract disorders	6 (<1)	3 (50)
Malignant disease	9 (<1)	4 (44)
Nutrition and blood	33 (2)	24 (73)
Musculoskeletal disease	56 (3)	28 (50)
Anticoagulants	161 (9)	16 (10)
Premedicants and analgesics*	854 (49)	0

*According to *British National Formulary.*
(Courtesy of Wyld R, Nimmo WS: *Br Med J* 296:744, March 12, 1988.)

on the day of or day after surgery. Withholding drugs from patients undergoing surgery may introduce variability in response during the perioperative period.

▶ It has always amazed me that, when you make a patient NPO, often they do not get their medicines, even some that you wish. I have now taken to writing "Nothing by Mouth Except Medicines" and say this specifically to the patient. As it is, when a patient takes the medicines and has increased anxiety, I worry that their level of anxiety will affect the drug's absorption pharmacokinetics and pharmacodynamics.—M.F. Roizen, M.D.

Approaches to Decreasing Anxiety

Reduction of Preoperative Anxiety: Music as an Alternative to Pharmacotherapy

Daub D, Kirschner-Hermanns R (Städtisch Klinikum Karlsruhe, West Germany)
Anaesthesist 37:594–597, 1988   3–2

It is generally believed that anxiolytic drugs are the best treatment for decreasing preoperative anxiety. However, it has been shown that a friendly staff, explanation of the procedure, and good organization also decrease preoperative anxiety, suggesting that preoperative anxiety is susceptible to treatment modalities other than drugs. Music therapy has a calming effect on brain-damaged children. However, its effectiveness in reducing anxiety during the preoperative period has not been evaluated.

In this study, 90 patients aged 15 to 65 years who were undergoing routine operations under general anesthesia were randomly assigned to 3 groups. Thirty patients did not receive any preoperative medication, 30 patients were given an intramuscular injection of thalamonal 1 hour before operation, and 30 patients listened to a Walkman tape player through ear phones to specially selected music, starting at least 45 minutes before operation. Only patients whose native tongue was German were included. All patients underwent psychometric testing 90 minutes before operation and 15 minutes before entering the operating room. On the evening of the day of surgery, each patient was asked to evaluate the preoperative period.

The patients assigned to the music group were an average of 8 years older than the thalamonal-treated group and about 6 years older than the control group. All 3 groups had comparable preoperative trait-anxiety. At the start of the preoperative period, state-anxiety in all 3 groups was still comparable, but it then increased in the thalamonal-treated group, decreased in the music-treated group, and remained unchanged in the control group. The differences in anxiety scores measured 15 minutes before entering the operating room between the 3 groups were statistically significant. Postoperatively, 26 of the 30 music-treated patients stated that they liked listening to music before the operation. Eleven patients had selected classical music and 19 selected light music. Patients who commonly listened to music for relaxation had lower anxiety scores than those who commonly listened to music for entertainment. That the music had been carefully selected to suit each patient's taste and personality added to an impression that the patient was not considered merely as an object to be operated on.

Carefully selected music used as premedication before operation significantly decreases preoperative anxiety.

▶ This is another article indicating the use of a nonpharmacologic approach to decreasing patient anxiety and, in other studies, analgesia.—R.D. Miller, M.D.

Effects of Mailed Preoperative Instructions on Learning and Anxiety
Mikulaninec CE (North Carolina Baptist Hosps, Winston-Salem, NC)
Patient Educ Counsel 10:253–265, December 1987   3–3

Surgical instruction after admission may be difficult to accomplish because of the patient's shortened length of stay, as well as the probable high level of anxiety that may be experienced after admission. Several studies have shown greater learning or better surgical outcomes when patients are given preadmission instruction in surgical exercises. A study was undertaken to determine the effects of mailing preoperative instructions on learning and anxiety compared with teaching performed by nurses after hospital admission.

Sixty-six patients aged 18–72 years who were to undergo elective general surgical procedures were sequentially assigned to 1 of 4 groups. Group 1 received an educational booklet, "Preparation for Surgery and Recovery," by mail 1 week before admission and also received the usual postadmission instruction by nurses; group 2 received only the preadmission booklet; group 3 received postadmission instruction; and group 4 received no instruction. All patients were either first-time surgery patients or those who denied having had instruction in surgical exercises with previous surgical procedures. At set times after hospital admission, all patients were assessed with 2 testing instruments, 1 of which was a researcher-devised checklist to measure behaviors (Fig 3–1). The Spielberger State Anxiety Inventory was also administered to assess the level of state anxiety.

All 3 groups that received teaching scored higher in terms of surgical exercise performance than those who had received no teaching, and all 3 forms of teaching were equally beneficial when compared with each other. There was no significant difference in anxiety level between groups.

Mailing preadmission material to elective surgical patients may be considered a viable alternative to postadmission instruction in surgical exercises. Mailing educational material to the home may offer advantages by promoting independent learning, reducing nursing time with regard to

Mikulaninec's Preoperative
Exercise Checklist

Previous Surgery   Yes   No
If yes, received previous instruction
in surgical exercises   Yes   No

Time begun_____

Time ended_____

I.D.#_____
Surgery_____
Age/Sex_____
Race_____
Education_____

Exercises	Sample Question	Behavior	Yes	No
DEEP BREATHING	Ask pt. to demonstrate deep breathing	1. Pt. places hand over abdomen or chest if incision will be abd. or chest		
		2. Pt. inhales slowly and deeply		
	Ask pt. how many times deep breathing should be done	3. Knows to deep breathe 3 times		
	Ask pt. to demonstrate coughing	4. Coughs deeply after deep breath		
	Ask how many times coughing should be done	5. Knows to cough several times		
	Ask how often deep breathing and coughing should be done	6. Knows to repeat deep breathing and coughing at least every two hours		
	Ask why these exercises should be done	7. Knows purpose of the exercises is to keep lungs functioning properly and prevent complications like pneumonia		
TURNING	Ask pt. to demonstrate turning	1. Demonstrate turning back to side or side to back or side to side		
	Ask: "How often?"	2. Knows to turn at least every two hours		
LEG EXERCISES	Ask pt. to demonstrate leg exercises	1. Bends leg fully (knee sharply bent)		
	Ask: "How often?"	2. Knows to perform once every hour		
FOOT EXERCISES	Ask pt. to demonstrate	1. Rotates ankle		
		2. Points toes 2-3 seconds, then relaxes		
		3. Dorsi-flexes foot 2-3 seconds, then relaxes		
	Ask: "How often?"	4. Knows to perform foot exercises once each hour		
	Ask: "Why?"	5. Knows purpose of bed exercises is to improve circulation/prevent complications		

a. Patient has/has not read the booklet, "Preparation for Surgery".
b. Instructions on surgical exercises received before contact with nurse researcher:

Fig 3–1.—Checklist to measure behaviors. (Courtesy of Mikulaninec CE: *Patient Educ Counsel* 10:253–265, December 1987.)

time spent in teaching surgical exercises after admission, and involving the family in the learning process.

▶ It is difficult to imagine that sending something in the mail will have useful educational and clinical results. Nevertheless, these results are encouraging.—R.D. Miller, M.D.

The Psychological Effects of Having a Contact-Person From the Anesthetic Staff

Elsass P, Deudahl H, Friis B, Møller IW, Sørensen MB (Rigshospitalet, Copenhagen)
Acta Anaesthesiol Scand 31:584–586, 1987   3–4

Preoperative information about anesthesia and surgical procedures does not always reduce a patient's anxiety. The supportive value of having a staff contact-person available for both cognitive and emotional support was investigated.

Identical questionnaires were administered preoperatively and postoperatively to 74 patients undergoing elective surgery. The course of anxiety was compared between patients who were given a 5-minute explanation as to where the anesthetic procedure would take place, how it would be administered, and how long it would take, and patients who received this information but also had an anesthetic nurse available for support during anesthesia and surgery preparation. These patients were also told that the nurse would be there when they awoke. These results were then compared with 3 previous studies.

Almost all patients found the preanesthetic explanation reassuring, but 84% of those who were also visited by an anesthetic nurse felt that this visit was more tranquilizing. The patients without staff contact-persons reported significantly more discomfort during preparation and awakening and significantly more side effects than those with a staff contact-person. The support of an anesthetic staff contact-person is more effective than either cognitive information or a tranquilizer in reducing patient anxiety.

▶ Rather than being described as having or not having a contact-person from the anesthetic staff, I think the 2 groups were different in that one had interviews by an anesthesiologist who may or may not have been involved in the patients' care, whereas the other group was interviewed by a nurse anesthetist who was directly involved in the patients' care. They found that patients had more anxiety in the group contacted by an anesthesiologist who may or may not have been giving them their anesthetic than in the group contacted by an anesthesiologist in the same category but that also was visited by a nurse anesthetist. Of interest is that the patients who saw the nurse anesthetist didn't have a changed anxiety score, but that the group that was seen by an anesthesiologist who may or may not have been involved in their care had increased anxiety as the time of the operation approached and even after the operation. I believe this has pertinence to those of us who see patients that we may not be giving anesthesia to versus those of us who require that the anesthesiologist giving the care is actually the one who sees the patients preoperatively.

I think this study needs to be repeated in a more defined way, looking at that problem to see whether it is indeed a problem, whether a 5-minute interview (the brief visit by the anesthesiologist) is really enough time, or whether other things should have been explained to the patient preoperatively. Was it the contact time with the nurse and physician versus the physician alone that was important, or was it that the physician was not the person who was administering their anesthesia that was important in allowing or in preventing the increase in anxiety? I don't think we know the answer to this question.—M.F. Roizen, M.D.

Consent

Surgical Informed Consent: What It Is and Is Not
Edwards WS, Yahne C (Univ of New Mexico)
Am J Surg 154:574–578, December 1987   3–5

The appropriate use of the informed consent interview can achieve better physician-patient relationships. Because few physicians are taught about informed consent during medical training, however, there are significant gaps in what physicians know about the process of informing their patients. A year-long study was undertaken to learn how well residents and faculty conduct informed consent interviews. Using an actress in the role of a patient, researchers videotaped unrehearsed consent interviews conducted by faculty and house staff. One surgeon was asked to give a poor interview; being cryptic, arrogant, and unsympathetic.

Many residents and staff understood the informed consent process well and conducted the simulated interviews appropriately, but whether they would have done as well in a real-life situation is unknown. Problems with the process include conflicting messages—from the courts, from within themselves, and from their peers—lack of time for dialogue with patients, and poor timing of the consent process. Some surgeons are biased toward surgery as the only satisfactory mode of treatment, and some believe that longevity should be the goal of treatment regardless of quality of life.

Surgeons should regard the informed consent process as an opportunity to communicate their personal concern for the patient as a human being rather than as a procedure to be performed. If the surgeon is sensitive to the patient's feelings, the patient-physician relationship can be strengthened.

▶ Multiple studies have been done indicating that most consents are rarely informed. This article offers some suggestions as to how informed consent can be improved.—R.D. Miller, M.D.

Anxiety and Informed Consent: Does Anxiety Influence Consent for Inclusion in a Study of Anxiolytic Premedication?
Antrobus JHL (General Infirmary at Leeds, England)
Anaesthesia 43:267–269, 1988   3–6

Sample selection for a clinical trial is biased if the variable under investigation influences patients to withhold consent to inclusion. Because studies of the efficacy of preanesthetic medication largely concern anxiolysis, it is important to determine whether anxiety can influence the granting of informed consent. Anxiety levels in patients who granted permission for inclusion in a hypothetical premedication study were compared with those of patients who withheld consent.

Forty-eight consecutive inpatients undergoing elective gynecologic surgery were studied. They completed 2 scales of anxiety: Spielberger's state-trait anxiety inventory and a 10-cm linear analog scale. A standardized explanation of the hypothetical premedication study was given, and the patients' consent was requested. Thirty-three granted consent, and 10 did not. Anxiety scores were found to be significantly higher for those withholding consent than for those granting it.

Patients with high levels of preoperative anxiety, who are in most need of anxiolysis, are more likely to withhold consent for inclusion in studies of premedication than are those with less anxiety. Thus, seeking informed consent introduces bias into studies of anxiolytic premedication.

► I think this article is important, as it approaches the question of how to get to study anxious patients who, as individuals, may be most in need of premedicants and, as a group, may be most in need of studies for premedication when they themselves opt out of studies of premedicants because of their anxiety. I think the gist of the article can be summarized by part of its last paragraph: "It is concluded from this study that patients with high levels of pre-operative anxiety who are most in need of anxiolysis are more likely to withhold consent for inclusion in studies of premedication than are those with less anxiety. It may be necessary, in order to establish efficacy in these patients, to proceed without obtaining their consent. Whether or not it is justified to do so must be judged by an independent ethical committee on the basis of specific proposals." I think this study highlights one of the hardest areas to examine and brings forth an ethical dilemma for which there is no solution at the present time. Before we go further on the ethical dilemma, I think that others should try to duplicate the data of Dr. Antrobus.—M.F. Roizen, M.D.

Testing

Operations Postponed by Anaesthetists: A Prospective Study
Whelan E, Gordon HL (Whiston Hosp, Prescot, England)
Ann R Coll Surg Engl 69:295–299, November 1987   3–7

The principal reasons for postponement of operations on the advice of the anesthetic staff were determined prospectively during a 12-month period. A mean 1.4% of 14,419 operations requiring general anesthesia were postponed. The greatest number of postponements occurred for patients with significant concurrent problems and for those scheduled for major and major plus procedures.

The main indication for postponement was cardiovascular problems, particularly hypertension, cardiac failure, and dysrhythmias. Anemia, chronic respiratory disease, and diabetes mellitus were the main noncardiovascular problems. Overall, 22% of the postponements were attributed to acute respiratory tract infections that occurred close to the time of planned surgery; 35% were attributed to medical problems detected for the first time on admission to the hospital (e.g., anemia, diabetes, and hypertension); 35% occurred because of chronic medical problems requiring further investigation or treatment; and the remaining postponements resulted from inadequate routine patient preparation.

An overall postponement rate of 1.4% appears to be an acceptable wastage rate, although efforts can be made to improve this figure. The following changes are recommended in the management of patients scheduled for elective surgery: standard screening at surgical outpatient clinics, assessment of patients with chronic problems on a day case basis 1–2 weeks before surgery, and use of "standby" waiting lists to allow the fullest use of operating time should a late postponement occur.

▶ This was accepted for publication because certain investigators are beginning to look into this costly and important practice. The conflict between patient welfare and inconvenience and cost is often difficult to resolve. This reviewer suspects that each hospital and the personalities in it will be more important than any general factors elicited by a study such as this.—R.D. Miller, M.D.

Physical Status Score and Trends in Anesthetic Complications
Cohen MM, Duncan PG (Univ of Manitoba)
J Clin Epidemiol 41:83–90, 1988

3–8

As deaths related to anesthesia have declined, nonfatal complications have gained importance as measures of the quality of care in this discipline. The American Society of Anesthesiologists' (ASA) Physical Status (PS) score is a composite evaluation of the patient's physical status that is unrelated to the patient's specific disease. The relationship of PS score and risk of nonfatal complications caused by anesthesia was investigated.

Anesthesiologists completed forms for 112,000 administrations of anesthetic, including information about the patient, anesthetic used, opera-

TABLE 1.—Intraoperative Complication Rate by ASA Physical Status (ASAPS-Specific Rate per 10,000 Anesthetics)

	ASAPS1	ASAPS2	ASAPS3	ASAPS4 & 5
Cardiac arrest	2.2	3.5	13.1	53.6
Arrhythmia	265.4	446.5	588.7	725.2
Hypotension	74.2	278.1	619.4	1197.7
Hypertension	18.5	83.0	188.6	214.5
Aspiration	4.3	6.2	9.7	20.4
Other respirtory	73.4	109.3	131.8	150.7
Drug	15.3	12.4	16.5	20.4
Surgical	21.6	19.6	42.1	97.0
Other	106.6	130.1	197.2	166.0

(Courtesy of Cohen MM, Duncan PG: *J Clin Epidemiol* 41:83–90, 1988.)

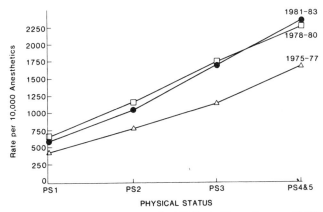

Fig 3–2.—Rate of intraoperative complications by ASA Physical Status Score per 10,000 anesthetics. (Courtesy of Cohen MM, Duncan PG: *J Clin Epidemiol* 41:83–90, 1988.)

tive procedure, and outcome. All postoperative complications were recorded and were evaluated by an anesthesia follow-up nurse. Complications were classified as major if they were life-threatening or if they significantly prolonged hospitalization and were classified as minor if they caused discomfort or inconvenience.

Physical Status-specific complication rates increased with increasing ASA physical status for 8 of 9 intraoperative complications (Table 1). Lower rates were seen from 1975 to 1977 than from 1978 to 1980 or 1981 to 1983 (Fig 3–2). Physical-Status 1 patients were more likely to have recovery room complications (Table 2). The risk of intraoperative or postoperative complications was increased in patients classified as PS2, PS3, or PS4 and PS5 combined (Tables 3 and 4). Physical Status-specific rates increased with increasing score and with operative time (Fig 3–3). The rate of all major postoperative complications increased with increasing PS scores (Fig 3–4).

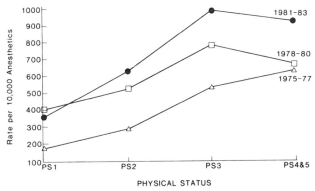

Fig 3–3.—Physical Status-specific rates for patients having at least 1 complication while in the recovery room. (Courtesy of Cohen MM, Duncan PG: *J Clin Epidemiol* 41:83–90, 1988.)

TABLE 2.—Recovery Room Complication Rate by ASA Physical
Status (ASAPS-Specific Rate per 10,000 Anesthetics)

	ASAPS1	ASAPS2	ASAPS3	ASAPS4 & 5
Cardiac arrest	3.0	3.0	13.1	17.9
Arrhythmia	19.7	73.1	157.4	201.7
Hypotension	156.6	170.1	206.3	176.2
Hypertension	33.8	116.3	189.2	120.0
Aspiration	1.8	1.7	5.1	7.7
Other respiratory	22.6	57.8	165.4	237.5
Drug	2.4	6.5	15.3	10.2
Surgical	17.7	23.5	50.0	46.0
Other	68.9	73.1	152.3	166.0

(Courtesy of Cohen MM, Duncan PG: *J Clin Epidemiol* 41:83–90, 1988.)

This ASA-PS classification appears to be independently predictive of intraoperative and major postoperative complications; however, when used alone, it is inadequate to predict anesthetic morbidity in the immediate postoperative period.

▶ This is an extremely important paper because of several aspects. First, it shows how a quality assurance program can be set up in a large hospital or university setting with essentially minimum costs and perhaps major benefit. Second, and equally important, it shows that in fact the ASA physical status score has not been subject to inflationary readings, at least in Winnipeg, for the period of 1975–1983 and that physical status scores are in fact correlated with intraoperative and serious postoperative adverse outcomes. It also shows that, although the number of intraoperative and minor recovery room complications such as nausea and vomiting or intraoperative hypotension are now greater than those in the years 1975–1977, the serious major postoperative complications such as myocardial infarction, nerve palsies, and respiratory compromise are all occurring less frequently now than in the past.

TABLE 3.—Postoperative Complication Rate by ASA Physical Status
(ASAPS-Specific Rate per 10,000 Anesthetics)

	ASAPS1	ASAPS2	ASAPS3	ASAPS4 & 5
Respiratory	1.2	6.7	11.9	17.9
M.I.	0.4	3.5	17.1	30.6
Other CVS	10.8	41.2	68.2	61.3
Venous	4.7	9.9	7.4	7.7
Arterial	2.0	16.6	55.1	71.5
Nerve palsy	1.0	1.7	1.7	7.7
Psychological	5.1	12.6	14.2	0
Awareness	4.9	8.4	8.0	12.8
Minor complications*	490.3	547.6	356.3	125.1

*Includes nauseas and vomiting, sore throat, back pain, muscular pain, mechanical, dental, eye, urinary, headache, and other.
(Courtesy of Cohen MM, Duncan PG: *J Clin Epidemiol* 41:83–90, 1988.)

Physical Status and Anesthetic Complications

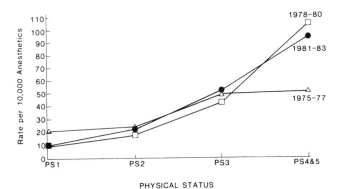

Fig 3–4.—Physical Status-specific rate for patients having at least 1 major postoperative complication. (Courtesy of Cohen MM, Duncan PG: *J Clin Epidemiol* 41:83–90, 1988.)

I think other interesting points of this article are that, if one looks at the number of patients who have myocardial infarctions, the incidence increases from 0.4 per 10,000 anesthetics for a patient with ASA physical status I to 30.6 for patients with ASA physical status IV and V. That is, 30 patients out of 10,000 will have a myocardial infarction, taking into account all ASA IV and V patients, as opposed to less than 1 per 10,000 if the patient has ASA physical status I. I recommend this paper be read by every anesthesiologist as I believe that it has information vital to us when patients ask about risk and that it is perhaps one of the key papers that I have been privileged to read in the last decade.—M.F. Roizen, M.D.

TABLE 4.—Relative Odds of Having a Complication: Crude and Adjusted Rates

	Crude relative odds (95% C.I.) re: ASAPS1	Adjusted* relative odds (95% C.I.) re: ASAPS1
Intraoperative		
ASAPS2:ASAPS1	1.81 (1.73, 1.90)	1.20 (0.99, 1.45)
ASAPS3:ASAPS1	2.83 (2.68, 2.98)	1.55 (1.08, 1.95)
ASAPS4 & 5:ASAPS1	4.07 (3.78, 4.40)	2.17 (1.50, 3.11)
Recovery room		
ASAPS2:ASAPS1	1.50 (1.40, 1.60)	0.98 (0.86, 1.14)
ASAPS3:ASAPS1	2.49 (2.32, 2.67)	1.05 (0.87, 1.25)
ASAPS4 & 5:ASAPS1	2.98 (2.66, 3.33)	0.67 (0.50, 0.91)
Postoperative major		
ASAPS2:ASAPS1	1.64 (1.19, 2.26)	1.33 (0.88, 2.00)
ASAPS3:ASAPS1	3.68 (2.67, 5.07)	2.26 (1.47, 3.48)
ASAPS4 & 5:ASAPS1	6.06 (3.96, 9.25)	3.82 (1.93, 7.58)

*Adjusted by logistic regression modeling for patient age, sex anesthetic technique, number of anesthetic drugs, experience of the anesthesiologist, length of anesthesia, whether procedure was major, intermediate, or minor, and whether procedure was elective or emergency.
(Courtesy of Cohen MM, Duncan PG: *J Clin Epidemiol* 41:83–90, 1988.)

Preoperative and Postoperative Medical Evaluation of Surgical Patients

Gluck R, Muñoz E, Wise L (Long Island Jewish Med Ctr, New York; State Univ of New York at Stony Brook)
Am J Surg 155:730–734, June 1988
3–9

Routine preoperative and postoperative medical evaluation by an internist has long been standard procedure in many institutions. However, today's rapidly changing health care reimbursement environment may affect the practice of using routine medical consultations. Because Medicare pays a set amount for each of 468 diagnosis-related groups (DRGs), it is likely that physician DRGs will create financial disincentives to obtain medical consultation for surgical patients. The cost-benefit ratio of routine preoperative and postoperative medical evaluation of surgical patients was examined.

The medical records of 70 randomly selected patients aged 40 years or older who underwent surgery during a 6-month study period were analyzed. The patients represented 4 different surgical disease categories, including major reconstructive vascular procedures, major small and large bowel procedures, cholecystectomy without common duct exploration, and major head and neck procedures. Each patient was independently graded for surgical risk according to the Anesthesiologists Physical Status Scale, which uses class 1 to denote normally healthy individuals, class 2 for patients with mild systemic disease, class 3 for patients with severe but not incapacitating systemic disease, class 4 for patients with incapacitating, life-threatening, systemic disease, and class 5 for moribund patients. Class 4 and class 5 patients were not included. All 70 patients underwent preoperative and postoperative medical evaluation. The number of recommendations made by medical consultants and the costs of consultation were tabulated and analyzed.

No preoperative or postoperative recommendations were made for any of the 12 class 1 patients. Only 8 preoperative and postoperative recommendations were made for 8 (30%) of the 27 class 2 patients, none of which were significant. However, 34 preoperative and postoperative recommendations were made for 30 (97%) of the 31 class 3 patients, 10 (33%) of which were significant.

Medical evaluation of low-risk surgical patients does not appear to affect outcome for these patients, and it appears that routine preoperative and postoperative medical evaluation could safely be omitted for class 1 and class 2 patients. However, medium-risk surgical patients appear to gain some benefit from preoperative and postoperative medical evaluation, and routine evaluation by an internist appears warranted for patients whose surgical risk is graded class 3 or higher.

▶ The physicians looked at the cost-effectiveness of preoperative and postoperative evaluation and found no benefit at all in evaluation of ASA class I and class II patients. Only when patients were class III or class IV did any benefit accrue. What is interesting is that, if they had done this evaluation looking at benefit-risk versus cost-benefit, they probably would have found that there was some risk to some of the recommendations in ASA class I or class II patients. Only when one examines class IV would there be a benefit. This obviously is speculative, but the data are nonetheless clear that no one in ASA class I and-class II received any benefit, and it was rare to have a benefit from preoperative "Medical Clearance" in the ASA class III patient.—M.F. Roizen, M.D.

Respiratory Criteria of Fitness for Surgery and Anaesthesia
Nunn JF, Milledge JS, Chen D, Dore C (Clinical Research Ctr, Harrow, England)
Anaesthesia 43:543–551, July 1988   3–10

Testing of preoperative pulmonary function is widely recommended, although there are few studies that provide a basis for interpretation of the results. The authors have previously reported the value of blood gases in predicting the requirement for postoperative ventilation. This study extends the series to 42 patients with severe chronic obstructive airway disease.

Fifty-three operations in 42 patients with forced expiratory volume in 1 second (FEV_1) of 1 L or less were retrospectively analyzed. Preoperative blood gas data and peak flow records were available for all patients.

Thirty-eight of 42 patients had uncomplicated anesthesia and surgery and normal postoperative periods. Four patients had artificial ventilation of the lungs. The best predictors of requirement for postoperative ventilation were the arterial PO_2 and dyspnea at rest.

Spirometric tests have limited value for screening; arterial blood gas tensions, particularly the PO_2 have much greater predictive value. The presence or absence of dyspnea at rest is also a useful predictor.

▶ The important message conveyed by this report is the absence of any test or symptom that contraindicates surgery. Identifying a single test or symptom that accurately predicts the need for postoperative mechanical ventilation also remains elusive. The authors emphasize the preoperative importance of dyspnea and arterial PO_2 in predicting the need for postoperative support of ventilation. It is reassuring that pulmonary function tests are not more informative than readily available data from arterial blood gases and physical examination. Nevertheless, I remain surprised that preexisting elevations in arterial PCO_2 did not correlate with the need for mechanical ventilation of the lungs independent of arterial oxygenation.—R.K. Stoelting, M.D.

The Poor Quality of Early Evaluations of Magnetic Resonance Imaging
Cooper LS, Chalmers TC, McCally M, Berrier J, Sacks HS (Harvard Univ; City Univ of New York; VA Med Ctr, Bronx, NY)
JAMA 259:3277–3280, June 10, 1988   3–11

Fifty-four articles on magnetic resonance (MR) imaging, published in English-language journals in 1980–1984, were reviewed using commonly accepted criteria of research methodology. Nearly two thirds of

TABLE 1.—Fourfold Table of Diagnosis Applied to Magnetic
Resonance Imaging*

Magnetic Resonance Image	Disease or Disorder	
	Present	Absent
Abnormal	True positive (a)	False positive (b)
Normal	False negative (c)	True negative (d)

*Sensitivity is calculated as a/(a + c); specificity as d/(b + d); positive predictive value, a/(a + b); and negative predictive value d/(c + d).
(Courtesy of Cooper LS, Chalmers TC, McCally M, et al: *JAMA* 259:3277–3280, June 10, 1988.)

the articles reviewed appeared in *Radiology* and the *American Journal of Radiology.*

Only 1 study gave evidence of prior planning by describing a protocol. Histopathologic findings were presented in only 22% of the articles. No article contained evidence of randomization of the sequence of the imaging procedures or blinding of the readers to other sources of information. There was some quantitation of the findings in 44% of articles. None of the articles included more than 5 of 10 procedures that were considered optimal, and there was no indication of improvement over time. Further, an understanding of the terms that should be used in MR studies requires visualization of the standard fourfold table (Table 1).

Health care professionals who pay for expensive diagnostic technology should require better research of its diagnostic efficacy. The need for proper quantitative methods is clear. Research in MR imaging has been limited largely to descriptive studies. None of the present studies can be considered a high-quality assessment by current criteria of research methodology (Table 2).

▶ I think this article is important for anesthesiologists, not because of the value of its articles of technology assessment pertinent to anesthesia, although MRI has some pertinence to anesthesia, but because of what it says about technology assessments and their quality. Because anesthesia is considered one of the high-tech specialties, I think we can do better at technology assessments and it is an ideal place for clinical studies to be done. It is from this type of analysis that one can get a benefit-risk ratio; that is, if you put capnography in your operating room, what are the chances of it leading to improvement of health versus the chances of it leading to the potential that you will harm someone? Is the rate of harm greater than the rate of benefit, or vice versa?

The fundamental concept and techniques in diagnostic test assessment are not complex, and the criteria for evaluating the literature are straightforward and few in number. Does the article include sensitivity, specificity, and appropriate statistical tests, blindness, and measured observer agreement? Does it have the predictive false-positive and predictive true-positive rates? It isn't hard to do good technology assessment, but it does require some planning. That only 20% of these studies had intact institutional review board approval probably indicates that these studies weren't well planned. Until physicians, as well

TABLE 2.—Criteria for Classifying Quality of Studies Assessing
Diagnostic Imaging Procedures*

Assessment Criteria	No. (%) of Articles (n = 54)
Evidence of research planning	
Prior protocol†	1 (2)
IRB approval only††	11 (20)
Neither§	42 (78)
Appropriate use of the terms sensitivity, specificity, positive or negative predictive value, false-positive or false-negative, and accuracy	
3 or more terms used†	10 (19)
1 or 2 terms used††	26 (48)
None§	18 (33)
Appropriate presentation of data described by each term	
2 or more terms†	20 (37)
1 term only††	12 (22)
None§	22 (41)
Appropriate calculation of the values for each of the described terms	
Done†	1 (2)
Not done§	53 (98)
Presentation of a "gold standard"	
Tissue diagnosis†	12 (22)
Other imaging procedure††	34 (63)
None§	8 (15)
Random order of imaging tests when comparing MRI with another procedure	
Done†	0
Not done§	54 (100)
Blinding of interpreter with regard to clinical history or other test results	
Done†	0
Not done§	54 (100)
Measurement of interobserver variability in reading images	
Done†	2 (4)
Not done§	52 (96)
Presentation of quantitative data, e.g., T_1 and/or full T_2 relaxation times	
Complete†	13 (24)
Partial††	11 (20)
None§	30 (56)
Appropriate statistical analysis of quantitative data	
Distribution curves with statistical analyses and/or ROC curves for each diagnosis†	0
Qualitative grouping as in a 2 X 2 table††	5 (9)
None§	49 (91)

*IRB, institutional review board; *MRI,* magnetic resonance imaging; *ROC,* receiver-operating characteristic.
†Fully satisfactory.
††Partially satisfactory.
§Unsatisfactory.
(Courtesy of Cooper LS, Chalmers TC, McCally M, et al: *JAMA* 259:3277–3280, June 10, 1988.)

as editors, demand appropriate evaluations be undertaken, publications without the above criteria and articles like the editorial in the *Mayo Clinic Proceedings* that says, "Don't confuse me with the facts; MRI is a good technology," will continue to be offered and the public may continue to believe that more expensive technology is better. The attitude expressed in those publications is that we don't need to evaluate benefit vs. harm in studies. Thus, new technologies will continue to be offered if those types of studies continue without a critical assessment of whether the technology creates more risk than benefit. Such studies will continue to have a persuasive and unhealthy effect on patient care and health care costs.

We as physicians need to do better and should demand better; it's not difficult. One can ask why technology assessments aren't better. I think there are several reasons, but the main one is that research funding for technology assessments is piddling compared with funding to look at the mechanism of disease. For instance, it is very difficult to get money to tell whether ST trend analysis or capnography is a benefit or a harm to patients, but it is very easy to get funding to look at the mechanism of myocardial ischemia intraoperatively. Because medical care involves both basic mechanisms of disease and clinical decision making, one would think that the clinical decision making and its basis, technology, would be allotted appropriate weight so that the art of clinical decision making can be made more scientific.—M.F. Roizen, M.D.

Prospective Assessment of a Protocol for Selective Ordering of Preoperative Chest X-Rays

Charpak Y, Blery C, Chastang C, Szatan M, Fourgeaux B (Hôpital St-Louis, Paris; Hôpital Rothchild, Paris)
Can J Anaesth 35:259–264, 1988   3–12

Numerous studies of the usefulness of routine preoperative chest x-ray examination suggest that the practice should be abandoned, but it continues in many institutions. According to a previously published protocol for selective ordering of 12 preoperative tests, the chest x-ray study is indicated in the presence of any lung, cardiovascular, or known malignant disease, in major surgical emergencies, for patients older than age 50 who smoke, for immunodepressed patients, and when there has been no previous health examination (e.g., for immigrants). The use of that protocol was evaluated.

During a 1-year study period, preoperative chest x-ray studies were ordered for 1,101 (28%) of 3,866 surgical patients. Abnormalities were found on 568 (52%) of the x-ray films, 133 (23%) of which had not been expected by anesthetists. However, the abnormal findings led to modification of medical decisions for only 51 patients. According to the anesthetists, 166 (15%) of the preoperative chest x-ray films were useful at some time during the patient's hospitalization. Only 2 of the 2,765 patients (72%) who did not have preoperative chest x-ray examinations would have benefited from such a study. Forty-four of the 3,866 patients died, but only 1 death occurred in a patient who did not have a preoper-

TABLE 1.—Complications Relating to Ordering of Preoperative Chest X-ray Examinations and Results

Preoperative chest x-rays

	Not ordered N = 2765	*Ordered and normal* N = 533	*Ordered and abnormal* N = 568
Peroperative complications	2.7%	6.7%	10.4%
Postoperative pulmonary complications	0.9%	12.0%	20.0%
Postoperative cardiac complications	0.7%	5.0%	14.0%
All complications	10.0%	39.0%	52.0%
Deaths	0.03%	1.6%	9.2%

(Courtesy of Charpak Y, Blery C, Chastang C, et al: *Can J Anaesth* 35:259–264, 1988.)

ative chest x-ray examination. However, this lack could not be linked to the death. The incidence of preoperative or postoperative complications in patients who did not have preoperative chest x-ray studies was lower than that in patients who did have preoperative chest x-ray studies (Table 1). The ordering of preoperative chest x-ray examinations was more predictive of perioperative complications than was an abnormal result in those who had preoperative x-ray examinations. Study of the rates of ordering for all indications according to protocol recommendations revealed an ordering rate of only 23% for immigrants without prior health examination (Table 2), but this was because most immigrants were pregnant women.

Routine ordering of preoperative chest x-ray studies can be abandoned without undesirable effects on patient care and outcome.

▶ We have now seen a large series of articles in the literature showing that selectively ordering tests based on history is the way you can eliminate between 40% and 60% of all tests without missing any significant abnormalities. In fact, in 3 studies, not only do you not miss significant abnormalities, but you improve the patient's health. This study points up another interesting problem. These people agreed on the indications for getting chest x-rays: cardiac disease, any lung disease, major surgical emergencies, malignancy, smoking in people aged more than 50 years, and immigrants without a prior health examination. Yet, with even those indications, 30% of the indicated chest x-rays were not ordered and approximately 30% of the chest x-rays that were obtained were not indicated. Whereas clinical judgment probably played a role in some of those decisions to order when not indicated and not to order when indicated, clearly errors played a role in some of them.

If there are this many errors in one set of indications for one laboratory test, can you imagine how many there will be when one looks at the whole range of 55 or so preoperative tests? That's why we have developed a computerized algorithm wherein the patients answer questions about their own history and the computer, using the same indication schemes that are indicated here and

TABLE 2.—Rates of Ordering for All Indications
Selected in Protocol

Indications	N	Ordering
Hypertension	336	57%
Ischaemic cardiopathy	152	82%
Nonischaemic cardiopathy	99	71%
Other cardiovascular diseases	149	46%
Asthma	112	29%
Chronic obstructive pulmonary diseases	117	79%
Other pulmonary diseases	214	71%
Major surgical emergencies	55	87%
Malignant diseases	268	81%
Smokers > 50 years old	203	74%
Migrants without prior health examination	120	23%

(Courtesy of Charpak Y, Blery C, Chastang C, et al: *Can J Anaesth* 35:259–264, 1988.)

that have been developed by myself and others over the last 10 years, indicates which laboratory tests should be obtained. I think we as physicians are going to start to see the benefits of studies like that of Charpak et al. be put to clinical use by both reducing the cost of care and improving the quality of it.— M.F. Roizen, M.D.

Evaluation of Coronary Artery Disease in Patients Having Noncardiac Surgery
Madlon-Kay R (Eisenhower Army Med Ctr, Fort Gordon, Ga)
South Med J 80:1366–1369, November 1987   3–13

Coronary artery disease is common in patients undergoing noncardiac surgery. Cardiology consultants are often asked whether a patient should have prophylactic coronary artery revascularization before surgery. Answering this question requires knowing which patients are at high risk. Exercise testing and a literature review were done to answer the question of who should undergo prophylactic revascularization.

In one study, 7 cardiac complications—1 fatal and 6 nonfatal infarctions—occurred in 96 patients without cardiac risk. Any test used to predict perioperative cardiac risk must justify its inconvenience and expense by proving that it adds to clinical variables. In a study of treadmill and arm exercise, patients with both an abnormal exercise electrocardiogram and impaired heart rate response had a 41% incidence of perioperative myocardial infarction; if only 1 of these parameters was abnormal, that incidence fell from 2% to 4%. In another study, age best discriminated between those at low and high risk; patients older than 70 years had a 19% complication rate, compared with a 1% rate for those younger than 70 years.

Radionuclide studies have also been done. In 1, the infarction rate was

0% in patients with an ejection fraction greater than 55% and 80% in those with ejection fractions less than 36%. However, in this study, radionuclide angiography was not assessed in a multivariate analysis with other clinical variables. In a study of exercise radionuclide angiography, only poor exercise capacity was predictive of cardiac complications, but these findings were limited by several factors.

Thallium scintigraphy was successfully used in 1 study to predict cardiac risk; only a reversible defect showed by thallium scan was correlated independently with ischemic complications. In another study, logistic regression analysis showed that a thallium scan of reversible defects was a far better predictor of risk than clinical or exercise parameters. However, thallium studies using oral dipyridamole are time consuming and unlikely to become popular. In addition, many false-positive results were obtained in these thallium studies. No controlled trial of coronary arteriography for risk assessment has been done.

Currently, there is no ideal test for preoperative cardiac risk assessment. A reasonable approach begins with the Goldman risk index. Exercise testing, radionuclide angiography, and thallium scintigraphy are not suitable screening tests for most patients.

▶ This is an excellent critical review of the available data; it appropriately comes to several conclusions. First, the value of exercise tests and dipyridamole thallium scanning remains doubtful because it has not been convincingly demonstrated that these are superior to history and other clinical data in determining risk or that intervention or increasing monitoring once you know about this risk is indeed a benefit to the patient. I strongly believe that, once you know about this risk, intervention can be beneficial. My own preference is that dipyridamole thallium scanning is an excellent way of confirming clinical knowledge, but unfortunately we don't have data on that at this time. Clearly, as the article states, any test used to predict perioperative cardiac risk must justify its expense, inconvenience, and, I might add, risk by proving that it adds significantly to the clinical variables already known. The second point they made that I think is important is that age and ejection fraction also appear to be extremely important risk factors for determining outcome, but we may not be able to change their effects.—M.F. Roizen, M.D.

4 Operating Room Environment

Patient's Welfare

Music During Regional Anesthesia: A Reduced Need of Sedatives
Walther-Larsen S, Diemar V, Valentin N (Univ of Copenhagen)
Reg Anaesth 13:69–71, April–June 1988   4–1

Several authors have reported their impression that the use of music or white noise during dental surgery was successful as an adjunct to regional anesthesia or as an independent anesthetic or sedative modality. However, the influence of music on the need for sedatives during regional anesthesia has not been studied. This study was done to test the validity of that impression.

The study population comprised 32 pairs of patients who were undergoing orthopedic or plastic surgical procedures under regional anesthesia. All patients were premedicated with 10–15 mg of orally administered diazepam. Half of the patients were allocated to a music group, and half, to a nonmusic group. The median interval between premedication and nerve block was 90 minutes for the music group and 65 minutes for the nonmusic group. Patients allocated to the music group were offered a portable recorder and a selection of music tapes to satisfy any taste. Droperidol (2.5 mg) was used as the first sedative, and diazepam (2.5 to 5 mg) was used for subsequent injections as needed. All patients were asked to complete a questionnaire after surgery to rate their satisfaction with the anesthesia.

Four (13%) of the 32 patients in the music group and 14 (44%) of the 32 patients in the nonmusic group requested sedatives. The difference was statistically significant. Almost all patients in both groups were satisfied with the anesthesia, but 12 patients in the music group and 5 patients in the nonmusic group indicated that they had felt anxious during surgery. The difference in reported anxiety levels was no doubt the result of drug-induced amnesia. However, this anxiety had not been obvious to observers during the anesthesia. It could not be determined whether the reduced consumption of sedatives in the music group was due to the calming effect of the music or whether the music merely served as a sound barrier to the traumatizing noises in the operating room.

Based on these findings, the use of music during regional anesthesia, particularly in outpatients, is highly recommended.

▶ We have found also that this technique works in our surgical operating rooms. Interestingly, we have music available in our labor and delivery suite for the use of the parturients, and I can't remember the patients commenting in a positive or negative fashion on its effect during labor and delivery. The only comment that comes to mind is that the older obstetricians prefer not to operate while listening to rock and roll!—G.W. Ostheimer, M.D.

Improved Recovery and Reduced Postoperative Stay After Therapeutic Suggestions During General Anaesthesia

Evans C, Richardson PH (United Med and Dental Schools of Guy's and St Thomas's Hosps, London)
Lancet 2:491–493, Aug 27, 1988   4–2

What a patient hears during general anesthesia may not be recalled after surgery, but some researchers have found that therapeutic suggestions do have an effect on postoperative recovery. The effect of therapeutic suggestions was tested in a double-blind, randomized, and placebo-controlled study.

Thirty-nine patients undergoing hysterectomy entered the trial. During surgery, a tape of advice and reassurance was played for 19 patients. A blank tape was played for those in the control group. Presurgical questionnaires assessed each patient's degree of anxiety. The nursing staff evaluated patient recovery, and the patients completed a postsurgical questionnaire. The preoperative mood in both groups was similar, and other variables showed no significant differences.

Those in the suggestion group had a postoperative stay that was 16% shorter than that of the control group (Fig 4–1). Gastrointestinal problems were significantly reduced in the suggestion group, and these patients were pyrexic for a significantly shorter period. Nurses rated most of the control patients as having an average or poorer than expected re-

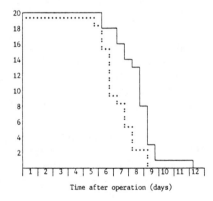

Fig 4–1.—Postoperative stay in hospital: *broken line,* suggestion group; *unbroken line,* control group. (Courtesy of Evans C, Richardson PH: *Lancet* 2:491–493, Aug 27, 1988.)

Number of patients still in hospital

Time after operation (days)

..............Suggestion group
_____Control group

Postoperative stay in hospital.

covery, whereas almost all of those in the suggestion group were thought to have a better than expected recovery.

Although patients in the suggestion group could not recall instructions, all but 1 guessed correctly that such a tape had been played. Some level of auditory perception is maintained during general anesthesia. The lowered stress brought about by reassurance and positive suggestions may affect the physical recovery from surgery.

▶ This is one of multiple articles indicating that nonpharmacologic approaches can influence postoperative narcotic utilization and overall well-being in the postoperative period.—R.D. Miller, M.D.

Effects of Sounds Presented During General Anaesthesia on Postoperative Course
Boeke S, Bonke B, Bouwhuis-Hoogerwerf ML, Bovill JG, Zwaveling A (Erasmus Univ, Rotterdam; Univ of Leiden; Univ Hosp, Leiden, the Netherlands)
Br J Anaesth 60:697–702, 1988   4–3

A randomized, double-blind study was undertaken to determine whether sounds presented during anesthesia could affect a patient's recovery. In all, 106 patients undergoing elective cholecystectomy were recruited for the trial. For 1 group, a tape of commentary on the patient's well-being and excellent outlook for recovery was played together with intervals of seaside sounds. Another group was given a combination of nonsense suggestions and seaside sounds. Seaside sounds alone were played for the third group, and patients in a fourth group were allowed to hear the usual, but amplified, noises of the operating room.

Patients were asked to rate their own sense of recovery from surgery. Nursing staff evaluations and length of hospital stay also were considered. No patients recalled events or sounds, and no group of patients had a significantly better outcome than others.

A number of factors may have influenced the lack of significant findings. It was theorized that the sounds may not have been striking enough, the operation may have been too uncomplicated to evoke responses in the patients, or the test methods were inadequate. Highly sensitive memory tests administered after anesthesia may be a better method of studying the phenomenon of intraoperative auditory registration.

▶ There is increasing concern about the overall environment in the operating room regarding sounds and issues that are discussed in terms of either conscious or subconscious perception by patients. That this study was unable to detect a difference does not mean that this whole issue is unimportant. Other studies clearly indicate that the sounds that are present in the operating room do have an influence on EEG and possibly even postoperative recovery. For example, a Beethoven sonata results in an EEG pattern completely different from that of the *1812* Overture at a similar anesthetic level. Clearly we are just scratching the surface of this important issue.—R.D. Miller, M.D.

Health Care Worker Protection

Risk to Surgeons: A Survey of Accidental Injuries During Operations

Hussain SA, Latif ABA, Choudhary AAAA (King Saud Univ, Abha, Saudi Arabia)
Br J Surg 75:314–316, April 1988   4–4

Eighteen surgeons reported 112 (5.6%) accidental injuries in a 1-year period when about 2,000 operations were carried out. Most were needle-stick injuries, but 4 surgeons reported being cut with a knife and 1 had a diathermy burn injury.

One fourth of the orthopedic operations were complicated by injury to the surgeon or assistant; the rate for general surgical procedures was 7%. The left hand was much more likely to be injured than the right, particularly the left index finger. Injuries occurred more often during longer operations and more frequently were incurred by surgical residents than by consultants with longer experience. Injuries occurred most often during closure of the wound. In 75% of the persons, no meaningful precautions were undertaken, such as changing gloves, rescrubbing, or applying antiseptic to the site of injury.

Accidental injuries seem to occur more often at the end of long operations, perhaps through a wish to finish the procedure quickly. Most needle-stick injuries occur as the needle emerges from the tissues, striking the overlying finger when not directly seen by the surgeon. Excessive fat tissue or inadequate assistance may sometimes be responsible. It might be best to use dissecting forceps in place of the fingers for manipulating the tissues while suturing.

▶ This is a restrospective study asking surgeons immediately after they have finished a case to report on when and where they got cut. Over 76% of operative injuries occurred while closing the wound, and most of them occurred in the left index finger, which alone accounted for more than one third of the needle sticks. Operations that lasted longer and operations that occurred at night had a higher incidence of association with glove perforations and accidental needle sticks than did those that occurred during the day or that were shorter. Almost all of the accidents were due to needle sticks. Very few, less than 4%, were due to knife cuts, and less than 1% were due to diathermy burns.

Although the data from a *British Journal of Surgery* study (Abstract 4–5) implied that about 50% of operations have an accidental glove perforation, the surgeons know about this only about one tenth of the time, as only 5.6% of the time did they know of an injury occurring or of a needle stick injury occurring. Perhaps most alarming was the cavalier attitude of the surgeons after they got stuck. Gloves were changed in only 25% of the cases, the surgeon rescrubbed in only 12% of the cases, and an antiseptic was applied to the site of injury or blood was squeezed out of it only 12% of the time. For only a little over 10% of the patients was a history taken to see whether the patient had a history of hepatitis B or other disease likely to be spread by this mechanism. In most cases the surgeons considered the injuries as trivial and disregarded them completely.

Is this another episode of us as physicians in general and specifically as surgeons believing we are immortal? I don't know, but I think we need better precautions regarding surgical wound behavior and we desperately need a vaccine to be developed for acquired immunodeficiency syndrome before we close wounds cavalierly. I believe that the risk of infection for anesthesiologists isn't much different from that for surgeons. The data say that we get hepatitis B as frequently as surgeons, which implies that we're as exposed and at risk for other diseases that have blood-borne transmission as their main vehicle. I think we are going to be in a major period of risk in the next several years, and I hope it lasts only that long. During that period, I wonder how many of us will routinely put on gloves to protect ourselves and how many will put on 2 sets of gloves.—M.F. Roizen, M.D.

Surgical Glove Perforations
Brough SJ, Hunt TM, Barrie WW (Leicester Gen Hosp, Leicester, England)
Br J Surg 75:317, April 1988   4–5

To prevent transmission of disease in either direction during surgery, it is necessary to have an intact barrier between the surgeon's hands and the patient's tissues. Of 339 gloves tested in a 1-month period, 37.5% were perforated. The rate for surgeons' gloves was 48.2%, and when mass closure was carried out, the rate was 73.5%. Fewer than half of the perforations were recognized by surgeons, and only 10% of scrub nurses recognized the occurrence of perforation (Tables 1, 2, 3, and 4).

The overall perforation rate of 37.5% in this study probably is an underestimate. The water inflation test used to detect perforations was 80% sensitive in identifying 25-gauge holes. Mass closure carries a high risk of glove puncture for the operating surgeon. Perforations incurred by scrub nurses appear related to handling of instruments and needles.

▶ This is a very interesting study in which, after a surgeon, his assistant, or the nurse finished an operation, the gloves were tested for leaks by simply filling them up with water and looking for the stream. Interestingly, 48.2% of surgeons' gloves and 42.5% of nurses' gloves (that is, gloves considered as a pair) were perforated. These rates were higher than that of the first assistant. The most common operations involving the perforations were closures that were

TABLE 1.—Surgeons' Gloves

	No.	Perforated pairs	χ^2 test
Mass closure operations	49	36 (73·5%)	
Other operations	63	18 (28·6%)	$P < 0.01$
Total	112	54 (48·2%)	
Known perforations		21	

(Courtesy of Brough SJ, Hunt TM, Barrie WW: *Br J Surg* 75:317, April 1988.)

TABLE 2.—Scrub Nurses' Gloves

	No.	Perforated pairs	χ^2 test
Mass closure operations	57	23 (40·4%)	
Other operations	63	28 (44·4%)	P = n.s.
Total	120	51 (42·5%)	
Known perforations		5	

*n.s., not significant.
(Courtesy of Brough SJ, Hunt TM, Barrie WW: Br J Surg 75:317, April 1988.)

TABLE 3.—First Assistants' Gloves

	No.	Perforated pairs	χ^2 test
Mass closure operations	45	15 (33·3%)	
Other operations	44	4 (9·1%)	P < 0·05
Total	89	19 (21·3%)	
Known perforations		8	

(Courtesy of Brough SJ, Hunt TM, Barrie WW: Br J Surg 75:317, April 1988.)

TABLE 4.—Second Assistants' Gloves

	No.	Perforated pairs	χ^2 test
Mass closure operations	14	2 (14·3%)	
Other operations	4	1 (25%)	P = n.s.
Total	18	3 (16·7%)	
Known perforations		0	

*n.s., not significant.
(Courtesy of Brough SJ, Hunt TM, Barrie WW: Br J Surg 75:317, April 1988.)

done with a cutting needle, in which 73.5% of gloves were perforated, as opposed to 28.6% when closures without a cutting needle were performed. Thus it is evident that the majority of known perforations occurred during closure.

Looking at the fact that between 0.1% and 2% of people who are stuck with needles from patients with AIDS become infected and assuming that a surgeon does roughly 200 operations a year, he or she will have 100 needle sticks a year through gloves and a chance roughly between 0.1% and 2% of being infected per year, if every patient operated on were HIV-positive. If the incidence of HIV positivity is 3% in the population, then the chance of being infected is 0.03% to 0.6% per year. If we assume it will take 10 years before a vaccine is available, an accumulative exposure rate would thus be between 0.3% and 6% risk of getting the virus. Clearly, if more than 50% of the hazard occurs during wound closure, something should be done during wound closure other than was done in this study in Great Britain.—M.F. Roizen, M.D.

▶ ↓ The following articles (Abstracts 4–6 and 4–7) should be read by all physicians who are involved in developing policies for protection of health care workers.—R.D. Miller, M.D.

Surveillance of Health Care Workers Exposed to Blood From Patients Infected With the Human Immunodeficiency Virus
Marcus R, CDC Cooperative Needlestick Surveillance Group (Center for Infectious Diseases, Atlanta)
N Engl J Med 319:1118–1123, Oct 27, 1988   4–6

Since 1983 the Centers for Disease Control (CDC) in cooperation with health care institutions throughout the United States have conducted ongoing national surveillance of health care workers to assess the risk of acquiring infection with the human immunodeficiency virus (HIV) after exposure to the blood or body fluids of patients infected with HIV.

As of July 31, 1988, 1,613 health care workers had been enrolled in the project, 1,201 of whom were exposed to blood from a patient infected with HIV or from a patient meeting the CDC case definition for acquired immunodeficiency syndrome. The exposed workers included 751 (63%) nurses, 164 (14%) physicians and medical students, 134 (11%) laboratory workers, and 90 (7%) phlebotomists. Of the 1,201 exposed workers, 962 (80%) received needlestick injuries, 103 (8%) were cut with sharp objects, 79 (7%) had contaminated open wounds, and 57 (5%) had contaminated mucous membranes. Thirty-seven percent of the 1,201 exposures could have been prevented if recommended infection-control precautions had been taken.

Four of 963 health care workers whose serum had been tested for HIV antibody at least 180 days after exposure tested positive, yielding a seroprevalence rate of 0.42%. Three of these 4 workers experienced an acute retroviral syndrome associated with documented seroconversion; the serum of the fourth worker was not available. Two of the seroconverted health care workers were injured by co-workers during resuscitation procedures. None of the 4 seroconverted workers had other risk factors for HIV infection.

Although the risk of seroconversion after documented exposure to the blood of patients infected with HIV is low, the need for compliance with recommended infection-control precautions to prevent exposure cannot be overemphasized.

Rates of Needle-Stick Injury Caused by Various Devices in a University Hospital
Jagger J, Hunt EH, Brand-Elnaggar J, Pearson RD (Univ of Virginia)
N Engl J Med 319:284–288, Aug 4, 1988   4–7

The acquired immunodeficiency syndrome (AIDS) epidemic has caused great concern among health care workers about risks, such as needle-

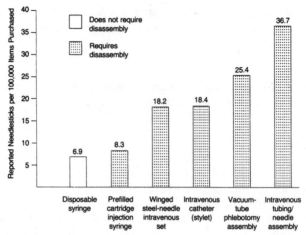

Fig 4-2.—Needle-stick injury rates per 100,000 items purchased, for 6 devices with needles. (Courtesy of Jagger J, Hunt EH, Brand-Elnaggar J, et al: *N Engl J Med* 319:284-288, Aug 4, 1988.)

stick injuries, in the hospital environment. In a 10-month period during 1986,there were 326 needle-stick injuries at a group of university hospitals, including 64% reported by nurses and nursing students and 20% by laboratory technicians and auxiliary radiology and respiratory therapy personnel.

About two thirds of the injuries occured in acute care units. The disposable syringe accounted for more injuries than any other device but had the lowest needle-stick rate (Fig 4-2). Rates were higher for devices requiring disassembly. Most incidents occurred when the devices were being prepared for disposal; only 17% occurred during actual use. Recapping was the most frequent mechanism of injury from disposable syringes. Most injuries with prefilled cartridge syringes were related to disassembly. Eight injuries involved intravenous catheters when difficulty occured in disposing of the stylet.

There is no single means of preventing needle-stick injuries. Optimally, needles would be replaced by other methods, or methods requiring fewer needles would be developed. This will require a sustained effort by both product manufacturers and the health care community.

Temperature Control

Spontaneous Post-anesthetic Tremor Does Not Resemble Thermoregulatory Shivering

Sessler DI, Israel D, Pozos RS, Pozos M, Rubinstein EH (Univ of California, San Francisco; Univ of Minnesota; Univ of California, Los Angeles)
Anesthesiology 68:843-850, January 1988   4-8

Although postanesthetic tremor is common during recovery from surgery, effective prevention and treatment await clarification of the mechanism of this tremor. In an effort to do this, electrical signals from muscles

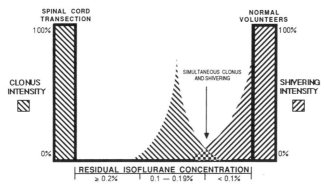

Fig 4–3.—Qualitative illustration suggesting possible recovery stages in patients who remain hypothermic during recovery from isoflurane anesthesia. Vertical axis on left indicates clonic tremor intensity, and includes control panel; vertical axis on right indicates intensity of normal shivering, and includes similar panel. Left control panel indicates that tremor in patients with spinal cord transections is completely clonic; panel to right indicates that spontaneous tremor in unanesthetized volunteers is normal shivering. Recovery, which is divided into 3 stages, is indicated on horizontal axis. At isoflurane concentration no greater than .2%, there is little muscular activity (both brain and spinal cord are "asleep"). At isoflurane concentrations between .1 and .19%, tremor is mostly clonic (brain is "asleep" and spinal cord is "awake," causing functional cord transection). When isoflurane concentration decreases to no greater than .1%, normal shivering predominates (both brain and spinal cord are "awake"). Both clonic tremor and normal shivering may occur simultaneously when isoflurane concentrations are near .1%. (Courtesy of Sessler DI, Israel D, Pozos RS, et al: *Anesthesiology* 68:843–850, January 1988.)

of surgical patients recovering from anesthesia were quantified, identified, and compared with those produced by pathologic clonus and cold-induced thermoregulatory shivering.

Electromyograms (EMGs) of 8 muscles were studied in 9 women recovering from isoflurane anesthesia, and the signals were compared with those of pathologic clonus induced by plantar flexion in unanesthetized patients with spinal cord transections and also with those of cold-induced shivering in normal anesthesia-free patients.

Analysis of EMG data in patients with postanesthetic tremor revealed 2 patterns: a tonic activity that did not resemble normal shivering and clonic activity similar to that produced by pathologic clonus. Tonic EMG activity also frequently contained a clonic component. During the later part of the recovery, hypothermic patients frequently exhibited no clinical or EMG evidence of muscular activity (Fig 4–3).

Normal thermoregulatory responses to cold are inhibited during recovery from general anesthesia. Generalized tremor is a combination of spontaneous clonus and a tonic activity different from that found in normal shivering.

▶ Postoperative tremor, especially following volatile, inhaled anesthetic is reasonably common and poorly understood. Clearly it is not always related to a decrease in body temperature. The authors are to be congratulated for pursuing this common and sometimes distressing postoperative event in some depth. Although they are presently identifying mechanisms, it is hoped that their future research will identify preventive measures.—R.D. Miller, M.D.

5 Anesthetic Techniques

Endotracheal Intubation

Use of a Lighted Stylet to Confirm Correct Endotracheal Tube Placement
Stewart RD, LaRosee A, Stoy WA, Heller MB (Univ of Pittsburgh; Ctr for Emergency Medicine, Pittsburgh)
Chest 92:900–903, November 1987   5–1

The threat of esophageal placement remains one of the most worrisome complications of endotracheal intubation. Prompted by encouraging results of guided orotracheal intubation using a rigid-wire lighted stylet, a technique was developed to confirm correct intratracheal placement of an endotracheal tube using a new flexible lighted stylet designed for nasotracheal intubation. With this technique, intratracheal placement of the light gives off an intense, circumscribed glow in the level of the laryngeal prominence and sternal notch, whereas the light is not usually seen or is perceived as dull and diffuse with esophageal placement. To determine whether these differences in transillumination of the soft tissues using the flexible lighted stylet can reliably be used to identify the position of an endotracheal tube at several sites in the upper airway, 35 volunteer intubators were asked to identify tube placement in 5 human cadavers of different body habitus. Endotracheal tubes were placed under direct vision at 3 sites: esophagus (20 cm from the teeth), trachea (20 cm from the teeth), and the right or left pyriform fossa.

In all, 168 placements were made in 40 trials. All but 1 of the 56 intratracheal placements were correctly identified; 1 was misidentified as esophageal by an inexperienced paramedic. Of 112 extratracheal placements, 1 was misidentified as intratracheal. The levels of experience or training bore no relationship to the ability of the intubator to identify correct placement. Average time for identification of intratracheal placement was 4.6 seconds.

The use of the flexible nasotracheal lighted stylet is a rapid and reliable method of confirming correct placement of endotracheal tubes. This method can reduce, if not eliminate, unrecognized esophageal intubation in the field, emergency department, intensive care unit, and operating room. Moreover, the device is inexpensive and reusable.

▶ The authors propose that capnometry is currently not practical in the critical care unit or emergency department and is not available to field personnel as a measurement to confirm tracheal placement of a tube. I agree that capnometry is not a practical measurement outside the hospital. Likewise, I disagree that this measurement is not available within the hospital where trained personnel should rely on a number of confirmatory observations (bilateral breath sounds, absence of gastric sounds, chest expansion, refilling of the reservoir bag, fogging in the tube) as well as capnometry to confirm accurate tracheal placement of the tube.—R.K. Stoelting, M.D.

A Comparison of Labetalol, Acebutolol, and Lidocaine for Controlling the Cardiovascular Responses to Endotracheal Intubation for Oral Surgical Procedures

Roelofse JA, Shipton EA, Joubert JJ de V, Grotepass FW (Univ of Stellenbosch, Cape Town, South Africa; Univ of The Orange Free State, Bloemfontein, South Africa)
J Oral Maxillofac Surg 45:835–840, October 1987   5–2

Hypertensive and tachycardic responses to laryngoscopy and tracheal intubation result from the increased sympathetic activity caused by stimulation of the upper respiratory tract. A comparison was made of the effects of labetol, acebutolol, and lidocaine on the hemodynamics of laryngoscopy and intubation during general anesthesia for oral surgical procedures.

All patients received premedication with Demerol and promethazine 60–90 minutes before anesthesia was induced. Eighty patients were divided into 4 equal groups. Patients in group 1 received labetalol, 1 mg/kg, as a bolus dose intravenously; patients in group 2 received acebutolol, 0.25 mg/kg, intravenously as a bolus dose; group 3 patients received lidocaine, 2 mg/kg, intravenously as a bolus dose; and group 4 served as a control group.

Lidocaine produced no significant variations in pulse rate, systolic, diastolic, and mean blood pressures when compared with the control values. Acebutolol had no significant effect on systolic, diastolic, and mean blood pressures until 4 and 5 minutes after intubation, when the systolic pressure dropped significantly and continued to drop even more significantly 10 and 20 minutes after intubation. Labetalol produced significant decreases in pulse rate and mean blood pressure 1 minute after a test dose was given. A significant decrease in pulse rate and systolic, diastolic, and mean blood pressures remained after intubation in patients given labetalol.

A preinduction dose of labetalol was more effective than acebutolol and lidocaine in attenuating pressor responses to instrumentation and intubation. Labetalol should be useful for patients at risk from the transient hypertension and tachycardia following intubation and instrumentation.

▶ This topic has been extensively investigated, and multiple different drugs have been proposed. In the rare case that pharmacologic protection is indicated, it is useful to select a drug that has a rapid onset and short duration and is equally effective against blood pressure and heart rate responses evoked by intubation of the trachea. Labetalol has many desirable characteristics, but it seems unlikely that the duration of this drug's effects would match the transient responses it is intended to attenuate.— R.K. Stoelting, M.D.

Predicting Difficult Intubation

Wilson ME, Spiegelhalter D, Robertson JA, Lesser P (Royal United Hosp, Bath, England; MRC Biostatistics Unit, Cambridge, England; Royal Naval Hosp, Plymouth, England)
Br J Anaesth 61:211–216, 1988   5–3

Failed or difficult intubation is a common cause of morbidity and mortality attributable to anesthesia. It would be useful if patients in whom intubation is likely to cause problems could be identified beforehand, so that a senior anesthesiologist could be at hand to deal with the problem. Although many features believed to hamper intubation have been described, a useful predictive rule has not yet been formulated.

In an attempt to identify features associated with difficult laryngoscopy, i.e., the inability to see even the arytenoids, a series of measurements of the head and neck were made in 633 patients who were undergoing routine surgery. Another 38 patients who had been difficult to intubate were also measured. The difficulty of laryngoscopy was assessed at intubation. Analysis of the data identified 5 useful risk factors measured at 3 levels of severity. No other factors improved the prediction. The predictive rule included body weight, head and neck movement, jaw movement, receding mandible, and buck teeth. These 5 risk factors were then tested prospectively for validation in 778 patients.

In the initial group of 633 patients, the incidence of difficult laryngoscopy was 9.3%. However, when the larynx was pushed backward to improve the view, the incidence of difficulty could be reduced to 5.9%. In the prospective study group of 778 patients, the incidence of difficult laryngoscopy was 1.5%. When the newly identified predictive rule was used to identify difficult intubation, 75% of the difficult laryngoscopies were accurately detected beforehand, but 12% of the uncomplicated laryngoscopies were falsely identified as difficult. Although a test that identifies 75% of difficult laryngoscopies appears valuable, the high number of false alarms may be unacceptable. Whether or not such a predictive rule would be helpful for identifying difficult intubations would depend on the staffing of hospitals.

Despite exploring many features, it was not possible to identify patients in whom laryngoscopy would be difficult without increasing the false alarm rate to an unacceptably high level. Because difficult intubations cannot yet be accurately predicted, anesthesiologists should practice simulated difficult intubations, or be able to do a simple cricothyroidotomy, if needed.

▶ The experienced anesthesiologist can instantly recognize the patient in whom tracheal intubation may be difficult. It is the unexpected difficult laryngoscopy that causes one to look retrospectively for findings that would have predicted this unexpected event. Even when the index of suspicion is high, there often is no logical approach other than to proceed. In many such instances, the anesthesiologist is able to achieve tracheal intubation, albeit with some extra effort. The important practice is to be prepared for the impossible tracheal intubation and have appropriate personnel and equipment immediately available.—R.K. Stoelting, M.D.

Difficulties With Tooth Protectors in Endotracheal Intubation
Aromaa U, Pesonen P, Linko K, Tammisto T (Helsinki Univ Central Hosp, Helsinki)
Acta Anaesthesiol Scand 32:304–307, 1988   5–4

To avoid litigation stemming from dental trauma during anesthesia, the use of tooth protectors has been advocated. However, tooth protectors are rarely used as they reportedly interfere with tracheal intubation. Because the degree to which tooth protectors hamper anesthesia has not been studied, the suitability of 3 different tooth protectors for routine use during endotracheal intubation was evaluated.

The study was done with 300 consecutive patients undergoing elective procedures requiring endotracheal intubation. Patients were randomly assigned to 1 of 4 groups of 75 patients each. In the first group, no tooth protector was used. In the second group, a Den-ex Teethprotector manufactured in Denmark was used. In the third group, a Camo SDI made in Sweden was applied, and in the fourth group, a Camo SDI from which 2.5 to 3 cm had been cut from its right end to facilitate intubation was used. The anesthesiologist assessed the preanesthetic dental status of the patient and reexamined the teeth during recovery. Dental status was defined as normal, high risk, or missing teeth. High risk teeth included serious caries, periodontal disease, restorations, crowns, and fixed partial dentures.

Intubation was not possible in 15 patients who had a Camo protector, in 8 patients with a Den-ex protector, and in 4 patients with a cut Camo protector in place. Lack of space within the oral cavity caused difficulty when guiding the endotracheal tube into the larynx in 44 patients in the Camo group, 19 patients in the cut Camo group, and 31 patients in the Den-ex group. In 50 patients, the protector had to be removed to enable intubation. Four patients sustained dental injuries, 2 losing a maxillary incisor despite the proper use of a Denex protector.

The design of currently available tooth protectors for use during anesthesia is not yet satisfactory because they interfere with intubation. However, despite certain disadvantages, tooth protectors should be used routinely in patients with vulnerable teeth.

▶ Detection of third heart sounds or detailed descriptions of diastolic murmurs by the anesthesiologists may impress a medical student but on a scale of 1 to 10 has modest practical importance when compared with the patient's dentition. Some dental injuries may be unavoidable. Nevertheless, routine preoperative evaluation of dentition plus discussion with the patient and documentation in the medical record have great practical value. Dental protectors are probably helpful in selected patients and deserve greater use than currently practiced.— R.K. Stoelting, M.D.

Spinal and Epidural Anesthesia

Spinal Anesthesia and Lumbar Lordosis

Logan MR, Drummond GB (Royal Infirmary, Edinburgh)
Anesth Analg 67:338–341, April 1988   5–5

Reportedly, posture during and after isobaric or hyperbaric intrathecal injections of local anesthetic solutions influences the spread of the resultant blockade. However, the assessor of the block in these studies was not blind to the patient position. A study was conducted to determine the effect of reducing lumbar lordosis by hip flexion on the extent of analgesic and anesthetic blockade and on cardiovascular side effects.

Forty patients aged 20–70 years were scheduled for elective surgery to the lower limb or perineum under spinal anesthesia. Patients were randomly assigned to a group that maintained 90 degrees hip flexion for 5 minutes after subarachnoid injection of the anesthetic solution, or to a group that was allowed to immediately lie supine with straight legs following injection. Each patient received 0.5% bupivacaine, 3 ml in 8% glucose, which was injected over exactly 20 seconds. Nerve blockade was assessesd by an observer who was blind to whether hip flexion had been maintained or not. Cephalad spread of analgesia, anesthesia, and degree of motor weakness in the legs was assessed at 5-minute intervals for 30 minutes. Arterial pressure and heart rate were recorded at baseline and at 5-minute intervals for 30 minutes thereafter.

The distribution of the upper extent of anesthesia in both groups showed bimodality 30 minutes after injection. Bimodality was more pronounced in the straight-hip group than in the flexed-hip group. In contrast, the upper extent of analgesia showed no statistically significant bimodality in either group. Four patients in the flexed-hip group did not attain full motor blockade of the lower limbs, whereas only 1 patient in the straight-hip group did not attain full motor blockade. Three patients in the flexed-hip group had inadequate blocks for surgery to the lower limbs and required general anesthesia. In 2 patients in the flexed-hip group typical postspinal headaches developed with photophobia and postural headache. Cardiovascular side effects were minimal and equal in both groups.

The technique of hip flexion during induction of spinal anesthesia to reduce lumbar lordosis does not significantly limit the height of anesthetic blockade, nor does it influence the cardiovascular effects of spinal blockade.

▶ Having assisted Dr. T. C. Smith with the original study of this nature utilizing hyperbaric tetracaine in the mid-1960's, I am delighted that his observations have withstood the test of time and have been corroborated by Logan and Drummond. It is unfortunate that the Scottish investigators did not evaluate 0.75% hyperbaric bupivacaine because 0.5% hyperbaric bupivacaine is not available in the United States at this time.—G.W. Ostheimer, M.D.

Incidence and Etiology of Failed Spinal Anesthetics in a University Hospital: A Prospective Study
Munhall RJ, Sukhani R, Winnie AP (Univ of Illinois, Chicago)
Anesth Analg 67:843–848, September 1988   5–6

Two recent retrospective studies of failed spinal anesthesic attempts reported variable results, with 1 hospital reporting a 17% failure rate. A prospective study was undertaken to provide more accurate data on the incidence of spinal anesthesia failure and on the factors that contribute to such failure.

During a 6-month period, 200 healthy consenting patients—146 males and 54 females aged 16–80 years—were scheduled for surgery under spinal anesthesia. Variables recorded for each patient were classified as demographic, anesthetic, and surgical. Anesthetic variables were further divided into technical and pharmacologic categories (table). The clinical efficacy of the spinal anesthetic was evaluated by recording the patient's subjective response to surgery and the need for supplemental agents to maintain patient comfort. Spinal anesthesia was classified as a failure if the surgical procedure could not be performed without changing to general anesthesia. Tetracaine was the spinal anesthetic agent used in all cases, with 142 patients receiving crystalline tetracaine, and 38 patients receiving a 1% tetracaine solution.

By the criteria defined for this study, spinal anesthesia failed in 8 (4%) of the 200 patients. Only 2 (25%) of the failures resulted from errors in technique; the other 6 failures (75%) resulted from errors in judgment involving 1 or more pharmacologic factors such as dosage, use of epi-

Factors Affecting Success or Failure of Spinal Anesthesia

Technical factors
1. Identification of subarachnoid space; related to training; ability to utilize different approaches
2. Documentation of free flow of CSF pre- and postinjection
3. Proper placement of catheter for continuous spinal technique
Pharmacologic factors (judgment error)
1. Selection of appropriate local anesthetic and addition of vasoconstrictor; depending on duration of surgery
2. Selection of appropriate dosage and baricity
3. Selection of appropriate position and interspace; depending on site of surgery
4. Selection of appropriate technique; single injection versus continuous catheter technique

(Courtesy of Munhall RJ, Sukhani R, Winnie AP: *Anesth Analg* 67:843–848, September 1988.)

nephrine, and positioning of the patient. Surgical procedures involving intraperitoneal manipulations accounted for 20% of the failures secondary to an inadequate level of surgical anesthesia.

High failure rates in patients having spinal anesthesia seem to be attributable directly to inadequate training. Many anesthesiology residency programs apparently fail to teach regional anesthesia properly.

▶ The authors' comment at the end of their paper reflects my opinion: "In summary, the present study indicates that at our institution [The University of Illinois, Chicago], a university teaching hospital, it is primarily errors in judgment in respect to pharmacologic factors, i.e., choice of drug, dose, and baricity, and proper positioning of the patient, that most commonly result in an unsatisfactory level and/or duration of block and spinal failure. Only with experience gained under the guidance of skilled teachers can the neophyte anesthesiologist develop not only the technical skills but, more important, the clinical judgment that results in a low incidence of failed spinals. Bridenbaugh [*Reg Anaesth* 7:26–28, 1982] recently reported the results of a survey of residency programs and the degree to which they are teaching regional anesthesia and concluded that many anesthesiology residency programs are failing to teach regional anesthesia. Without this experience it is no wonder that the failure rates of spinal anesthesia (and other regional technique) are high and, of course, with such high failure rates anesthesiologists are reluctant to use spinal anesthesia even when indicated. We believe that the low incidence of failed spinals in our study is related to the extensive clinical experience in regional anesthesia gained by residents at our institution."—G.W. Ostheimer, M.D.

Unexpected Cardiac Arrest During Spinal Anesthesia: A Closed Claims Analysis of Predisposing Factors
Caplan RA, Ward RJ, Posner K, Cheney FW (Univ of Washington)
Anesthesiology 68:5–11, January 1988   5–7

A review of 900 closed insurance claims for major anesthetic complications occurring in an 8-year period disclosed 14 patients who sustained sudden cardiac arrest during spinal anesthesia. The victims had an average age of 36 and were relatively healthy. All of them were resuscitated, but 6 incurred severe neurologic damage and died in the hospital. Only 1 survivor became independent in daily self-care.

All but 1 of the arrests occurred after surgery was in progress. The most frequent early clues to arrest were bradycardia and cyanosis (table). Both diagnosis and initiation of cardiopulmonary resuscitation were prompt (Fig 5–1). The usual duration of external heart massage was 15 minutes or less. Most patients received ephedrine and atropine initially and bicarbonate and epinephrine later.

The inconsistent finding of cyanosis in these patients suggests that respiratory insufficiency may go unnoticed. A pulse oximeter therefore should be in place when sedatives are given, or if it is difficult for any reason to communicate with the patient. It seems wise to administer epi-

Initial Clues of Arrest (No. of Patients)			
	1st Clue	2nd Clue	Combined Incidence
Bradycardia	7	2	9
Hypotension	2	6	8
Cyanosis	4	3	7
Loss of consciousness	1	1	2
Asystole	0	2	2

(Courtesy of Caplan RA, Ward RJ, Posner K, et al: *Anesthesiology* 68:5–11, January 1988.)

nephrine early in the treatment of sudden bradycardia, and a full resuscitating dose should be given immediately when cardiac arrest is recognized.

▶ This article and the accompanying editorial by Dr. Keats (*Anesthesiology* 68:2–4, January 1988) are required reading by the practicing anesthesiologist. Although it seems that there was a reasonable response by the anesthetist when the bradycardia and hypotension developed, one wonders whether the

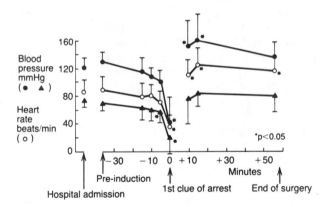

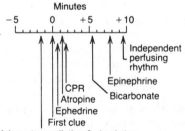

Fig 5–1.—Composite display of vital signs *(upper graph)* and key events *(lower graph)* in 14 patients with cardiac arrest during spinal anesthesia. Systolic blood pressure, *closed circles;* diastolic blood pressure, *closed triangles;* heart rate, *open circles.* $*P < .05$ versus hospital admission values. (Courtesy of Caplan RA, Ward RJ, Posner K, et al: *Anesthesiology* 68:5–11, January.)

development of a cardiac arrest could have been prevented by more vigilance. All too often, after the administration of a spinal anesthetic, attention to the patient may be diminished because it is felt that the anesthetic level will not change much during the operative procedure. There is excellent evidence that the level of sympathetic blockade will continue to ascend during the early part of the operative procedure and the patient's response may be modified by the administration of intraoperative sedatives, narcotics, or both.

I completely agree with the recommendation of the authors that a pulse oximeter is essential whenever sedative effects are administered or when the ability to communicate with the patient is impaired for whatever reason. I also agree that epinephrine should be considered when the standard treatment of increased fluid infusion and ephedrine is not improving the hemodynamic status of the patient. However, I would urge the listener not to use a full resuscitative dose of epinephrine to treat developing hypotension and bradycardia. One tenth milligram of epinephrine may be all that would be necessary in this circumstance to initiate an increase in pulse and blood pressure. However, if cardiopulmonary arrest develops, then a full resuscitative dose 0.5–1.0 mg of epinephrine must be administered immediately. Although I agree with Dr. Keats that immediate and effective action must be initiated, I do want to raise a note of caution about the overaggressive use of epinephrine, just as he has raised a caution about the overutilization of ephedrine.

Since the appearance of the article and the accompanying editorial, I have become aware of several instances in which anesthesiologists or residents have administered epinephrine with the development of hypotension, bradycardia, or both during a spinal or epidural anesthetic when ephedrine might have been the better drug of choice. The result has been severe hypertension in several instances from the utilization of large doses of epinephrine. I certainly agree that, if a diminution in blood pressure and heart rate does not respond to an adequate dose of ephedrine, epinephrine should be administered. However, the inappropriate use of epinephrine can lead to disastrous effects from severe hypertension and, perhaps, intercerebral hemorrhage.

I am in complete agreement that the universal practice of providing intraoperative sedation by intravenous sedatives and narcotics may not be entirely appropriate in all cases. Finally, I agree that institution of closed chest cardiac massage and positive pressure ventilation is essential at the time of an apparent cardiac arrest and open cardiac massage must be considered earlier during resuscitation in the operating room. Continued studies like this, as Dr. Keats says, will create a new awareness of the problems facing the anesthesiologist even in rare instances, and the ultimate result will be better patient care.— G.W. Ostheimer, M.D.

The Effect of Rotation of an Epidural Needle: An In Vitro Study
Meiklejohn BH (Leicester Royal Infirmary, Leicester, England)
Anaesthesia 42:1180–1182, 1987   5–8

Some authors suggest that rotation of the epidural needle may increase the risk of dural puncture; others advocate rotation of the needle through

270 degrees, with aspiration every 90 degrees, in case the flow of cerebrospinal fluid is prevented by a flap of dura. A study was undertaken to test whether this procedure risks puncturing the dura.

Technique.—Sections of the thoracolumbar dural sac were obtained from 3 adult spines at postmortem examination. The sacs were divided into anterior and posterior strips and segmented. Initial measurements were made for segments from each dural sac using a needle weighted until dural puncture occurred without needle rotation. Smaller weights were used while the needle was rotated clockwise. The weight and rotation required to puncture the dura were recorded.

Forty segments were tested from 3 sacs. For all 3 dural sacs there was a highly significant inverse correlation between the amount of rotation and the weight required to puncture the dura. Significantly less weight was required to puncture when the needle was rotated than when it was not.

Because inadvertent dural puncture can be a life-threatening complication, all possible steps should be taken to avoid it. Based on these results, it is recommended that, once the needle has been inserted into the epidural space, it should not be moved except to remove it.

▶ Your editor initially learned to identify the epidural space with a short, straight, beveled, winged (Salt-MacIntosh) needle. This sharp-edged needle would easily perforate the dura upon rotation and, therefore, was not to be rotated upon placement in the epidural space. Subsequently, when using the Huber tip modification of the winged Tuohy (Weiss) needle I would rotate the needle 90 degrees to place my catheter cephalad or caudad in the epidural space. Unfortunately, I realized this was fraught with the possibility of dural puncture when it occurred on occasion. Therefore, your editor is in agreement with the author that once the needle is placed in the epidural space, it should not be rotated. Rotation and aspiration through the needle does not guarantee that the point of the needle is not going to end up in a vein or the subdural or subarachnoid space. The wall of a vein or a flap of tissue could prevent aspiration regardless of where the tip of the needle is placed.—G.W. Ostheimer, M.D.

Inadvertent Subdural Injection: A Complication of an Epidural Block
Lubenow T, Keh-Wong E, Kristof K, Ivankovich O, Ivankovich AD (Rush Presbyterian St Luke's Med Ctr, Chicago)
Anesth Analg 67:175–179, February 1988   5–9

The subdural space is generally thought to exist in the cerebral meninges. However, it may extend down into the spinal segment of the meninges, causing unexpected sensory, sympathetic, and motor blocks when local anesthetics are inadvertently deposited there. To determine the incidence of inadvertent subdural block, data on 2,182 epidural injections given in a 30-month period were analyzed. All of the patients had low back pathology.

Patients who experienced any untoward or unpleasant side effects from

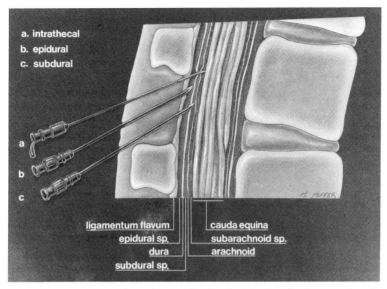

Fig 5–2.—Relative position of intrathecal, epidural, and subdural needle placement. If needle is in subdural space, with dura straddling bevel, some of local anesthetic may be deposited in subdural space and some, in epidural space. (Courtesy of Lubenow T, Keh-Wong E, Kristof K, et al: *Anesth Analg* 67:175–179, February 1988.)

the injection were identified for follow-up. A subdural block was defined as an extensive neural block in the absence of subarachnoid puncture out of proportion to the amount of local anesthetic injected. Eighteen patients met the criteria for an incidence of 0.82%. Cadaveric dissection also was done to clarify further the presence and anatomical position of the subdural space (Fig 5–2).

Subdural injection is a complication of epidural block that seems more common than has previously been recognized. An earlier report estimated the incidence of subdural block to be 0.1%, much lower than the incidence of 0.82% found in this large series.

▶ I agree!—G.W. Ostheimer, M.D.

Anatomical Re-Evaluation of Lumbar Dura Mater With Regard to Postspinal Headache: Effect of Dural Puncture
Dittmann M, Schäfer H-G, Ulrich J, Bond-Taylor W (Kreiskrankenhaus, Bad Säckingen, West Germany; Univ Hosp of Basel, Switzerland)
Anaesthesia 43:635–637, 1988   5–10

Although spinal anesthesia has been used for 100 years, the debate over what causes the typical postspinal headache continues. Leakage of cerebrospinal fluid (CSF) through the spinal needle hole in the dura has been implicated as a likely cause of postspinal headaches. The gross

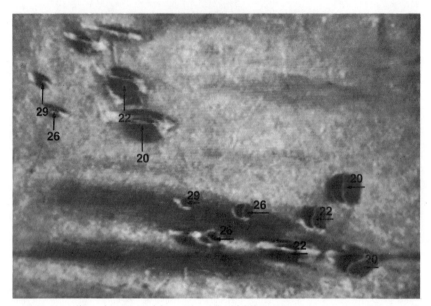

Fig 5–3.—Effects of puncture of dura with needles of different sizes. Punctures in *top left* are made with needle bevels as parallel as possible to dural fibers and those in *upper row* in *bottom right* with bevels rotated through 90 degrees. "Tin-lid" effect can be seen clearly and is *arrowed*. Numbers refer to needle sizes. (Courtesy of Dittmann M, Schäfer H-G, Ulrich J, et al: *Anaesthesia* 43:635–637, 1988.)

structure of dura mater in the lumbar region was examined and the effect of dural puncture with needles of different sizes was assessed.

Fresh cadaver specimens of dura were punctured with 20-, 22-, 26-, and 29-gauge Quincke needles, with their bevels held as parallel as possible to the dural fibers, and the resultant holes were examined. The needle bevels were then rotated 90 degrees and reintroduced through the dura. The effect of penetration of the dura in areas of different thickness was also studied.

Contrary to statements in earlier reports, the texture of dura mater, particularly the arrangement of the elastic fibers, was not uniform, and the thickness of the dura varied from 0.5 mm to almost 2.0 mm. A "tin-lid" phenomenon was observed with each needle size (Fig 5–3). The perforation resembled the top of a tin that had been almost completely opened, but with the lid hinged at 1 point. This phenomenon was also observed when the needle bevels had been turned 90 degrees, although the holes were then somewhat rounder.

When a needle was inserted through a thick part of the dura, the hole tended to be ellipsoid but shrank a short time later. However, when the same size needle penetrated a thinner part of the dura, the resultant hole was larger and tended to shrink much more slowly. Even with 20-gauge needles, the "tin-lid" phenomenon could effectively close the hole in the dura.

The findings of this study may explain why some patients, particularly the elderly who physiologically have a lower CSF pressure, do not experience postspinal headache despite the use of large-gauge needles.

▶ The debate continues over whether spinal needles should be inserted parallel to the dural fibers or at a right angle to the direction of the fibers. In this study, the size and shape of a hole depended to a lesser extent on the direction of the needle. The shape of the holes were found to be either round or ellipsoid. The most important factor, in the opinion of these authors, is the size of the needle that perforates the dura in producing a postdural puncture headache. Your editor looks forward to the next study dealing with this issue, which we will present in the YEAR BOOK OF ANESTHESIA.—G.W. Ostheimer, M.D.

Epidurally Administered Halothane Vapor Potentiates Mepivacaine-Induced Epidural Anesthesia: A Report of 10 Cases
Suwa K (Univ of Tokyo)
J Anesth 2:90–93, 1988   5–11

Animal experiments have shown that inhalational anesthetics have some effect on the spinal cord. It was theorized that, owing to their gaseous state, inhalational anesthetics might be better diffused into epidural space than conventional liquid anesthetics and, if so, that injection of halothane vapor into epidural space might induce epidural anesthesia faster than conventional local anesthetics. This concept was tested in 10 patients who underwent major intra-abdominal procedures.

General anesthesia was induced with thiopental and was maintained with 66% nitrous oxide and 0.27% enflurane, combined with epidural anesthesia using mepivacaine, 1 mg/minute, and halothane vapor, 1.5 ml/minute. Halothane vapor was prepared by drawing air or nitrous oxide into a 50-ml glass syringe in which a few milliliters of liquid halothane had been placed in advance.

A 4-hour anesthesia required 360 ml of 30% halothane vapor, which is equivalent to about 120 ml of pure halothane vapor or 0.5 ml of liquid halothane. Compared with a group of 10 patients who underwent similar operations and received similar general anesthesia combined with conventional epidural anesthesia using mepivacaine alone, the time required for awakening in the halothane group was significantly shorter. However, contrary to expectation, onset of anesthesia in the halothane group was not substantially faster. Furthermore, sterile injection of halothane vapor was not easily accomplished and had to be considered less than ideal.

Although the results of this study confirm that halothane vapor can be injected into epidural space and can achieve epidural anesthesia without major side effects, the usefulness of this technique and its potential advantages over conventional epidural anesthesia remain to be explored.

▶ Your editor could not believe this study when he first read it and felt there must have been a misprint in that halothane vapor was injected into the epidural space! Regardless of the findings of the author, the potential for disaster surrounds this experiment. Did the author consider the possibility of having an intravenous injection of the gaseous vapor that could result in a massive air embolism? I can't believe this study ever got through an institutional review board. Hopefully, no other investigators will follow up on evaluating the usefulness of this technique and its potential advantages over conventional analgesia and anesthesia.—G.W. Ostheimer, M.D.

Peripheral Nerve Blocks

Anterior Approach to Celiac Plexus Block During Interventional Biliary Procedures
Lieberman RP, Nance PN, Cuka DJ (Univ of Nebraska Med Ctr, Omaha; Omaha VA Hosp)
Radiology 167:562–564, May 1988   5–12

A small percentage of patients undergoing percutaneous biliary procedures may experience severe pain. Celiac block was used as a means of relieving this pain, employing an anterior approach. The advantage of this method is that it can be performed, if needed, during the procedure. A posterior block must be done before the start of the procedure, without knowing whether the block will be necessary.

Among 65 biliary procedures on 36 patients, 18 celiac blocks were performed. Fluoroscopy guided the choice of a skin puncture site on the anterior abdominal wall. The physician injected 40 ml of 0.5% lidocaine into a site over the L-1 vertebra, using a 20-gauge needle 15 cm long. Patient behavior and comments were used to evaluate the block's effectiveness. Investigators also reviewed computed tomography scans and ultrasound examinations of the patients for possible complications.

Ten celiac blocks offered very good to excellent pain relief, 1 reduced pain but was not able to make the patient comfortable, and 6 blocks had little or no effect. One patient could not be evaluated. The main side effect was hypotension. No patient experienced damage to internal organs from the needle.

The success rate reported for posterior block is higher than that in this anterior block trial. A different placement of the needle or a larger amount of anesthetic might have given relief to more patients. With these technical modifications, the anterior approach, which is faster, easier, and less painful than posterior block, might prove to be the analgesic method of choice in such procedures.

▶ This article was accepted because it appears in a journal not likely to be read by anesthesiologists. That the success is higher with a posterior block makes this reviewer question whether the anterior block approach to the celiac plexus should be adopted.—R.D. Miller, M.D.

TABLE 1.—Results of Clinical Study

	Group A (Prilocaine only; n+18)		Group B (Prilocaine and Atracurium; n=18)		Significance of difference between means
	Range	Mean	Range	Mean	
Ease of reduction (0 = impossible; 10 = very easy)	0–10	6	3–10	8·4	$p < 0.025$
Time to return of fine movement (min)	1–20	4·8	12–45	25·8	$p < 0.001$
Pain scores (0 = painless; 10 worst pain imaginable):					
Prior to injection	1–8	4·1	1–10	4·8	N.S.*
10 min after injection	0–2	0·5	0–2	0·5	N.S.*
During reduction	0–7	1·8	0–4	0·6	$p < 0.05$
Post-reduction film:					
Unacceptable	2		0		
Acceptable	4		6		
Good/anatomical	12		12		

*N.S., not significant.
(Courtesy of McGlone R, Heyes F, Harris P: *Arch Emerg Med* 5:79–85, 1988.)

The Use of a Muscle Relaxant to Supplement Local Anaesthetics for Bier's Blocks
McGlone R, Heyes F, Harris P (General Infirmary, Leeds, England; Hull Royal Infirmary, Hull, England; Derbyshire Royal Infirmary, Derby, England)
Arch Emerg Med 5:79–85, 1988   5–13

Because the Bier's block technique provides poor muscle relaxation in patients requiring reduction for wrist fracture, the effect of the addition of atracurium, which provides full neuromuscular block for no more than 35 minutes, was evaluated in 4 volunteers. A clinical study of 36 patients with wrist fractures was then carried out. Patients were randomized to receive either prilocaine alone or prilocaine with atracurium (Table 1).

TABLE 2.—Suggested Dosage for Upper
Limb Bier's Blocks (Torda and
Klonymus, 1967)

Muscle relaxant	Dose (mg)
Tubocurarine	1
Gallamine	10
Succinylcholine	4
Decamethonium	0·2
(Atracurium	2)

(Courtesy of McGlone R, Heyes F, Harris P: *Arch
Emerg Med* 5:79–85, 1988.)

As expected, return of fine-motor control was delayed in the group receiving atracurium. Three patients in this group also had transient difficulty with focusing. Because of significant pain relief and increased muscle relaxation in the atracurium group, reductions were easier to perform. Reduction initially failed because of lack of relaxation in 2 patients in the prilocaine-only group. Suggested dosages for upper limb Bier's blocks are given in Table 2.

The addition of atracurium to Bier's block is suggested in a selected group of patients—particularly in heavily built adults with significant displacement at the fracture site—before reduction of wrist fractures.

▶ This is certainly an interesting concept. Certainly there is no doubt that the atracurium must diffuse to the neuromuscular junction and produce partial paralysis. We have all known that the closed arm technique can be used for evaluating onset and duration of neuromuscular blockade. As a result, these findings are no surprise. The application of well-known information to the clinical setting is certainly encouraging. These authors suspect that this is an extremely useful technique.—R.D. Miller, M.D.

Clinical Pharmacokinetics of Carbonated Local Anesthetics II: Interscalene Brachial Block Model

Sukhani R, Winnie AP (Univ of Illinois, Chicago)
Anesth Analg 66:1245–1250, December 1987   5–14

Carbonated local anesthetics have shorter latency periods than the equivalent hydrochloride salts when used for brachial plexus anesthesia. A double-blind study was done to determine whether lidocaine carbonate produces a similar increase in dermatomal spread compared with lidocaine hydrochloride.

Thirty healthy adults undergoing upper extremity surgery under interscalene brachial plexus block were studied. The effects of lidocaine carbonate and 1.1% and 1% lidocaine hydrochloride were compared. Epinephrine was added to both solutions before injection.

Compared with lidocaine hydrochloride, lidocaine carbonate produced a 38% reduction in onset time and a pronounced increase in the extent of anesthesia. Lidocaine carbonate produced surgical anesthesia of the upper extremity, including the hand, in 87% of the patients, whereas lidocaine hydrochloride produced comparable anesthesia in 53% of the patients. Supplemental blocks were required in 66% of the patients who received lidocaine hydrochloride and in only 25% of those who received lidocaine carbonate.

In this series, lidocaine carbonate provided a clinically significant reduction in latency and an increase in the spread of anesthesia when compared with lidocaine hydrochloride.

Comparison of Bupivacaine and Alkalinized Bupivacaine in Brachial Plexus Anesthesia

Bedder MD, Kozody R, Craig DB (Univ of Manitoba)
Anesth Analg 67:48–52, January 1988   5–15

The role of alkalinization of bupivacaine 0.5% on clinical efficacy, onset, and regression in patients undergoing upper extremity surgery with subclavian perivascular brachial plexus blockade was investigated in 60 patients with American Society of Anesthesiologists classifications I and II. By random assignment, 30 patients received bupivacaine 0.5%, 3 mg/kg, and 30 received alkalinized bupivacaine 0.5%, 3 mg/kg. Onset and regression of sensory blockade were determined by pinprick in the C4–T2 skin dermatomes. Motor blockade was evaluated by using a scheme of proximal to distal muscle group paralysis.

Time to onset of sensory blockade and time to peak sensory effect did not differ significantly between the 2 groups. Also, no difference in time to onset of motor blockade or time to peak motor effect was noted. Regression of postoperative sensory and motor blockade also was comparable in both groups.

Alkalinization of bupivacaine 0.5% solutions does not seem to confer any added clinical benefit in subclavian perivascular brachial plexus blockade when compared with commercially available bupivacaine.

▶ Discussion continues about whether carbonization is equivalent to the addition of sodium bicarbonate to alkalinize local anesthetics. For the basis of this discussion, let us assume for lidocaine that carbonation and alkalinization are equal. Clearly, lidocaine's onset and spread is enhanced with carbonation or alkalinization. The same is not true with alkalinized 2-chloroprocaine.

There have been conflicting reports with the use of alkalinized bupivacaine. Hilgier demonstrated that alkalinization of bupivacaine solution increased onset and prolonged duration of sensory blockade. However, Bedder et al. did not find any clinical advantage to alkalinization of bupivacaine. Caution must be used when alkalinizing bupivacaine because a very small additional amount of sodium bicarbonate could result in precipitation. This does not occur with the addition of varying amounts of sodium bicarbonate solution to lidocaine. There-fore, it would seem that the alkalinization or carbonization of lidocaine en-hances its clinical applicability in regional block, whereas 2-chloroprocaine and bupivacaine are not given any increased advantage over the standard solutions and, in fact, may become a problem because of their precipitation after the ad-dition of sodium bicarbonate. The verdict on mepivacaine is still to be announced.— G.W. Ostheimer, M.D.

Comparison of Lidocaine and Prilocaine for Intravenous Regional Anesthesia

Bader AM, Concepcion M, Hurley RJ, Arthur GR (Harvard Univ; Brigham and Women's Hosp, Boston)
Anesthesiology 69:409–412, September 1988 5–16

There has been a great deal of controversy over which anesthetic is the most appropriate for intravenous regional anesthesia (IVRA). Lidocaine is probably the most widely used, but prilocaine appears to be better tol-erated than lidocaine with regard to systemic toxicity. When equal doses of both these agents are given for regional blockade, circulating prilocaine concentrations are lower than circulating lidocaine levels, sug-gesting that prilocaine may offer a particular advantage in IVRA. Al-though prilocaine has been associated with methemoglobin formation, the doses of prilocaine required to produce clinically significant prilocaine levels are much larger than the dose used in IVRA. This study was done to compare the efficacy and safety of equal doses of lidocaine and prilocaine for IVRA.

The study was done with 21 patients who were scheduled for hand surgery under IVRA. Eleven patients with a mean age of 56 years were randomly assigned to IVRA using prilocaine, and 10 patients with a mean age of 50 years were assigned to IVRA using lidocaine. Venous blood drug levels were measured before tourniquet deflation and at 1, 3, 5, 10, 30, 60, 90, and 120 minutes thereafter. Times to onset of anesthe-sia to pinprick and resolution of analgesia were also assessed and re-corded.

Onset of anesthesia to pinprick was essentially the same for both drugs, as were time to resolution of anesthesia and total tourniquet times. Mean peak venous blood concentrations were 1.60 mg/ml for lidocaine at 3 minutes after tourniquet deflation and 0.70 mg/ml for prilocaine at 5 minutes after tourniquet deflation. Prilocaine blood levels were signifi-cantly lower than lidocaine blood levels from 3 to 120 minutes following tourniquet deflation. In the prilocaine-treated patients, methemoglobin levels increased significantly from 0.5% to 3% at 60 minutes after tour-niquet deflation, whereas the lidocaine-treated patients showed no change in methemoglobin levels. The highest methemoglobin level mea-sured in any patient was 3.2%. (Cyanosis occurs when approximately 10% of the hemoglobin present is oxidized to methemoglobin). At 90 minutes after tourniquet deflation, methemoglobin levels were returning toward the control value. Side effects in both groups were minimal. No patient demonstrated cyanosis.

Prilocaine and lidocaine are comparable in terms of onset, duration, and quality of anesthesia when used for IVRA. However, the significantly lower blood prilocaine levels may indicate a greater margin of safety for this agent as compared with lidocaine. The methemoglobinemia observed with prilocaine was not clinically significant.

▶ Prilocaine is an excellent drug for intravenous regional anesthesia (IVRA) and other peripheral nerve blocks. However, the possibility of methemoglobinemia has caused anesthesiologists to disregard this drug in practice, which is unfortunate because its physicochemical characteristics make it a very safe local anesthetic. Hopefully, there will be a renewed interest in this local anesthetic before it becomes financially unfeasible for continued commercial production.— G.W. Ostheimer, M.D.

Central Nervous System Complications After 6,000 Retrobulbar Blocks
Nicoll JMV, Acharya PA, Ahlen K, Baguneid S, Edge KR (King Khaled Eye Specialist Hosp, Riyadh, Saudi Arabia)
Anesth Analg 66:1298–1302, December 1987   5–17

Life-threatening complications can result from spread of local anesthetic to the central nervous system after retrobulbar injection. Six thousand consecutive patients had retrobulbar anesthesia for eye surgery using a standard percutaneous inferotemporal approach. Most anesthetics consisted of a combination of 2% lidocaine, 0.5% bupivacaine, and hyaluronidase.

Sixteen patients (1 in 375) had signs of direct spread of anesthetic to the central nervous system, ranging from drowsiness and vomiting to seizures, unconsciousness, and cardiopulmonary arrest. None of the patients died, although several were apneic for varying periods and 3 became comatose. Symptoms could not be related to the dose of anesthetic or the experience of the anesthesiologist. No technical factors could be implicated. Symptomatic treatment with atropine, oxygen, fluids, and the head-down position were usually sufficient. When the patient was stable and anesthesia remained adequate, surgery proceeded.

If promptly recognized and treated, central spread of local anesthetic after retrobulbar injection should not entail great danger. The exception is asystole. This block remains a safe and effective form of anesthesia for ophthalmic surgery. Costs are minimal, and perioperative morbidity is relatively infrequent.

▶ This is an excellent review of the problems with retrobulbar block. This block was used by ophthalmologists and anesthesiologists in only ophthalmic or ophthalmic and otolaryngologic hospitals for many years. The utilization of regional anesthetic techniques for day surgical patients, which in some institutions comprise the majority of surgical cases, has led to a resurgence of interest by anesthesiologists in these techniques. Because of the medicolegal situation in many states, surgeons are reticent to do major blocks other than local infiltration for their surgical procedures and prefer to have anesthesiologists perform the block. It behooves the anesthesiologist to become familiar with blocks that were not previously utilized in their institutions because the economics of day surgical care is dependent upon the anesthesiologist being conversant in all forms of regional and general anesthesia. Studies such as this demonstrate that regional anesthesia can be successfully administered to a wide range of patients with little morbidity and mortality. Large studies of this type should be extended to other blocks commonly used for day surgical and in-house patient procedures in order to establish the safety of various blocks.—G.W. Ostheimer, M.D.

6 Anesthesia for Certain Types of Surgery

Cardiopulmonary Bypass

Cerebral Microembolism During Cardiopulmonary Bypass: Retinal Microvascular Studies In Vivo With Fluorescein Angiography
Blauth CI, Arnold JV, Schulenberg WE, McCartney AC, Taylor KM (Hammersmith Hosp, London; Moorfields Hosp, London)
J Thorac Cardiovasc Surg 95:668–676, April 1988   6–1

Systemic microembolism is a risk of cardiopulmonary bypass, but the consequences of microembolism in the systemic microcirculation during bypass are not completely understood. Fluorescein angiography was used to assess the incidence of microembolism in the retina during cardiopulmonary bypass and to quantify retinal microembolic events with reference to bypass time, arterial line filtration, and psychometric testing. Angiographic and histologic findings after bypass were correlated with those in an animal model.

Twenty-one patients having elective cardiopulmonary bypass underwent retinal fluorescein angiography 5 minutes before bypass was discontinued. Control angiograms were obtained before operation and, in 5 patients, immediately before bypass. Results were correlated with those of an animal study. Patients also took 4 psychometric tests before and after operation.

After 31–67 minutes of cardiopulmonary bypass, all of the patients had retinal microvascular occlusions, indicating microembolism. Before surgery, patients had normal retinal perfusion. During bypass, patients had a mean of 3.5 blocked arterioles of less than 50 μm caliber and a mean of 6.3 focal areas of capillary nonperfusion per 30-degree field of retina centered on the macula. There was partial reperfusion with occlusions in 4 of 5 (80%) patients 30 minutes after bypass; at a median of 8 days after surgery, only 2 of 16 (12%) patients had persistently occluded retinal vessels. The total microembolic count was not correlated with bypass time nor was it reduced by arterial line filtration in a subgroup of 11 patients. Retinal microvascular occlusions were more numerous in patients with psychometric deficits. Retinal histologic studies in a dog model of cardiopulmonary bypass revealed intravascular platelet-fibrin microaggregates 20 to 70 μm in diameter and focal ischemic changes in 7 of 9 dogs.

There is a high incidence of microvascular occlusion in the internal carotid artery during bypass that is consistent with microembolism. The hypothesis that cerebral microembolism is an important etiologic factor in neuropsychologic impairment after cardiopulmonary bypass remains to be proved.

▶ This technique may be analogous to the precordial Doppler in detecting venous air embolism, i.e., microemboli are detected more often than postoperative symptoms would suggest. Indeed, the authors emphasize that the clinical significance of their findings is uncertain. Failure of arterial line filtration to alter the incidence of microembolism further questions the significance of these microemboli.—R.K. Stoelting, M.D.

The Effect of Arterial Filtration on Reduction of Gaseous Microemboli in the Middle Cerebral Artery During Cardiopulmonary Bypass
Padayachee TS, Parsons S, Theobold R, Gosling RG, Deverall PB (Guy's Hosp, London; London Bridge Hosp, London)
Ann Thorac Surg 45:647–649, June 1988   6–2

The incidence of major neurologic damage after cardiac surgery and cardiopulmonary bypass (CPB) has been reduced significantly during recent years. However, up to 70% of all patients undergoing CPB show subtle postoperative impairment of cerebral function, which has been attributed to inadequate cerebral perfusion and microembolic phenomena. To reduce the number of circulating gaseous microemboli, filtration of arterial blood during CPB has been suggested, but its value has been disputed. This study was done to determine the effect of including an arterial filter in a CPB circuit incorporating a bubble oxygenator.

Eighteen patients aged 43 to 65 years and undergoing CPB were randomly assigned to either CPB without an arterial filter, CPB with a 40-μm filter, or CPB with a 25-μm filter. Transcranial Doppler ultrasound was used throughout CPB to monitor middle cerebral artery blood velocity. Doppler signals were recorded onto a stereo cassette tape. The number of microemboli was expressed as the microembolic index (MEI).

Controls had the highest incidence of gaseous microemboli at both low and high oxygen flow rates. At low oxygen flow rates, the 25-μm arterial filter reduced the MEI by 100% and the 40-μm filter reduced the MEI by 99%. However, at high oxygen flow rates, the 25-μm filter reduced the MEI by 100% and the 40-μm filter reduced the MEI by 60% to 100%.

An additional study of vented hearts in 3 patients undergoing cardiac valve operations showed that trapped air inside the heart may be responsible for the origin of gaseous microemboli.

A 25-μm arterial filter placed in the CPB circuit effectively reduces the number of gaseous microemboli in the middle cerebral artery.

▶ In contrast to the preceding report (Abstract 6–1), these data suggest that arterial filters are effective in reducing the incidence of microemboli during and after cardiopulmonary bypass. For the anesthesiologist, an important message remains: microemboli, with or without arterial filters, can occur. Understanding this risk is a valid reason to avoid the administration of nitrous oxide to these patients.—R.K. Stoelting, M.D.

Postoperative Effects of Intrathecal Morphine in Coronary Artery Bypass Surgery

Vanstrum GS, Bjornson KM, Ilko R (Mercy Hosp and Med Ctr, San Diego)
Anesth Analg 67:261–267, March 1988   6–3

A randomized, double-blind trial was devised to evaluate the effectiveness of intrathecal morphine in coronary artery bypass (CAB) surgery. Spinal opiates have been widely used for postoperative pain, but their benefits and risks in CAB surgery have not been documented.

Thirty patients undergoing elective CAB surgery entered the study. Group I (16 patients) received 1 ml of 0.05 morphine through lumbar puncture with a 22-gauge or 25-gauge needle. The 14 controls (group II) were given a placebo, 1 ml of saline. A record was kept of the amount of

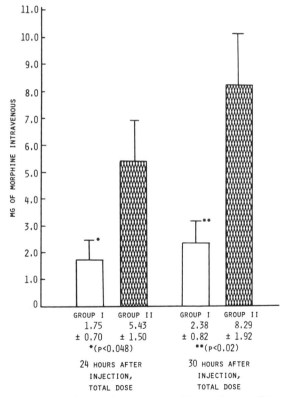

Fig 6–1.—Postoperative supplemental intravenous morphine requirements. Data were recorded 24 and 30 hours after intrathecal injection. Group I received intrathecal morphine, 0.5 mg; group II received intrathecal saline. (Courtesy of Vanstrum GS, Bjornson KM, Ilko R: *Anesth Analg* 67:261–267, March 1988.)

intravenous morphine sulfate administered postoperatively as needed for pain (Fig 6–1).

Group II required a significantly greater amount of morphine than group I, both 24 hours and 30 hours after the intrathecal injection. Patients receiving the placebo needed more antihypertensive drugs in the period after surgery. Five patients in group I did not require either morphine or nitroprusside postoperatively, but all of the controls needed 1 or both drugs. No important side effects were seen in either group.

Although the benefits of intrathecal morphine seem clear, the risks of a lumbar puncture do exist. Respiratory depression or arrest and urinary retention can occur, but are avoidable with certain precautions. To avoid a spinal hematoma, surgery should be postponed if the tap is difficult or bloody. Spinal narcotics have been used on approximately 1,000 patients during a 3-year period and no neurologic complications have occurred.

▶ The differences between study groups for postoperative intravenous morphine or nitroprusside requirements are not impressive. As the authors recognize, the benefits of this approach may not be sufficient to warrant the theoretic risks of postheparinization lumbar epidural hematoma. Based on the magnitude of these beneficial effects, it would seem unlikely a fully informed patient would consent to intrathecal morphine even when the risk of hematoma is a remote and theoretic risk.—R.K. Stoelting, M.D.

Magnesium and Coronary Revascularization
Harris MN, Crowther A, Jupp RA, Aps C (St Thomas' Hosp, London)
Br J Anaesth 60:779–783, 1988   6–4

It is well established that hypomagnesemia has a negative effect on the cardiovascular system. Previous studies have confirmed that extracorporeal hemodilution decreases plasma magnesium levels. The effect of intraoperative administration of magnesium chloride on plasma Mg levels and sinus rhythm following coronary artery bypass grafting was studied in 20 patients without cardioplegic arrest.

Nine patients with a mean age of 58.4 years were given 16 mmole of MgCl in 10 ml of water, and 11 patients with a mean age of 61.9 years had only 10 ml of water injected into the venous side of the extracorporeal circuit during the first aortic cross-clamp period of cardiopulmonary bypass. All patients also received 20 mg of furosemide administered concomitantly with MgCl or placebo. Plasma Mg and potassium levels and urinary Mg excretion were measured before operation and at regular intervals thereafter for up to 24 hours after operation. The electrocardiogram was recorded continuously in the postoperative period. Twelve-lead electrocardiograms were obtained before and 6 and 24 hours after operation, and QT intervals corrected for heart rate were calculated at regular intervals.

One patient in the control group and 2 patients in the Mg group had no arrhythmia during the 24-hour study period. One patient in each group had atrial fibrillation. Five (45%) patients in the control group and 4 (44%) patients in the Mg group had atrial extrasystoles. Seven (64%) patients in the control group and 2 (22%) in the Mg group had frequent ventricular arrhythmias. This difference was statistically significant.

In the control group, mean plasma Mg concentrations were significantly lower after operation than before and remained below normal throughout the study period. In the Mg-treated group, mean plasma Mg concentrations were elevated until 1 hour after operation, after which they remained within normal limits for the duration of the study. Urinary Mg excretion was higher in the Mg-treated group, with 58% of the administered Mg excreted within the first 24 hours.

Intraoperative administration of Mg may reduce the incidence of potentially serious ventricular arrhythmias after coronary bypass operations.

▶ Explanations for cardiac dysrhythmias following cardiopulmonary bypass are often complex and reflect multiple mechanisms. Certainly, electrolytic disturbances, particularly potassium, are a common consideration. Based on the present data, magnesium should also be considered.—R.K. Stoelting, M.D.

Hormonal and Metabolic Changes During Hypothermic Coronary Artery Bypass Surgery in Diabetic and Non-diabetic Subjects
Crock PA, Ley CJ, Martin IK, Alford FP, Best JD (Univ of Melbourne; St Vincent's Hosp, Fitzroy, Australia)
Diabetic Med 5:47–52, January 1988   6–5

Diabetic patients have coronary artery disease of greater severity and at a younger age than do nondiabetic persons and have an increased risk of operative mortality and morbidity when undergoing coronary artery bypass grafting (CABG). In addition, CABG under hypothermic anesthesia is a major physical stress associated with a period of diabetic destabilization because of increased stress hormones and hypothermia. The hormonal and metabolic changes of non–insulin-dependent diabetic patients and nondiabetic patients were compared.

The 3 groups studied were 8 nondiabetic patients, 8 patients with non–insulin-dependent diabetes mellitus given a glucose pump priming solution, and 8 comparable diabetic patients given a nonglucose infusion. No significant differences in stress hormone responses between the diabetic and nondiabetic patients were noted, with epinephrine concentrations rising by tenfold, norepinephrine by fourfold, and cortisol by twofold to threefold. Glucagon values increased significantly during bypass in diabetic patients who did not receive a glucose prime. Comparably marked hyperglycemia was observed in both glucose-primed groups during bypass; exclusion of glucose from the prime in diabetic patients prevents this increase. After surgery, the rise in insulin in the glucose-primed diabetic patients contrasted with the slower rise in the non–glucose-primed diabetic patients who were also hyperglycemic at this stage.

Diabetic patients had stress hormone responses to hypothermic CABG similar to those in nondiabetic patients. Increased stress hormones and hypothermia impair the disposal of glucose given in the priming solution, resulting in intraoperative hyperglycemia. When glucose is omitted from this solution, hyperglycemia develops after surgery because of persistently elevated stress hormones and a poor endogenous insulin response.

▶ Patients with diabetes mellitus undergoing cardiopulmonary bypass present a unique challenge for maintenance of normal blood glucose concentrations. Even in the absence of diabetes, the hormonal stress response to cardiopulmonary bypass and hyperthermia interfere with glucose homeostasis. For these reasons, continuous insulin infusions may deserve consideration in the management of patients with diabetes undergoing operations requiring cardiopulmonary bypass.— R.K. Stoelting, M.D.

Bladder Temperature as an Estimate of Body Temperature During Cardiopulmonary Bypass
Bone ME, Feneck RO (London Chest Hosp, London)
Anaesthesia 43:181–185, March 1988   6–6

The safe duration of circulatory arrest during open heart surgery is limited by the viability of the central nervous system, which is dependent on the temperature of the brain at the moment the blood flow is stopped. A major risk during the transition phases of cooling and rewarming is the development of large thermal gradients in the body tissues, which may imply slow heat transfer and an increased risk of imbalance between metabolite supply and demand. Accurate estimates of core body temperature are important during cardiopulmonary bypass, but yet there is no ideal site for estimates of body core temperature. Bladder temperature, as measured by the recently developed thermistor-tipped urinary catheter, was compared with esophageal, nasopharyngeal, rectal, and cutaneous temperatures in 33 patients during cardiopulmonary bypass. Two groups of patients were investigated: those who underwent cardiopulmonary bypass at 28 C and those who underwent cardiopulmonary bypass without active whole body cooling but with simple drift of temperature to approximately 34 C.

The bladder site was warmer than all other monitored sites in the prebypass period and showed the least variation in temperature. The rate of change of bladder temperature during cooling and rewarming was significantly lower than for esophageal and nasopharyngeal temperatures but was greater than or similar to the rate of change of rectal and cutaneous temperatures. In addition, bladder temperature monitoring was satisfactory in 5 patients monitored after the operation in the intensive care unit.

Bladder temperature appears to offer a convenient estimate of core body temperature in patients who undergo cardiac surgery. It is also a safe, convenient, and accurate method of measuring temperature during surgery and in the intensive care unit.

▶ Monitoring body temperature at more than 1 site during cardiopulmonary bypass may have unique importance in preventing undesirable temperature changes after bypass. Minimization of the temperature difference between core tissues and peripheral tissues is likely to be associated with the least downward drift of temperature in the postoperative period. Indeed, drug-induced peripheral vasodilation with nitroprusside or isoflurane may minimize peripheral hypothermia that is likely to accompany low cardiac output. The observation that bladder temperature was warmer than other monitored sites suggests this site may serve as a measure of core body temperature.—R.K. Stoelting, M.D.

Nerve Injury and Musculoskeletal Complaints After Cardiac Surgery: Influence of Internal Mammary Artery Dissection and Left Arm Position
Roy RC, Stafford MA, Charlton JE (Wake Forest Univ; Univ of Newcastle upon Tyne, England)
Anesth Analg 67:277–279, March 1988   6–7

Some studies have reported upper extremity nerve injury after cardiac surgery. Whether dissection of the internal mammary artery (IMA) and the position of the left arm are related to the frequency of neurologic dysfunction and musculoskeletal problems after cardiac surgery was investigated in 200 patients scheduled for medial sternotomy and cardiopulmonary bypass. Patients were classified into 4 groups: group A, scheduled for left IMA harvest, had the left arm abducted 90 degrees; group B also had the left arm abducted 90 degrees but had no IMA harvest; group C had the left arm at the side and left IMA harvest; group D had the left arm at the side without IMA harvest.

Complete data for 162 patients were reported. There were 16 upper extremity nerve injuries. Twelve of these involved the brachial plexus: 7 were left-sided, 4 were right-sided, and 1 was bilateral. There were 4 peripheral left-sided nerve injuries in patients whose brachial artery was not cannulated. No patient had significant functional disability. Thirty-nine percent of patients with IMA grafts had musculoskeletal complaints or neurologic dysfunction or both, compared with 17% without IMA grafts. However, when upper extremity nerve injuries alone were compared, there was no difference attributable to IMA harvesting. Arm position was not a factor.

There was a 10% incidence of upper extremity nerve injury after cardiac surgery; IMA dissection, arm position, and internal jugular vein catheterization were not influential.

▶ Nerve injuries involving the brachial plexus are often assumed to reflect improper positioning of the extremity during surgery. The demonstration that a substantial incidence of upper extremity nerve injury follows cardiac surgery and is not influenced by arm position is important information when such an unfortunate event occurs despite appropriate intraoperative precautions.—R.K. Stoelting, M.D.

Venous Admixture to Radial Artery Blood Samples During Cardiopulmonary Bypass

Aronson S, Neff WA, Slogoff S, Keats AS (Texas Heart Inst, Houston)
Chest 92:836–838, November 1987   6–8

In patients undergoing coronary artery bypass, blood drawn from the left radial artery was highly unsaturated (oxygen tension [PO_2], 35 mm Hg) when blood entering the aortic cannula had a PO_2 of 290 mm Hg at a perfusion pressure of 35 mm Hg and flow of 50 ml/kg per minute. The difference in PO_2 decreased with increasing perfusion pressure and was identical only when the left arm was repositioned. It was hypothesized that impaired venous return from an extremity during low arterial perfusion pressure could result in venous admixture to radial artery samples by blood being drawn through the capillary bed or venoarterial shunts or both. Thirty patients undergoing cardiopulmonary bypass were studied to determine the circumstances during which venous admixture to radial artery blood could occur during cardiopulmonary bypass. The roles of arterial-to-venous pressure gradient, the duration of increased venous pressure, and volume of blood withdrawn on the difference in PO_2 between radial artery and arterial oxygenator samples were investigated.

The relationship between PO_2 for the radial artery and oxygenator did not change when venous pressure was 80% of arterial; however, when venous pressure equaled arterial pressure, radial artery PO_2 progressively decreased to 45 ± 26 mm Hg. Desaturation of radial artery blood also occurred with increased duration of venous obstruction and occurred immediately if the arterial tree was emptied after occlusion.

Venous admixture to arterial blood samples may occur during little or no flow in the radial artery, as a result of transcapillary aspiration of deep venous blood. Values for PO_2 under these circumstances can grossly underestimate aortic PO_2. This phenomenon may produce a potential source of error in measuring arterial oxygen tension when perfusion pressure is low and venous pressure is high, such as during cardiopulmonary resuscitation, cardiac tamponade, and profound right heart failure, as well as during obstructed venous return during cardiopulmonary bypass.

▶ A low PO_2 in a blood sample drawn from an arterial site may be viewed, in retrospect, to indicate unrecognized esophageal placement of the endotracheal tube. In this regard, the potential for venous contamination of an arterial sample during cardiopulmonary resuscitation is an important concept to consider, especially when all other evidence indicates the tube was properly placed in the trachea.—R.K. Stoelting, M.D.

Evidence for Involvement of Hypocapnia and Hypoperfusion in Aetiology of Neurological Deficit After Cardiopulmonary Bypass

Nevin M, Colchester ACF, Adams S, Pepper JR (St George's Hosp, London; Atkinson Morley's Hosp, London)
Lancet 2:1493–1496, Dec 26, 1987   6–9

It was observed that most patients were being hyperventilated accidentally before going on bypass. Severe hypocapnia and large fluctuations in $PaCO_2$ and jugular bulb pressure soon after the start of bypass were noted. A study was done to investigate whether there is a relationship among preoperative perfusion pressure, CO_2 changes, and postoperative neuropsychometric deficit.

Arterial and jugular bulb pressures and blood gas tensions were recorded for 65 patients undergoing coronary artery graft surgery. Routine perioperative monitoring was used with the first 35 patients. For the next 30 patients, who were similar in age and other variables, special measures were used to maintain normocapnia by continuous monitoring during surgery. On the third day after surgery, clinical neurologic deficits were observed in 46% of the patients in the first group and in 27% of the patients in the second group. Psychometric deficits were noted in 71% and 40%, respectively.

On analysis of recorded data, more than half of the patients in the first group were hypocapnic immediately before onset of cardiopulmonary bypass. Those with postoperative deficits differed from the others in this group in having had greater changes in $PaCO_2$ after onset of bypass and lower cerebral perfusion pressures in the first 10 minutes after bypass, usually because of an increase in cerebral venous pressure.

Accidental hyperventilation before perfusion and rises in cerebral venous pressure because of fluctuations in $PaCO_2$ immediately after onset of perfusion may contribute importantly to the development of postoperative neuropsychometric deficit. If these findings are confirmed, cardiac units will have to work harder to maintain normocapnia throughout surgery.

▶ Microemboli have been most often incriminated as causes of neurologic dysfunction following cardiopulmonary bypass. Hemodilution and hypothermia are believed to offset any potential hazard of a decreased cerebral blood flow associated with reduced perfusion pressures. The role of hyperventilation of the lungs and associated increased cerebral venous pressure before cardiopulmonary bypass has not been commonly considered in calculating cerebral perfusion pressure; perhaps it should.—R.K. Stoelting, M.D.

Loss of the Somatosensory Evoked Response as an Indicator of Reversible Cerebral Ischemia During Hypothermic, Low-Flow Cardiopulmonary Bypass
Wilson GJ, Rebeyka IM, Coles JG, Desrosiers AJ, Dasmahapatra HK, Adler S, Feitler DA, Sherret H, Kielmanowicz S, Ikonomidis J, Gatley RAA, Taylor M (Hosp for Sick Children, Toronto; Univ of Toronto)
Ann Thorac Surg 45:206–209, February 1988   6–10

Hypothermic cardiopulmonary bypass with reduced extracorporeal flow rate (EFR) has made possible the performance of many intracardiac repairs, but what minimum EFR is necessary to maintain cerebral function remains a question. The somatosensory evoked response (SSER) as a monitor of cerebral protection during nonpulsatile, hypothermic cardiopulmonary bypass was assessed in 13 dogs. Extracorporeal flow rate thresholds for loss of SSER were determined by stepwise reduction of the EFR from 2.0 to 0.25 L/minute/m^2 at perfusion temperatures of 35 C, 30 C, 25 C, and 20 C. Testing began at 35 C in 6 dogs in group I and at 20 C in 7 dogs in group 2. Immediately on loss of SSER, defined as a decrease of 80% or more in the amplitude of the somatosensory evoked potentials, EFR was restored to 2.0 L/minute/m^2.

The EFR threshold for loss of cortical SSER ranged between 0.25 to 0.75 L/min/m^2 from 20 C to 35 C. However, SSER was always restored on return of EFR to 2.0 L/minute/m^2, indicating that loss of SSER was a completely reversible ischemic phenomenon. The EFR threshold for loss of SSER was equivalent in both groups at 35 C, but at lower temperatures, group 1 thresholds were significantly higher than those in group 2. The initial ischemic insult at 35 C for group 1 caused neurophysiologic changes, such as depletion of cortical energy reserves, which diminished subsequent tolerance to ischemia at lower temperatures. In contrast, group 2 dogs had EFR thresholds similar to those of group 1 at 35 C in spite of previously having undergone ischemic insults at 20 C to 30 C.

Loss of SSER is a warning of reversible cerebral ischemia. A normal state of electrocortical function can be preserved, even with transient ischemic loss of cortical SSER, provided that adequate EFR is restored immediately on loss of SSER and EFR manipulations are conducted under moderate hypothermia (less than 30 C). The SSER monitoring is a useful measure of cerebral function during low-flow, hypothermic cardiopulmonary bypass.

▶ Local custom and scientifically unsubstantiated practices often determine the flows, perfusion pressures, or both that are considered acceptable during cardiopulmonary bypass. Recognition that somatosensory evoked potentials are useful in recognizing reversible cerebral ischemia during hypothermic cardiopulmonary bypass will make possible the evolution of logical guidelines for desirable perfusion pressures.—R.K. Stoelting, M.D.

Beneficial Effects of Endotracheal Extubation on Ventricular Performance: Implications for Early Extubation After Cardiac Operations
Gall SA Jr, Olsen CO, Reves JG, McIntyre RW, Tyson GS Jr, Davis JW, Rankin JS (Duke Univ)
J Thorac Cardiovasc Surg 95:819–827, May 1988   6–11

Early endotracheal extubation after uncomplicated cardiac operations appears to shorten intensive care unit stays, decrease postoperative medication requirements, lessen cardiopulmonary morbidity, and improve patient comfort without increasing the incidence of pulmonary complications. However, resistance to this technique remains. To evaluate the effects of early extubation on postoperative cardiac performance, 7 men aged 28–56 years were studied. Six had undergone elective coronary artery bypass grafting and 1 had an isolated repair of an asymptomatic secundum atrial septal defect.

The average cardiopulmonary bypass time was 105 minutes with a mean aortic cross-clamp time of 40 minutes. Postoperative cardiac performance was measured with left ventricular (LV) micromanometers that had been placed during operation, LV minor axis dimension crystals, and left atrial and intrapleural pressure catheters. Physiologic data were obtained during operation, during controlled mandatory ventilation in the intensive care unit, and during spontaneous respiration immediately after extubation.

None of the patients died during operation, and none had perioperative myocardial infarction. Early endotrachial extubation to spontaneous breathing was associated with improved cardiac performance, which resulted from enhanced ventricular filling. Improved cardiac performance was documented by a significant decline in intrapleural pressure and a significant increase in LV end-diastolic diameter, ejection diameter shortening, stroke work, and increased cardiac output.

Early extubation in postoperative patients who undergo uncomplicated cardiac surgical procedures enhances cardiac performance and should be adopted as the standard of current care.

▶ Tracheal intubation has many desirable effects in the early postoperative period following cardiopulmonary bypass. The changes described by the authors of this study seem low on the priority list if one is looking for reasons for early extubation of the trachea.—R.K. Stoelting, M.D.

Binding of Fentanyl and Alfentanil to the Extracorporeal Circuit
Hynynen M (Helsinki Univ Central Hosp)
Acta Anaesthesiol Scand 31:706–710, 1987   6–12

When a patient is connected to a cardiopulmonary bypass (CPB) system, there is a decrease in the plasma opiate concentration because of the dilution effect of priming volume, lung sequestration, decreased elimination, and possibly the adsorption of the drug to the CPB apparatus. The adsorption of fentanyl and alfentanil by CPB circuits using either a bubble or a membrane oxygenator was studied.

Adsorption of the analgesics to the CPB equipment was measured in vitro by adding either fentanyl or alfentanil to the priming solution, which was either saline or a mixture of saline and blood. Opiate concentrations were determined during a 60-minute operation of a closed CPB system. In another trial, the CPB circuit was primed with fentanyl or alfentanil, which was circulated for 10 minutes before the equipment was connected to patients undergoing cardiac surgery with high-dose opiate anesthesia.

Sixteen patients scheduled for coronary surgery were anesthetized with fentanyl; 11 similar patients received alfentanil. Six patients from each group were connected to the CPB system primed with no opiates; the remainder were placed on the systems primed with either fentanyl or alfentanil.

In the in vitro study, 29% of the predicted fentanyl levels and 80% of

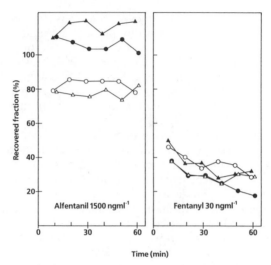

Fig 6–2.—Fractions of calculated alfentanil (1,500 ng/ml) and fentanyl (30 ng/ml) concentrations recovered in prime solutions during 60-minute circulation in closed cardiopulmonary bypass system. Each *line* represents single experiment. Constitution of prime in experiments with bubble oxygenator is indicated as follows: *white circle*, without blood; *black circle*, with blood; and that with a membrane oxygenator as follows: *white triangle*, without blood; *black triangle*, with blood. (Courtesy of Hynynen M: *Acta Anaesthesiol Scand* 31:706–710, 1987.)

the alfentanil levels were recovered when saline prime was used regardless of whether the equipment was a bubble or a membrane oxygenator. When blood was added, fentanyl levels were similar to those with saline alone, but with alfentanil, recovery exceeded the calculated concentrations (Fig 6–2). When patients were connected to the CPB system, priming with the analgesics prevented the sharp reduction in opiate concentration that is normally seen at initiation of CPB.

In a clinically relevant dose range, a smaller percentage of alfentanil than of fentanyl is adsorbed by CPB apparatus. Addition of the opiates to the priming solution maintains a high level of plasma opiate concentration at initiation of CPB.

▶ Loss of drug into the cardiopulmonary bypass circuit represents a route of drug uptake that is not often considered. This drug loss resembles insulin adsorption into the delivery system, which has been long recognized to decrease the amount delivered to the patient. Unlike insulin delivery, loss of drug into the cardiopulmonary bypass circuit is often offset by hypothermia and reduced drug requirements.—R.K. Stoelting, M.D.

Effect of Hypothermic Hemodilutional Cardiopulmonary Bypass on Plasma Sufentanil and Catecholamine Concentrations in Humans
Okutani R, Philbin DM, Rosow CE, Koski G, Schneider RC (Harvard Univ; Massachusetts Gen Hosp, Boston)
Anesth Analg 67:667–670, 1988   6–13

High doses of fentanyl or sufentanil are commonly used for induction and maintenance of anesthesia during cardiopulmonary bypass (CPB). Previous studies have shown that plasma levels of fentanyl are decreased sharply with initiation of CPB and continue gradually to levels lower than can be ascribed to hemodilution alone. This phenomenon has been attributed to increases in a variety of hormones and is considered a hormonal stress response. Sufentanil is reportedly more effective than fentanyl in decreasing this hormonal stress response before, but not during, CPB. The effect of hypothermic hemodilutional CPB on plasma sufentanil and catecholamine concentrations was assessed.

Forty patients undergoing elective coronary artery surgery were randomly assigned to 1 of 4 treatment groups, with each group receiving different doses of sufentanil for anesthesia induction. The patients in all 4 groups were comparable for age, sex, degree of disease, preoperative medications, and operative procedure. All patients were cooled during CPB to 25 C. Radial arterial blood samples for determination of plasma concentrations of sufentanil and catecholamine were collected before CPB, during CPB at 15, 30, 45, and 60 minutes, during rewarming, and 15, 60, and 240 minutes after CPB.

There was an initial significant decrease in sufentanil levels in all 4 groups following institution of CPB. However, plasma levels of sufentanil were stable during the remainder of the hypothermic period. Sufentanil plasma levels were increased significantly with rewarming in all 4 groups when compared with those measured at 45 minutes of CPB. Immediately after CPB, sufentanil plasma levels were increased further in all 4 groups, approaching plasma sufentanil levels of the pre-CPB samples. Catecholamine responses to CPB were similar in the 2 groups that received the higher doses of sufentanil. There was a wide variability in individual norepinephrine responses in these 2 groups. A statistically significant increase in epinephrine was noted with rewarming, but individual changes in plasma sufentanil and epinephrine levels were not correlated significantly.

Sufentanil disposition during hypothermic CPB differs from that of fentanyl, as no measurable metabolism or excretion of sufentanil appears to occur during CPB.

▶ Adequacy of anesthesia as produced by inhaled or injected drugs is difficult to quantitate during cardiopulmonary bypass. It is a long-standing clinical impression that anesthetic requirements are reduced during and following cardiopulmonary bypass. This is fortuitous considering the reductions in plasma drug concentrations associated with institution of bypass and subsequent rewarming. The role of hypothermia and a lingering effect on rewarming presumably play some role in reduced anesthetic requirements.— R.K. Stoelting, M.D.

Effects of Nitrous Oxide on Coronary Perfusion After Coronary Air Embolism

Tuman KJ, McCarthy RJ, Spiess BD, Overfield DM, Ivankovich AD (Rush-Presbyterian-St Luke's Med Ctr, Chicago)
Anesthesiology 67:952–959, December 1987   6–14

Coronary air embolism may complicate bypass surgery. Even a small amount of air in the left side of the heart and coronary arteries may impair cardiac function. Because nitrous oxide also causes myocardial dysfunction, its use may accelerate dysfunction or ischemia when coronary air embolism is present. The cardiac effects of coronary air embolism with and without nitrous oxide were compared in swine.

Cardiac output, systemic arterial perfusion pressure, and coronary perfusion pressure declined after coronary air embolism. Left ventricular contractile force decreased as end-diastolic pressure increased. All parameters returned toward baseline when nitrous oxide was discontinued. However, if ventilation with nitrous oxide continued, animals died within 2–4 minutes. Regional myocardial ischemia and arrhythmia were more evident in animals given nitrous oxide.

These findings suggest that nitrous oxide be avoided after cardiopulmonary bypass is discontinued. A risk of coronary air embolism remains present then, and it is a potentially devastating occurrence when nitrous oxide is present.

▶ Unsuspected air in the coronary circulation introduced at the time of bypass grafting may be a more common cause of myocardial dysfunction following cardiopulmonary bypass than is generally recognized. The magnitude and duration of this cause of "postpump failure" can be easily minimized by avoiding the use of nitrous oxide.—R.K. Stoelting, M.D.

Carotid Endarterectomy

The Appropriateness of Carotid Endarterectomy
Winslow CM, Solomon DH, Chassin MR, Kosecoff J, Merrick NJ, Brook RH (Rand Corp, Santa Monica, Calif; Univ of California, Los Angeles; Fink and Kosecoff, Inc, Santa Monica, Calif)
N Engl J Med 318:721–727, March 24, 1988   6–15

The number of carotid endarterectomies performed annually in the United States has dramatically increased during recent years. However, there is controversy over the appropriateness of the indications for this procedure. The literature was reviewed to identify the circumstances under which carotid endarterectomy was considered beneficial and a list of 864 possible indications was compiled. A panel of nationally known experts was asked to rate the appropriateness of each indication, using a modified Delphi technique. The panel's ratings were then used to determine the appropriateness of carotid endarterectomy in a random sample of 1,302 patients, aged 65 years or older, residing in 3 selected geographic areas, including an urban area, a rural area, and a mixed urban/rural area. The appropriateness rating was based on the results of angiographic assessment, estimated surgical risk, and, when applicable, whether the operation had been performed on the carotid artery ipsilateral or contralateral to the cerebral hemisphere associated with the patient's symptoms. Carotid endarterectomies done in patients with minimal stenosis and with no ulcer on carotid angiography, or in those who were at high surgical risk were never rated appropriate.

Using this rating process, 35% of the patients had carotid endarterectomy for appropriate reasons; 32%, for equivocal reasons, and 32%, for inappropriate reasons. Fifty-four percent of all procedures were done in patients who had no transient ischemic attacks in the carotid distribution. Also, 9.8% of the patients had major postoperative complications, defined as stroke with residual deficit at hospital discharge or death within 30 days of operation.

Carotid endarterectomy was highly overused in the 3 geographic areas studied. No surgeon whose major complication rate exceeds 8% should perform carotid endarterectomy under any circumstances.

▶ The gist of this article is that at least 30% of carotid endarterectomies are inappropriate, but the gist of that statement depends a lot on the quality of what they define as inappropriate. One of the things that they defined as inappropriate was high medical risk. I personally don't believe that is inappropriate, as more than 50% of the patients for whom we have administered anesthesia for carotid surgery are in that category and we have less than a 3% morbidity among that group of patients. What they have shown is that, where people don't perform many carotid endarterectomies a year, the risk is much greater than that of the large published series from universities or major clinics. For example, they found an average of 9.8% serious morbidity, meaning either mortal event or stroke with major residual deficit on discharge from the hospital. That compares with less than 3% of the series in which I am personally involved or have seen from major universities, whereas those series from community hospitals where surgeons who do carotid endarterectomies are performing the surgery 10 to 25 times per year have been in the 10% to 16% range.

I think that, like most things, the more you do of something, the better you get at it, up to a point. However, 4 factors accounted for three fourths of all inappropriate procedures, and I think one cannot help but agree with at least some of those 4 factors. Operations on arteries with minimal stenosis and no ulceration accounted for 48% of the inappropriate procedures. Operations on completely occluded vessels accounted for 6%. Thus, one cannot argue with at least 54% of the operations that were judged inappropriate. I do argue with the category of operations on patients at high surgical risk because of their medical conditions, as I have stated above. In addition, the operation on arteries contralateral to the hemisphere associated with symptoms when the ipsilateral artery has severe stenosis may be related to the fact that at least several surgeons I know believe that clearing the least risky artery first lowers morbidity for operations on the higher risk artery. I think it is hard to argue with the conclusion that, if you have a rate of complications exceeding 8% in your individual practice position, perhaps you should not be involved in caring for patients undergoing carotid endarterectomy. If, on the other hand, you have a rate of less than 8%, you should get a concentration of all the other patients.

Such a statement also means that we should do something to determine the outcome of our patients at the time they leave the hospital. It also means something I believe in deeply: that there is a team providing care for the patient and that less than optimal surgery or less than optimal anesthesia or less than optimal internal medical care all reflect on the other medical specialties, and that an individual whose practice pattern doesn't fit the team's practice pattern may not help patient outcome, no matter how good the individual practice is when divorced from the team.—M.F. Roizen, M.D.

Operative and Long-Term Results of Staged Contralateral Carotid Endarterectomy: A Personal Series
Morrow CE, Espada R, Howell JF (Baylor College of Medicine, Houston)
Surgery 103:242–246, February 1988   6–16

The operative risks and the proper interval for patients undergoing staged contralateral carotid endarterectomies remain uncertain. The long-term incidence of stroke after bilateral carotid endarterectomy is also unknown. The results of staged contralateral carotid endarterectomies done by 1 surgeon in a consecutive series of 89 patients were analyzed.

The 34 women and 55 men, aged 37 to 81 years, underwent the procedures from 1966 to 1985. There were no deaths after a first or contralateral carotid endarterectomy. Three minor and 1 major cardiovascular accidents, for an incidence of 4%, occurred after a first procedure, whereas only 1 major cardiovascular accident, for an incidence of 1%,

TABLE 1.—Complications in 89 Patients Treated by Staged
Bilateral Carotid Endarterectomy

Complication	First carotid endarterectomy No. of pts	Contralateral carotid endarteretomy No. of pts
Minor CVA	3*	0
Major CVA	1	1*
Hematoma	1	2
Hoarseness	1	1
Vocal cord paralysis	2	1
Marginal mandibular (VII) nerve weakness	1	0
Postendarterectomy hypertension (>200/100 mm Hg)	33	62

CVA, cerebrovascular accident.
*One patient suffered mild CVA after first endarterectomy and major CVA after contralateral endarterectomy.
(Courtesy of Morrow CE, Espada R, Howell JF, et al: *Surgery* 103:242–246, February 1988.)

TABLE 2.—Postoperative Hypertension According to Interval Between First and Contralateral Carotid Endarterectomy

Interval between first and contralateral carotid endarterectomy (wk)	No. of pts	Postendarterectomy hypertension (>200/100) No. of pts (%)			
		None	First carotid endarterectomy only	Contralateral carotid endarterectomy only	Both carotid endarterectomies
1	19	4 (21)	2 (10)	7 (37)	6 (32)
2	12	2 (17)	1 (8)	7 (58)	2 (17)
3	6	2 (33)	0 (0)	2 (33)	2 (33)
4	12	3 (25)	2 (17)	6 (50)	1 (8)
>4	40	9 (22)	2 (5)	14 (35)	15 (38)
Total	89	20 (22)	7 (8)	36 (40)	26 (29)

(Courtesy of Morrow CE, Espada R, Howell JF, et al: *Surgery* 103:242–246, February 1988.)

occurred after a contralateral carotid endarterectomy (Table 1). Postendarterectomy hypertension occurred in 33 (37%) of the patients after a first operation and in 62 (70%) of the patients after a contralateral carotid endarterectomy (Tables 2 and 3).

The staged contralateral carotid endarterectomy can be safely done with a stroke mortality approaching 1%. Postendarterectomy hypertension, although more common after the contralateral procedure than after the first operation, has no correlation with the interval between procedures. After a staged bilateral carotid endarterectomy, only 1% of patients had transient ischemic attack symptoms, but 6% suffered a late stroke.

▶ This is an excellent and interesting study of 89 patients with bilateral carotid endarterectomies done by 1 surgeon over a 20-year period. The stroke rate of 4% after the first carotid and 1% after the second carotid is about what the literature would say occurs in university centers, but I thought the most interesting part of this study was the postoperative hypertension and late results. Roughly 37% of the patients had postendarterectomy hypertension after their first operation, as did 70% after the second operation. Whether these patients

TABLE 3.—Postendarterectomy Hypertension and Neurologic Complications According to Preoperative Blood Pressure

Preoperative blood pressure	No. of pts	First carotid endarterectomy			Staged contralateral carotid endarterectomy		
		Postoperative hypertension No. of pts (%)	Minor CVA	Major CVA	Postoperative hypertension No. of pts (%)	Minor CVA	Major CVA
Hypertensive group (>150/90)	65	26 (40%)	3	1	47 (72%)	—	1
Normotensive group (<150/90)	24	7 (30%)	—	—	15 (62%)	—	—

CVA, cerebrovascular accident.
(Courtesy of Morrow CE, Espada R, Howell JF, et al: *Surgery* 103:242–246, February 1988.)

had restricted fluid or whether the hypertension caused or resulted in serious problems is not clear from this study, but almost all of the complications occurred in patients who were hypertensive and also had preoperative hypertension. The preoperative hypertension was judged by blood pressure greater than 150/90, and the postoperative hypertension was classified as being greater than 200/100. All 5 of the neurologic complications occurred in patients with preoperative hypertension, and 4 of the 5 complications occurred in patients who also had postoperative hypertension.

The low stroke rate after the second carotid indicates that a staged carotid endarterectomy can be done safely, but the high percentage of patients with hypertension means that the anesthesiologist should look for this, and perhaps prophylactic treatment for hypertension with something like an esmolol or a labetolol drip as one goes to the recovery room might be indicated were you to have a similar patient group. We found that continuance of preoperative hypertensives and restriction of fluid during the operation are major factors that have reduced the incidence of postoperative hypertension in our anecdotal series.

The other interesting part of this paper relates to the late outcome. Of the 89 patients, 4 died of stroke at operation, and 5 had major cerebral vascular accidents 1, 6, 8, 9, and 12 years after bilateral carotid endarterectomy. Other causes of late death included myocardial infarction in 7 patients, malignant conditions in 4 patients, congestive heart failure in 1 patient, and unknown causes within the follow-up period in 11 patients. Even though it is clear that the natural history of these patients cannot be defined, because more than a third of them had transient ischemic attacks (TIAs), and one can expect a 10% stroke rate per year in TIA patients, the incidence of stroke seems to have been reduced, even if one looks at just preventing stroke in those patients with TIAs compared with the operative follow-up results. With a mean follow-up of more than 5 years, approximately 17 of the patients with TIAs would have been expected to have experienced strokes during that period.—M.F. Roizen, M.D.

The Risk of Perioperative Stroke in Patients With Asymptomatic Carotid Bruits Undergoing Peripheral Vascular Surgery
Gutierrez IZ, Barone DL, Makula PA, Currier C (VA Med Ctr, Buffalo; State Univ of New York at Buffalo)
Am Surg 53:487–489, September 1987   6–17

Perioperative stroke after peripheral vascular reconstruction in patients without previous neurologic symptoms is a dreaded complication. Asymptomatic internal carotid artery disease that may predispose a patient to this complication may be manifested by a carotid bruit. The incidence of perioperative stroke was studied in patients who had asymptomatic carotid bruits.

Three hundred male patients underwent 374 peripheral vascular reconstructive procedures. Before surgery, they had GEE-OPG assessment of any incidental asymptomatic carotid bruits found by auscultation. A bruit was considered hemodynamically significant if the OPG test result proved positive. Seventy-four patients (24.7%) had 118 carotid bruits.

Twenty-five (22.3%) of the 112 bruits studied by OPG were hemodynamically significant. Three perioperative strokes occurred, yielding an incidence of 0.8%.

The strokes occurred only in patients with hemodynamically significant bruits, yielding an incidence of perioperative strokes in such patients of 16%. Strokes occurred within 24–48 hours after surgery. All 3 patients who sustained perioperative strokes had undergone reconstructive surgery for aortoiliac occlusive disease. All 3 patients had had bilateral carotid bruits, and in 2, the dense cerebral infarcts were ipsilateral to the hemodynamically significant carotid bruits.

A perioperative stroke incidence of 16% was found among patients who had positive OPG test results on their carotid bruits. A subgroup of patients with asymptomatic carotid bruits was identified as being significantly at risk for perioperative stroke.

▶ This article comes on the heels of others in the literature (namely, Barnes et al: *Surgery* 90:1075–1083, 1981; and Ropper et al: *N Engl J Med* 307:1388–1390, 1982) that show that asymptomatic carotid bruits are a risk factor for cardiac deaths but not for stroke. In this article the authors show that, in fact, asymptomatic carotid bruits can be extremely hemodynamically significant and can lead to a stroke rate for other vascular procedures that is as high as 16% compared with a stroke rate of 0% in patients with carotid bruits that are not hemodynamically significant. In this category, the classification of hemodynamically significant or insignificant was made by "GEE-OPG" studies. The OPG result was considered positive if there was a systolic pressure index less than 0.69 or if there was a difference of 5 mm Hg between the 2 eyes. In their laboratory this was associated 95% of the time with a significant stenotic lesion or total occlusion of the internal carotid arteries as verified by angiography and occurred when there was greater than 75% reduction in the cross-sectional area of the carotid.

Thus, the study differs from other studies because it implies that, once a carotid bruit is seen, one should not just think of coronary artery disease as a major risk factor but should also evaluate whether the carotid bruit is the result of a hemodynamically significant internal carotid lesion, as it was in approximately 20% of patients in this study.—M.F. Roizen, M.D.

Continuous Electroencephalographic Monitoring During Carotid Endarterectomy
McFarland HR, Pinkerton JA Jr, Frye D (St Luke's Hosp, Kansas City, Mo)
J Cardiovasc Surg 29:12–18, January–February 1988   6–18

Earlier studies in which continuous EEG was used for intraoperative monitoring during carotid endarterectomy (CE) showed good correlation between cerebral blood flow and EEG changes. Conversely, measurement of the internal carotid artery stump pressure was unreliable as an indicator of decreased regional cerebral blood flow. During a 10-year study pe-

TABLE 1.—Carotid Endarterectomy: EEG Changes
During Carotid Clampings*

	No.	(%)
1. Ipsilateral attenuation	20	(39)
2. Ipsilateral slowing with attenuation	11	(21)
3. Ipsilateral slowing without attenuation	7	(14)
4. Bilateral attenuation	2	(4)
5. Bilateral slowing with attenuation	5	(10)
6. Bilateral slowing without attenuation	5	(10)
7. Contralateral slowing without attenuation	1	(2)
Total	51	(100)

*Changes occurred in 51 of 386 EEGs.
(Courtesy of McFarland HR, Pinkerton JA Jr, Frye D: *J Cardiovasc Surg* 29:12–18, January–February 1988.)

riod, EEG monitoring was used as the sole determinant for carotid shunting during CE in 377 patients.

The patients, 239 (63%) men and 138 (37%) women aged 33–89 years, underwent 427 CE procedures. Indications included transient ischemic attack in 307 (72%) patients, reversible ischemic deficit or stroke in 66 (15%), and asymptomatic bruit with high-grade stenosis of an internal carotid artery in 54 (13%). Continuous EEG monitoring was performed during 392 procedures, and EEG change during carotid artery clamping (Table 1) was the sole determinant for the use of a temporary carotid shunt.

Three (0.7%) patients died during the early postoperative period, but none had had operative EEG changes or had received a shunt during CE. Eleven (2.5%) patients had strokes; 2 (0.5%) of those strokes occurred during operation and 9 (2.0%) occurred in the early postoperative period. The combined morbidity/mortality in this study population was 2.8%. Fifty-four patients who underwent CE under EEG monitoring received temporary shunts because EEG changes suggested cerebral ischemia. None of these 54 patients died, but 6 (11%) experienced permanent neurologic deficits; all 6 patients had contralateral internal carotid artery occlusion before CE.

Intraoperative EEG recordings were interpreted after operation by an experienced electroencephalographer who considered the EEG changes in 3 patients to be insignificant. The other 51 tracings (13%) showed focal EEG changes that were correlated well with neurologic deficits occurring during operation. However, stump pressure measurements were not correlated with either EEG changes or neurologic deficits, as more than half of the 59 patients who had stump pressure of 25 mm Hg or less had no EEG changes, received no shunt, and experienced no neurologic deficits.

Continuous intraoperative EEG monitoring during CE effectively determined significant cerebral ischemia and the need for using a carotid shunt. Intraoperative EEG monitoring improved the neurologic outcome in the patients studied.

TABLE 2.

New Postoperative Neurologic Problem

		+	–
EEG	+	6	45
	–	5	330

Sensitivity = 6/11 = 55% at worst; predictive positive rate = 6/56 = 10.8% at worst; specificity = 330/335 = 98.5% at worst; predictive negative rate = 330/380 = 87% at worst.
(Data from McFarland HR, Pinkerton JA Jr, Frye D: *J Cardiovasc Surg* 29:12–18, 1988.)

▶ The most important information in this article is the description of the EEG changes one should expect if there is cerebral ischemia after temporary occlusion of the carotid artery. Fifty-one of 386 EEG tracings were considered ischemic (13%). The most common pattern was ipsilateral attenuation (decreased amplitude), which was seen in 39% of ischemic EEG tracings. Ipsilateral attenuation with associated ipsilateral slowing (decreased frequency) occurred in another 21%; 14% had ipsilateral slowing without attenuation. Also seen, though less frequently, were bilateral attenuation (4%), bilateral slowing with (10%) and without (10%) attenuation, and contralateral slowing without attenuation (2%). Shunting resolved these ischemic changes 96% of the time.

Of the patients whose carotid flow was "shunted" because these EEG changes were judged ischemic in the operating room, 6 (11%) had permanent neurologic damage. The stroke rate for all operations was 2.5%. The authors make the claim that, because the incidence of stroke is low when they use the EEG, the EEG is a vital monitor. They argue that EEG monitoring warns the surgeons that cerebral ischemia is occurring promptly enough so as to allow timely placement of a shunt to restore blood flow.

Although acute placement of a shunt reversed ischemic EEG changes 96% of the time, at no time did the authors demonstrate that, once the EEG is changed, their intervention results in better outcome for their patients. The data they have, as in Table 2, show that the sensitivity is at least 55% for the EEG for the detection of perioperative neurologic deficit (the EEG demonstrates an abnormality 55% of the time the patient does). The 2 patients who awoke with new neurologic deficits had intraoperative EEG ischemia. Of the other 9 patients with postoperative strokes (at 1 hour to 12 days), only 4 had intraoperative EEG ischemia. We may speculate that these were thrombotic complications (only 1 of the 9 had routine antiplatelet therapy); still we are left without proof of the EEG's value in improving neurologic outcome.

Fifty-five percent is not very good; in fact, the positive predictive rate, that is, how likely a patient with an abnormal EEG is to have a stroke, was 10.8%. Its negative predictive rate (how likely one is to end up neurologically intact with a normal intraoperative EEG) is only 87%. This contradicts much of what is known about EEG. Electroencephalography is supposedly a very sensitive monitor but not specific because electrical failure of neurons occurs at a higher blood flow than that necessary to prevent neuronal death. The data in this article do not demonstrate this.

I believe we need a major study to look at the overall sensitivity and specificity of the EEG in a randomized controlled study to see whether this technology does improve outcome. Until then, it is my feeling that the EEG probably does improve outcome, but not because it improves neurologic outcome. Rather, I believe that having EEG confirmation of a level of cerebral blood flow sufficient to sustain electrical activity allows the clinician to avoid vasoconstrictors and in fact to lower the blood pressure. The EEG guides afterload reduction, thereby protecting the heart, the organ responsible for the greatest rate of morbidity and mortality in patients undergoing carotid endarterectomy.—M.F. Roizen, M.D.

Neurosurgical

The Acute Cerebral Effects of Changes in Plasma Osmolality and Oncotic Pressure
Zornow MH, Todd MM, Moore SS (Univ of California, San Diego, La Jolla)
Anesthesiology 67:936–941, December 1987   6–19

It is generally accepted that a decrease in plasma oncotic pressure may result in the development of peripheral edema. However, the effect of a hypo-oncotic state on brain water content is less well understood. Using hollow-fiber plasmapheresis to manipulate plasma composition, the effects of acute changes in plasma osmolality or colloid oncotic pressure on the EEG, regional cerebral blood flow, intracranial pressure, and brain tissue specific gravity were studied in rabbits.

Fifteen anesthetized, neurologically normal New Zealand white rabbits were studied. Rabbits in which either osmolality or oncotic pressure was decreased by plasma replacement with an appropriate solution were compared with control animals in which these variables remained constant. Rabbits in which plasma osmolality was decreased by 13 ± 6 mOsm/kg showed evidence of significant increase in cortical water content, whereas a 65% decrease in oncotic pressure failed to produce any change. No significant differences were found in mean arterial pressure, central venous pressure, regional cerebral flow, or EEG among the groups. Intracranial pressure rose in all groups, but the largest increase—8.1 ± 4.4 mm Hg—occurred in animals whose osmolality was decreased. The rise in intracranial pressure in rabbits rendered hypo-oncotic was no different from that in the control group (Fig 6–3).

An acute fall in oncotic pressure does not promote a rise in cerebral water content in uninjured brains. Unlike peripheral tissues, the presence of the blood-brain barrier with its small pore size and limited permeability may enhance the importance of osmolality and minimize the role of oncotic pressure in determining water movement between the vasculature and brain tissue.

▶ These data are potentially very useful in guiding the clinician in decisions regarding type and amount of volume replacement in neurosurgical patients. It is

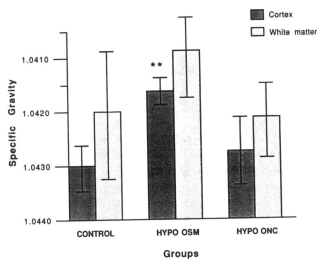

Fig 6–3.—Cortical and white matter specific gravities of 3 groups upon completion of plasmapheresis. Note: The greater the specific gravity, the lower the water content (i.e., brain tissue with specific gravity of 1.0430 contains less water than tissue with specific gravity of 1.0417. **$P < .01$ vs. other groups. (Courtesy of Zornow MH, Todd MM, Moore SS: *Anesthesiology* 67:936–941, December 1987.)

important to remember, however, that these data are for neurologically normal animals. Would these data be the same for brain-injured patients?—R.K. Stoelting, M.D.

Incidence and Cardiac Effects of Systemic Venous Air Embolism: Echocardiographic Evidence of Arterial Embolization via Noncardiac Shunt
Gottdiener JS, Papademetriou V, Notargiacomo A, Park WY, Cutler J (Washington VA Med Ctr, Washington DC; Georgetown Univ)
Arch Intern Med 148:795–800, April 1988   6–20

Central nervous system dysfunction in venous air embolism can result from air entering the arterial circulation. The frequency of systemic venous and paradoxical embolization was defined in a study of several medical and surgical procedures with which this has been associated.

The patient population consisted of 10 persons undergoing upright neurosurgical procedures under general anesthesia, 12 patients having epidural anesthesia, and 10 patients having pacemaker insertion. With the use of 2-dimensional and pulsed-wave Doppler echocardiography, the frequent presence of air in the right heart chambers of the patients was documented. Also, the presence of air in the left atrium and left ventricle via noncardiac shunt was noted in 1 patient. Experimental studies in dogs confirmed paradoxical air embolism in the absence of anatomical communications between right and left heart chambers. Systemic venous air also caused a dose-dependent increase in pulmonary artery pressure and diastolic flattening of the ventricular septum with increase in left ventricular filling pressure, despite preserved systolic function.

Venous air embolism may begin a series of pathophysiologic events that result in pulmonary hypertension, pulmonary arteriovenous shunting with hypoxemia, and systemic arterial air embolization through noncardiac right-to-left shunt. The use of echocardiography with Doppler during procedures associated with a high risk of air embolization allows immediate identification of venous and paradoxical air embolization and characterization of its pathophysiology.

▶ This article adds the diagnostic criteria of the diastolic flattening of the ventricular septum on echocardiography to the sign of systemic arterial air embolization via noncardiac shunt. I think the other major addition that this article makes is the relative safety of epidural anesthesia in nonpregnant individuals, as in none of the 12 patients was air embolization documented during epidural anesthesia as it was in 43% of pregnant women in the report by Naulty et al. (*Anesthesiology* 57:410–412, 1982).—M.F. Roizen, M.D.

Venous Air Embolism, Hypotension, and End-Tidal Nitrogen
Matjasko MJ, Hellman J, Mackenzie CF (Univ of Maryland, Baltimore)
Neurosurgery 21:378–382, September 1987   6–21

The precordial Doppler detector is the most sensitive means of diagnosing venous air embolism. However, false results lead many clinicians to depend on end-tidal gas measurements to verify embolism in the operating room. A decrease in end-tidal carbon dioxide is more sensitive than an increase in end-tidal nitrogen in laboratory studies, but the latter change occurs earlier.

The effects of bolus and infusion venous air embolism were studied in supine, anesthetized dogs. The emboli were administered in random order (1–2.5 ml/kg per minute). Changes in precordial Doppler sounds occurred in all animals at all doses. During bolus embolism, the end-tidal nitrogen increased before the end-tidal carbon dioxide declined, as well as during infusion embolism of 1 mg/kg per minute. At larger infused doses, both parameters changed simultaneously.

An increase in end-tidal nitrogen is a sensitive sign of venous air embolism, even in the presence of marked systemic hypotension. A delayed decrease in end-tidal nitrogen can be confusing if the initial rise is missed, or if air is aspirated from a central venous catheter. If the anesthesiologist eliminates leaks and stabilizes gas flow and anesthetic depth, an increase in end-tidal nitrogen signifies venous air embolism. The end-tidal carbon dioxide may decline in the absence of venous air embolism as a result of blood loss or a sudden decline in cardiac output secondary to surgical manipulation.

▶ Clinically, early recognition of venous air embolism requires appreciation of the characteristics of patients at risk and a high index of suspicion. In contrast to capnography, it seems unlikely that measurement of end-tidal nitrogen concentrations will ever achieve frequent application even considering its possible value in recognizing venous air embolism.—R.K. Stoelting, M.D.

Effect of the Trendelenburg Position on the Distribution of Arterial Air Emboli in Dogs
Butler BD, Laine GA, Leiman BC, Warters D, Kurusz M, Sutton T, Katz J (Univ of Texas, Houston; Univ of Texas, Galveston)
Ann Thorac Surg 45:198–202, February 1988   6–22

A rationale for the use of the Trendelenburg position (TP) in arterial air embolism is based on the concept of air buoyancy, which suggests that bubbles will tend to float away from the dependent regions of the body. The efficacy of the TP in venous air embolism with circulatory arrest or extremely low flow conditions is not in question because bubbles tend to rise in a stagnant fluid volume. However, for the TP to be effective in preventing the distribution of arterial gas bubbles to the brain, the force of buoyancy would have to exceed the opposing force of the arterial blood flow when the heart is ejecting. To test the hypothesis that TP would prevent arterial bubbles from entering the carotid arteries, the effects of buoyancy on the distribution of arterial gas bubbles were investigated in in vitro and in vivo techniques in dogs.

In the in vitro studies, a simulated carotid artery preparation was used to determine the effects of bubble size and vessel angle on the velocity and direction of bubble movement in flowing blood. Whereas larger bubbles increased in velocity in the same direction as the blood flow at 0-, 10-, and 30-degree vessel angles and decreased when the vessel was positioned at 90 degrees, smaller bubbles did not change velocity from 0 to 30 degrees, but increased in velocity in the same direction as blood flow at 90 degrees. In the in vivo studies, the effects of the 0-, 10-, 15-, and 30-degree TP on the distribution of arterial bubbles into the carotid arteries were examined in 10 anesthetized dogs. Regardless of the degree of TP, the bubbles passed into the carotid artery simultaneously with passage into the abdominal aorta.

The force of buoyancy does not overcome the force of arterial blood flow, and the TP does not prevent arterial bubbles from reaching the brain.

▶ It is common practice for cardiac surgeons to request the "head down" position as part of "air maneuvers" before allowing ejection of blood into the aorta after closure of a cardiotomy. These data suggest that any residual air is likely to enter the aorta when left ventricular ejection ensues. The message would seem to be to remove all significant air before allowing the aortic valve to open, regardless of body position.—R.K. Stoelting, M.D.

Urologic

Ethanol Monitoring of Irrigating Fluid Absorption in Transurethral Prostatic Surgery

Hahn RG (Huddinge Univ Hosp, Huddinge, Sweden)
Anesthesiology 68:867–873, June 1988   6–23

Absorption of irrigating fluids used in transurethral resection of the prostate (TUR) can suddenly cause a variety of symptoms, including apprehension, confusion, hypertension, blurred vision, renal insufficiency, or circulatory shock. Although the mortality for this syndrome has decreased with the introduction of nonhemolytic irrigating fluids, symptoms from irrigant fluid absorption still occur in 5% to 10% of all patients who undergo TUR. A method was developed for the continuous monitoring of irrigant solution absorption during TUR by measuring ethanol absorption from these fluids in expired breath (EB).

The validity of this new method was assessed by examining the relationship between EB-ethanol$_A$ and several common indices of irrigant absorption in 50 men (mean age, 69 years) who were undergoing TUR for benign prostatic hypertrophy under epidural anesthesia. The irrigant used for TUR was 1.5% glycine + 2% ethanol in water. The EB-ethanol$_A$ was measured with an Alcolmeter at 10-minute intervals, and the readings were compared with serum sodium and serum glycine levels, and with the absorbed volume of irrigant solution.

There was a direct relationship between EB-ethanol$_A$ and changes in serum glycine concentrations, and an inverse relationship between EB-ethanol$_A$ and changes in serum sodium concentrations. The cumulative absorbed volume of irrigating solution could be predicted from a single EB-ethanol$_A$ reading at the end of each 10-minute interval. Extravasation of irrigating fluid was indicated by a persistent stable or increasing EB-ethanol$_A$ after the use of irrigant had been discontinued.

Monitoring of EB-ethanol$_A$ is a simple and inexpensive technique for measuring irrigant fluid absorption during TUR.

▶ This is an intriguing method of monitoring vascular absorption of irrigating fluid. It is unlikely, however, to find common use in centers where TUR of the prostate is a surgical procedure of brief duration. Furthermore, analysis of serum sodium concentrations gives similar information and, in occasional patients at risk, may be repeated at short intervals. Perhaps the most memorable finding is that the bladder mucosa is impermeable to ethanol.—R.K. Stoelting, M.D.

An Assessment of Prostatectomy for Benign Urinary Tract Obstruction: Geographic Variations and the Evalution of Medical Care Outcomes

Wennberg JE, Mulley AG Jr, Hanley D, Timothy RP, Fowler FJ Jr, Roos NP, Barry MJ, McPherson K, Greenberg ER, Soule D, Bubolz T, Fisher E,

Malenka D (Dartmouth College; Harvard Univ; Maine Med Assessment Program, Augusta, Me; Univ of Massachusetts; Univ of Manitoba; et al)
JAMA 259:3027–3030, May 27, 1988   6–24

There is considerable variability between communities in the rates of prostatectomy performed in the treatment of benign prostatic hypertrophy. In an effort to understand how clinical decisions contribute to these striking geographic variations, the theories underlying the decision-making process for recommending prostatectomy to patients were reviewed.

Whereas regulatory rules require that the efficacy of new drugs must be confirmed before they are approved for widespread use in medical practice, surgical procedures are not easily subjected to regulation, as there are no scientifically valid standards available on which to base a decision to perform prostatectomy. Therefore, the following 4 steps for the systematic assessment of prostatectomy were used: evaluation of the published literature and current opinion, analysis of insurance claims data, interviews with patients and their physicians, and analysis using a decision model.

It appears that the unwanted variations in prostatectomy rates between geographic areas are because of a lack of precise information on the risks and benefits of the procedure, an inappropriate belief that the operation prolongs life, and an inability to evaluate whether the patient's preference for treatment outcome was integrated with the surgeon's preferences and recommendations.

The development of a standard procedure for informed-patient decision making was recommended. The decision to undergo prostatectomy should be dependent on how the patient values specific outcomes and his attitude toward risk. Cohorts of patients who choose operation and of those who choose watchful waiting should be followed to evaluate and compare clinical outcomes. The results of those evaluations could then be used to update the information presented to patients as part of the decision-making process. Such a systematic updating process would introduce an element of self-correction into the informed-patient decision procedure.

▶ The third of 3 extremely provocative articles (Abstracts 6–24 through 6–26) summarizes the results of a prostatectomy assessment project and discusses the approach this group thought viable for reducing uncertainty about appropriate care. There are some surprises from this review, which was based on data for operations occurring in Maine and Manitoba in the mid-1970s.

First of all, the authors found that open prostatectomy, which clearly has fallen on disuse, appeared to have better outcomes than did the transurethral operation. They proposed that a randomized clinical trial may someday be needed to resolve the clinical controversy if it persists after nonexperimental studies that better characterize the issue are also performed. Who would have thought an open procedure would lead to less morbidity? Clearly, surgical morbidity in both open and closed prostatectomy overwhelms anesthetic morbidity. Second, the authors found a need to focus attention on new methods of informing patients of their options and to assess treatments according to the patient's initial preferences for possible outcomes and alternate choices, that is, the need to assess the process of watchful waiting versus prostatectomy using the quality of life measures and looking at whether patients really do benefit from this operation or the benefit is greater than presumed. Clearly many operations fit into the characteristic of a surgical procedure of which the major benefit is to reduce symptoms and improve the quality of life. To transurethral resection of the prostate could be added coronary artery bypass operations (other than for left main disease), angioplasty, cholecystectomy, hysterectomy, total knee and hip replacements, and perhaps lens extraction, for which the primary, if not the exclusive, objective is improvement in the quality of life.

My overall impression after reading these 3 articles and digesting them is that we may be on the verge of a new era in which computerization of data allows us to talk to patients about risk and to quantify the risks of having surgery with any one surgeon-anesthesiologist combination versus watchful waiting under the aegis of any one urologist or internist. However, I find it hard to believe that we've educated even a relatively small fraction of the public enough to make these decisions rationally and in the time frames in which they need to be made. Heck, sometimes I even have great problems in deciding whether to have coffee or Diet Pepsi or to go swimming or cut the grass! For me to try at one time to discuss with my doctor the decision to have prostatectomy in which there is a 93% chance of a better outcome but a 7% chance of a worse outcome, and that my longevity will be decreased by 1.01 months by having the operation but my quality of life, based on the average of other people who have had this operation, will be improved by 2.94 life-adjusted months, when all I'm really trying to do is to get rid of some mild incontinence and the pain when I have retention, seems to me a major step for which I am not sure the public is ready. I think these are provocative and important articles, but like the Studebaker when it first came out, it may be too early to implement them and implementation of the ideas presented in these 3 articles may be more than 20 years off.—M.F. Roizen, M.D.

Watchful Waiting vs. Immediate Transurethral Resection for Symptomatic Prostatism: The Importance of Patients' Preferences
Barry MJ, Mulley AG Jr, Fowler FJ, Wennberg JW (Harvard Univ; Univ of Massachusetts; Dartmouth College)
JAMA 259:3010–3017, May 27, 1988   6–25

Prostatectomy for benign prostatic hypertrophy is performed for 2 reasons, namely, to prevent future morbidity and mortality and to reduce symptoms. However, although there is little disagreement on the need to operate on patients with chronic urinary retention or other severe symptoms of prostatism, there is considerable disagreement over the theory that prostatectomy extends life expectancy among patients with milder symptoms. As far as the relief of symptoms is concerned, the decision to operate should be dependent largely on a particular patient's expectations.

A decision-analysis model was developed to help the surgeon make the decision to recommend either prostatectomy or watchful waiting to men with prostatism but without signs of chronic retention. A starting age of 70 years was selected for a "base case" to estimate expected utility on index symptoms for either strategy. The data used in this analysis were taken from the medical literature, Medicare claims, and patient interview studies.

In this base-case analysis in 70-year-old men, immediate operation resulted in the loss of 1 month of life expectancy. When adjustments were made for quality of life, immediate operation was favored with a net utility benefit of 2.94 quality-adjusted life-months. However, the net utility benefit was even higher for men who were already impotent before operation, as they did not lose utility for the complication of postoperative impotence.

These results demonstrated a small improvement in the prognosis for quality of life if immediate operation was selected over watchful waiting. However, the analysis was particularly sensitive to the degree of postoperative disutility attributable to the index symptoms of prostatism. The patient's own preference should be the key factor in deciding whether or not to recommend prostatectomy to that patient.

▶ In the second article in a series, the authors (this time the group is headed by Barry and Mulley, with Fowler and Wennberg as coauthors) use decision analysis and patient preferences to decide whether surgery is indicated. They use a prototypical 70-year-old man and find that immediate surgery results in an average loss of 1.01 months of life expectancy due to perioperative mortality, but when adjustments were made for quality of life, immediate surgery was favored with a net benefit of 2.94 quality-adjusted life months. In fact, the entire analysis is heavily weighted on patients' regard for or disutilities in quality of life measurements with symptoms of mild incontinence, impotence, and pain.

Perhaps the most important implication from this article is that there is a dominance of these utility factors to determine whether one should undergo an operation or not. Thus there can be no truly definitive list of indications that can be promulgated and readily reviewed retrospectively to decide on appropriateness of a surgical (or nonsurgical) recommendation. It is almost as if patients must be asked about their preferences for outcomes, and these will differ for patients with similar medical histories, findings from physical exams and laboratory studies, and symptom levels. For procedures in which the preventive component dominates thinking, such as cholectomy for cancer of the bowel, a uniform threshold for surgery based on objective criteria that can be reviewed retrospectively seems feasible, the authors added. However, they wrote that, when operations that carry risks are undertaken primarily to improve the quality of life, the threshold should appropriately vary from patient to patient according to the strength of their feelings about the symptoms and their attitudes toward risks. Thus what we are seeing is perhaps an increasing burden or responsibility for the physician to discuss risk and the patient utility with the patient before an operation.

Although it is not proposed here, we might be hearing at some point in the future that a patient's medical history is fed into a computer, which gives a relative risk ratio based on outcome for that individual's surgeon and the surgical milieu, including hospital and anesthesiologist. The surgeon can then discuss this with the patient, the patient then can weigh the benefits that he sees and risks that he has, and from that decision a statistical decision on whether he should undergo or not undergo surgery comes forth. The patient might even be shown interviews of patients who underwent this procedure, their results, and their feelings about the symptoms afterwards. What it then comes down to is a complex decision based on the patient's feelings of the utilities, or weights, of certain outcomes. Are patients intelligent enough to make these types of decisions? I don't know, but I don't think so at this time. We have editors of *The Wall Street Journal* who can't understand the importance of a randomized clinical trial in determining whether a drug benefit happens and believe that patients with acquired immunodeficiency syndrome should just be allowed to choose any drug and don't understand how that would impede the progress of developing useful drugs. If we have intelligent people like that having problems with these decisions, what will the common folk who are less educated in medicine than the science editors of *The Wall Street Journal* do to try to understand the benefits of these procedures?—M.F. Roizen, M.D.

Symptom Status and Quality of Life Following Prostatectomy
Fowler FJ Jr, Wennberg JE, Timothy RP, Barry MJ, Mulley AG Jr, Hanley D (Univ of Massachusetts; Dartmouth College; Maine Med Assessment Program, Augusta, Me; Harvard Univ)
JAMA 259:3018–3022, May 27, 1988   6–26

There is much professional uncertainty concerning the appropriate method for treating benign prostatic hypertrophy because the subsequent reduction in symptoms and improvement in quality of life after prostatectomy have not yet been documented conclusively. To estimate the probability for symptom relief and improvement in the quality of life, and to evaluate patient concern about the symptoms of prostatism, patients were interviewed before and after undergoing prostatectomy for benign prostatic hypertrophy.

The preoperative interview included questions about the patient's past history of prostate symptoms and how much he was bothered by his symptoms. Three postoperative interviews, scheduled 3, 6, and 12 months after operation included questions on current symptom status, postoperative complications, and on how much the patient was bothered by the recuperation process. Of 318 patients who completed the initial interview, 263 completed all 3 postoperative interviews.

Prostatectomy effectively reduced symptoms in 93% of the patients with severe preoperative symptoms and in 79% of those with moderately severe preoperative symptoms. There was also improvement in the quality of life associated with the operation, but only for patients who had acute urinary retention or other severe preoperative symptoms. However, 7% of those with severe symptoms and 5% of those with moderately severe symptoms before operation reported severe symptoms 1 year after operation. Patients with similar postoperative symptoms were bothered to a considerably different degree by their symptoms.

The data from this analysis underscore the importance of patient participation in the decision to perform prostatectomy for benign prostatic hypertrophy.

▶ The first article in a series of 3 by the same authors reports the results of a patient survey regarding quality of life. Patients who had severe symptoms or acute retention did benefit in a reduction of symptoms and experienced quality of life improvements as rated by standards about their activities, general health index, and mental health index. Those with moderate or mild symptoms and without acute retention did not have a statistically significant improvement in the indices of quality of life. In fact, short-term complications of varying severity occurred in 24% of patients, with 12% having to be readmitted to the hospital on an acute basis within 3 months of surgery, and another 3% having to be admitted within the next 9 months with symptoms related to the prostatectomy. Unfortunately, there is no control group in these studies to show what would have happened if the patients had only been followed by watchful waiting: that is, would these problems and the mortality have been increased, or would the quality of life have decreased if only watchful waiting had been employed?

The authors then make the point that, because it is the quality of life indices that prostatectomy for benign prostatic hypertrophy improves, and not mortality or any other vital function, patients should be allowed to weigh their appraisal of the benefits in considering surgery and it should be the patient's "utility" or weight of benefits that governs the decision to operate or not to operate. Although it is a nice theory, no data have been presented that show it should be the case or that in fact patients can do it well without emotional biases, or for that matter, whether the emotional biases relate to a patient's own quality of life indices after surgery. It is interesting that, of the 471 patients asked to participate, 55 were eliminated from analysis because they had elevated creatinine or blood urea nitrogen levels or the presence of hydroureter. Those are conditions in which prostatectomy is shown to save renal function. In addition, 61 patients who had postsurgical pathology reports indicating malignancy of the prostate were removed from analysis as well. Thus it is not clear what the natural role of the operation would have been if one had included these cases.—M.F. Roizen, M.D.

Extracorporeal Shock Wave Lithotripsy in Traumatic Quadriplegic Patients: Can It Be Safely Performed Without Anesthesia?
Spirnak JP, Bodner D, Udayashankar S, Resnick MF (Case Western Reserve Univ)
J Urol 139:18–19, January 1988   6–27

Early clinical experience indicates that patients with traumatic spinal cord injury and renal stones are being treated successfully with extracorporeal shock wave lithotripsy (ESWL) under general or regional (spinal or epidural) anesthesia. Five patients with traumatic quadriplegia underwent ESWL under local field block or no anesthesia.

Ten ESWL treatments were performed on 8 kidneys. In 3 patients, 7 treatments were performed successfully without use of local, regional, or general anesthesia. The other 2 patients were able to distinguish sharp from dull sensations on preoperative skin testing and were treated after a 0.25% bupivacaine field block. All 5 patients received supplemental doses of diazepam and fentanyl and were monitored closely by an anesthesiologist for signs and symptoms of autonomic dysreflexia.

Varying degrees of hypertension occurred in all 5 patients, but this was significant only in 2 and responded to hydralazine intravenously. The complete clinical syndrome of autonomic dysreflexia did not occur. Three patients were free of stones, and 2 had insignificant residual caliceal fragments.

Extracorporeal shock wave lithotripsy may be performed safely in patients with traumatic quadriplegia without the added risk of general or regional anesthesia provided that they are monitored closely by an anesthesiologist for signs and symptoms of autonomic dysreflexia.

▶ Actually, the use of monitored anesthesia care in patients undergoing lithotripsy who do not have neurologic damage is increasing in popularity.—R.D. Miller, M.D.

Comparative Evaluation of General, Epidural and Spinal Anaesthesia for Extracorporeal Shockwave Lithotripsy
Rickford JK, Tytler JA, Speedy HM, Lim M (St Thomas's Hosp, London)
Ann R Coll Surg Engl 70:69–73, 1988   6–28

Patients who are treated for renal stone disease by extracorporeal shock waves, a treatment in use since 1980, may be given general, epidural, or spinal anesthesia. Various complications can result from whatever form of anesthesia is chosen, but no comparative evaluation of the various types has been reported.

The results with each method of anesthesia were evaluated in 61 patients of similar age, weight, and height who underwent extracorporeal shock wave lithotripsy. Epidural anesthesia was used for 22 patients; spinal, for 19; general, for 20. Blood pressure was automatically recorded before the procedure and several times during treatment (Fig 6–4). The patients were then asked to respond to 2 questionnaires (table).

Blood pressure changes were most marked in the general anesthesia group. Several patients who received general anesthesia experienced hypotension after immersion in the bath. In all 3 groups, decreases in systolic and diastolic pressure were associated with placement in the hoist, but the pressure rose again after immersion in the patients who received

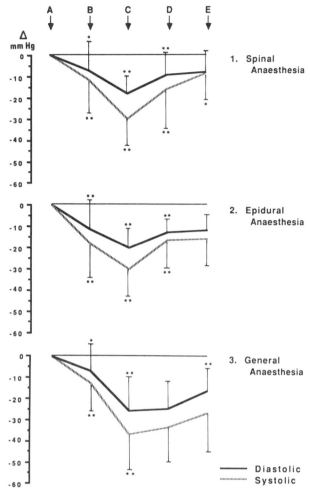

Fig 6–4.—Changes (mean ± SD) in systolic *(broken line)* and diastolic *(solid line)* blood pressure during stages of treatment. A, preinduction. B, postinduction. C, after placement in hoist. D, after immersion in bath. E, 5 minutes after beginning of extracorporeal shock-wave lithotripsy. *Asterisk* indicates $P < .05$ compared with value for preceding stage; *double asterisk, $P < .01$.* (Courtesy of Rickford JK, Tytler JA, Speedy HM, et al: *Ann R Coll Surg Engl* 70:69–73, 1988.)

epidural and spinal anesthesia. Thus, patients who receive general anesthesia must be carefully watched because of the chance of hypotension.

Nausea, vomiting, and sore throat were the most common complaints among patients who received general anesthesia. Backache and urinary retention were problems often experienced by those who received epidural anesthesia. Headaches were reported with great frequency by patients who received spinal anesthesia: 53% listed this complaint on the second postoperative questionnaire, compared with only 18% and 11% of the patients who received epidural and general anesthesia, respectively.

The 2 methods of regional anesthesia provide the advantage of patient

Results From First and Second
Postoperative Questionnaires

	Group (n)		
	SA (19) %	EA (22) %	GA (20) %
Nausea and vomiting[1]	21.1	27.3	50
Abdominal pain[1]	36.8	45.5	25
Backache[1]	36.8	45.5	20
Headache[1]	10.5	18.2	15
Urinary retention[1]	0	27.3	0*
Headache[2]	52.6	18.2	11.1*
Sore throat[2]	15.8	4.6	44.4*
Preference for[2] alternative technique	31.6	31.8	27.8

Note.—SA, spinal anesthesia; EA, epidural anesthesia; GA, general anesthesia; [1] first questionnaire; [2] second questionnaire.
*$P < .01$.
(Courtesy of Rickford JK, Tytler JA, Speedy HM, et al: *Ann R Coll Surg Engl* 70:69–73, 1988.)

cooperation during extracorporeal shock wave lithotripsy, but both may necessitate additional drug therapy for pain. More than a third of the patients in the epidural anesthesia group received supplementary treatment, compared with only 10.5% in the spinal anesthesia group. Preparation time for general anesthesia was 19.7 minutes; for spinal anesthesia, 27.8 minutes; for epidural anesthesia, 43.4 minutes. On the whole, general and epidural anesthesia are both suitable choices for extracorporeal shock wave lithotripsy. Although spinal anesthesia has some advantages, the high frequency of postanesthesia headaches make it less desirable than the other 2 methods.

▶ This is an interesting comparison in the United Kingdom; however, in the United States monitored anesthesia care is also being used increasingly.— R.D. Miller, M.D.

Laryngeal

The Helium Protocol for Laryngotracheal Operations With CO_2 Laser: A Retrospective Review of 523 Cases

Pashayan AG, Gravenstein JS, Cassisi NJ, McLaughlin G (Univ of Florida)
Anesthesiology 68:801–804, May 1988   6–29

Since the introduction of CO_2 laser for laryngeal surgery, reports of indirect ignition of the endotracheal tube in an oxygen- and nitrous oxide-enriched atmosphere have stimulated the pursuit of various forms of prevention. A protocol was developed for the use of helium in anesthetic/ventilatory gases that prevents fires during CO_2 laser resection of airway lesions.

During a 5-year study period, 148 patients underwent 523 laryngotracheal procedures using the helium protocol for CO_2 laser resection of tissue. Anesthesia was induced either by intravenous injection of thiopental, methohexital, or ketamine, or by halothane/nitrous oxide inhalation. Special unmarked polyvinyl chloride tracheal tubes without a barium stripe were used for all procedures. Mechanical ventilation was initiated after tracheal intubation, nitrous oxide was discontinued, and helium in a concentration of 60% was added to the anesthetic gas mixture. The tracheas of 233 patients were intubated through tracheostomy stomas, wheras 290 patients had orotracheal intubation. As part of the protocol, CO_2 laser power density was limited to 1,992 W/cm^2 and the surgeon applied the laser beam only in a series of short, repeated bursts to resect tissue.

The protocol was adhered to in 522 of the 523 procedures, and all lesions were successfully resected without fire or complications related to the protocol. However, 1 flash fire occurred when the protocol was not followed after a tracheal tube cuff had been accidentally punctured by the laser, causing a significant gas leak and difficulty with ventilation. The anesthesiologist tried to remedy the problem and filled the breathing bag by pushing the oxygen flush valve without notifying the surgeon, who continued the laser resection. Laser exposure was immediately stopped when the flash fire occurred, and the patient sustained no ill effects. Fiberoptic laryngoscopy revealed minimal scarification at the site of the fire, but the patient remained asymptomatic at follow-up 3 months later.

The helium protocol, which prevents plain, unwrapped polyvinyl chloride tracheal tubes from igniting during CO_2 laser operations, appears to be a safe alternative for laser microsurgery of laryngotracheal lesions.

▶ There are undeniable merits in using helium as part of the delivered gases during anesthesia for CO_2 laser surgery. Anyone asked to give advice for purchase of equipment to use in the "laser room" should consider an anesthesia machine with a helium flowmeter. This is also likely to be a popular machine for those with young children who enjoy balloons at their birthday parties.— R.K. Stoelting, M.D.

Orthopedic

Prospective, Multi-Centre Trial of Mortality Following General or Spinal Anaesthesia for Hip Fracture Surgery in the Elderly
Davis FM, Woolner DF, Frampton C, Wilkinson A, Grant A, Harrison RT, Roberts MTS, Thadaka R (Christchurch Clinical School, Christchurch, New Zealand; Nelson Hosp, Nelson, New Zealand; Royal Perth Hosp, Perth, Australia; Dunedin Hosp, Dunedin, New Zealand; Auckland Hosp, Auckland, New Zealand)
Br J Anaesth 59:1080–1088, September 1987   6–30

Reports of hospital mortality after surgical correction of fracture in the upper femur in the elderly have varied from 2.7% to 28%. It has been suggested that subarachnoid block is associated with a lower incidence of

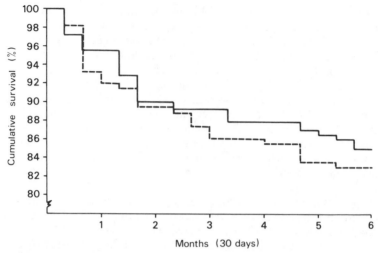

Fig 6–5.—Cumulative mortality over first 6 months after surgery. There were no differences between 2 anesthetic groups (*solid line*, general anesthesia; *dashed line*, subarachnoid block). (Courtesy of Davis FM, Woolner DF, Frampton C, et al: *Br J Anaesth* 59:1080–1088, September 1987.)

early mortality than general anesthesia in these patients. A large randomized trial was designed to examine the effect of anesthesia on mortality in the elderly.

A group of 538 elderly patients scheduled to undergo internal fixation for fracture of the upper femur were randomized to either receive subarachnoid block or narcotic-relaxant anesthesia. Patients who died within the first month after surgery were autopsied to confirm cause of death where possible.

There was no significant difference in mortality between the 2 anesthesia groups at 28 days or at 6-month follow-up (Fig 6–5). A delay to surgery of more than 24 hours following admission was associated with early mortality.

▶ There is a suggestion that regional anesthesia with associated postoperative analgesia and reduced incidence of thromboembolism may result in improved outcome compared with general anesthesia in similar patients. Clearly, many individual and unpredictable patient characteristics and events will eventually determine outcome. It is reasonable to speculate that choice of anesthetic technique could play an important role in some patients. It seems equally unlikely that the superiority of one approach over another for all patients undergoing a given operation will be convincingly demonstrated. The well-trained and experienced anesthesiologist will make all approaches acceptable and, hopefully, equally safe.—R.K. Stoelting, M.D.

Serum Myoglobin Following Tourniquet Release Under Anaesthesia
Laurence AS, Norris SH (Sheffield Univ, Sheffield, England)
Eur J Anaesth 5:143–150, 1988   6–31

Prolonged ischemia from pneumatic tourniquets used during certain orthopedic procedures may cause some muscle damage. Whenever a muscle is damaged, myoglobin is released into the circulation. Other studies have shown that suxamethonium, when given as part of an anesthetic regimen, increases serum myoglobin levels in some patients. Serum myoglobin levels were compared before and after deflation of a pneumatic tourniquet, and whether suxamethonium administration would further increase serum myoglobin levels was investigated.

Of 34 patients aged 16 to 65 years who underwent elective nerve and tendon reconstructions that required application of a pneumatic limb tourniquet, 17 received general anesthesia without suxamethonium, whereas the other 17 patients were given suxamethonium as part of the anesthetic regimen. Four patients required reapplication of the tourniquet 10 to 15 minutes after release because the surgical procedure could not be completed within the allotted time. Blood samples for myoglobin measurement were collected before anesthesia and at regular intervals thereafter.

In patients who did not receive suxamethonium, tourniquet times of up to 2.5 hours were not associated with any detectable muscle damage, as determined by minimal serum myoglobin changes after tourniquet release. Serum myoglobin levels rose immediately after suxamethonium administration in 8 of 17 patients, with peak concentrations occurring 20 to 40 minutes after injection but returning to normal within 2 hours after anesthesia induction. None of the patients had a rise in serum myoglobin levels after tourniquet release. Three of the 4 patients who required reapplication of the tourniquet had increased serum myoglobin levels after the second deflation. This increase was statistically significant.

Pneumatic tourniquets appear to cause no detectable ischemic damage for up to 2.5 hours with or without the use of suxamethonium as part of the anesthetic regimen. However, reapplication of a pneumatic tourniquet after a short period of reperfusion appears to cause some muscle damage and may be inadvisable.

▶ The role of volatile anesthetics in accentuating myoglobin release evoked by succinylcholine needs to be considered. For example, in pediatric patients, the combination of halothane and succinylcholine is associated with accentuated myoglobin release. Nevertheless, the importance of myoglobin release, if any, remains undetermined.—R.K. Stoelting, M.D.

Outpatient

Automated Three-Part Leukocyte Differential Counts in the Preoperative Evaluation of Ambulatory Surgery Patients
Kalish RJ, Goldberg G, Roberts K, Schwartz S, Iorio C (State Univ of New York, Syracuse; Cigna Healthplan, Phoenix)
Arch Pathol Lab Med 111:1155–1157, December 1987   6–32

There is controversy over the value of preoperative laboratory screening tests for asymptomatic patients undergoing elective surgery. The benefits of preoperative 3-part differential cell counts were evaluated in patients undergoing minor ambulatory elective surgery.

Two-hundred ninety-five patient specimens were randomly selected to assess the clinical value of the Coulter-S-Plus V 3-part leukocyte differential cell count in preoperative evaluation for ambulatory surgery. Patient charts were reviewed and adverse outcomes were recorded.

Of the 295 scheduled operations, 28 were cancelled and 7 patients were hospitalized after surgery. Only 2 of these 35 patients had abnormal differential cell counts; both were detected using default criteria. In these patients, surgery was cancelled because of upper respiratory tract infection. Overall, only 5% of patient samples resulted in machine-generated flags, perhaps because the population studied was relatively healthy.

These data might be construed as an argument against doing any differential cell counts in this patient population. Because white blood cell abnormalities are rare in this group, an extremely large patient study would be required to ascertain whether the screening differential could detect an abnormality not apparent from quantitative red blood cell, white blood cell, and platelet parameters. Estimates that the use of the 3-part differential cell count could decrease the number of manual differential cell counts by 65% may be high. However, in an identified patient population, screening differential cell count can result in significant cost savings without adversely affecting patient care.

▶ I think this paper nicely shows in a relatively small sample that an automated system looking at white cell differentials was as good as a manual system and, if you will, condemns the point that differentials are needed for preoperative evaluation. In fact, I think the telling point in this paper comes in a statement used in the discussion: "Admittedly, one could use our data to argue against doing any kind of differential count at all in this select group of patients." This is the statement that I believe is most truthful. We shouldn't even worry about whether one can do it by machine or manually. It is not needed at all. I think that we as physicians should do what is needed to decrease unnecessary medical care, that is, medical care that does not add to patient benefit and only increases patient risk, through the iatrogenic disease the follow-up tests create, and our malpractice risk, through lack of notation in the chart. If one absolutely needs a differential because the surgeons require it, then use the automated system, as it will save over 65% of the cost of the differential done manually. But we probably don't need the differential count at all except in symptomatic patients, and that is what the data from this study show.—M.F. Roizen, M.D.

Which Intravenous Induction Agent for Day Surgery? A Comparison of Propofol, Thiopentone, Methohexitone and Etomidate

Heath PJ, Kennedy DJ, Ogg TW, Dunling C, Gilks WR (Addenbrooke's Hosp, Cambridge, England; Med Research Council Biostatistics Unit, Cambridge, England)
Anaesthesia 43:365–368, 1988   6–33

Propofol has been studied extensively in day case anesthesia, but most studies comparing the effectiveness of propofol against standard anesthetic induction agents have not been blind. The induction characteristics, postoperative sequelae, and recovery with propofol, thiopental, methohexital, and etomidate were compared in 80 day patients undergoing vaginal abortions; the assessors did not know which agent was being administered.

The study was done with 4 age-matched groups of 20 women each. No premedication was prescribed, and each patient was given intravenous alfentanil 7 μg/kg via the dorsum of the nondominant hand. The anesthetic induction agents used were either 2.5% thiopental, 5 mg/kg; 1% propofol, 2.5 mg/kg; 1% methohexital, 1.5 mg/kg; or 0.2% etomidate, 0.3 mg/kg, with supplements of the same agent given as required. Because of standard practice, 1 ml of 1% lidocaine solution was added to propofol and methohexital, but not to thiopental or etomidate. Patients were allowed to breathe a mixture of 70% nitrous oxide in oxygen spontaneously. No oxytocic drugs were administered.

Methohexital and etomidate caused more side effects than either propofol or thiopental. Etomidate was associated with a significantly higher incidence of spontaneous movement on induction, muscle twitch, tremor, and pain at the injection site than the other 3 agents. The incidence of restlessness in the recovery room was also higher with etomidate. Thiopental and propofol were considered to be the better induction agents, whereas propofol produced the best recovery of the 4 agents. The mean immediate recovery times for propofol and methohexital were significantly shorter than those for the other 2 agents.

▶ All factors considered, propofol is as good as any currently available drug for induction of anesthesia and is probably superior to most, especially if repeated doses are required. The need for rapid and predictable recovery from the effects of injected anesthetic drugs administered to outpatients will most likely result in propofol becoming the most frequently utilized induction drug in this setting.—R.K. Stoelting, M.D.

Effects of Eliminating Nitrous Oxide in Outpatient Anesthesia
Melnick BM, Johnson LS (Univ of Pittsburgh; Magee-Women's Hosp, Pittsburgh)
Anesthesiology 67:982–984, December 1987   6–34

The most common complications of outpatient general anesthesia are nausea and vomiting; nitrous oxide is implicated in these complications. The incidence of postoperative nausea and vomiting, other common postoperative complications, and intraoperative recall were compared in healthy female patients undergoing minor surgical procedures when anesthesia was used with and without nitrous oxide.

Sixty ambulatory female patients were divided into 2 groups according to odd or even year of birth. Group I received isoflurane in oxygen, and group II received isoflurane in nitrous oxide and oxygen in concentrations appropriate for the surgical procedures. Patients were evaluated for pain, nausea, vomiting, and level of consciousness at 15-minute intervals. One day postoperatively, patients were questioned about pain, nausea, and recall.

The groups were comparable in levels of consciousness at all time intervals and in numbers of patients complaining of pain. In group II, 25% of patients had nausea and vomiting, compared with 3.6% in group I. Patients with emetic symptoms had a significantly longer recovery-room stay. No patient recalled any events between anesthesia and awakening in the recovery room.

Elimination of nitrous oxide from isoflurane/oxygen anesthesia for minor outpatient procedures in healthy women significantly decreases the incidence of postoperative nausea and vomiting without increasing the risk of intraoperative awareness. It must be remembered, however, that severe postoperative pain can also influence emetic symptoms.

▶ There is much controversy in the literature about the effects of eliminating nitrous oxide and the role of nitrous oxide in causing postoperative nausea and vomiting. This study, which essentially looks at the patient group where no confounding variables such as laparoscopy and insufflation of CO_2 into the belly are used, indicates that nausea and vomiting is more common in the nitrous oxide group. But once again, the numbers are small.

If one uses meta-analysis, which is essentially combining the smaller studies that are done into significant groups, there is clearly an indication that nitrous oxide, when confounding variables are removed, is associated with increased nausea and vomiting. But the confounding variables are strong enough that in most practice situations the addition of nitrous oxide probably has no major influence on the overall incidence of nausea and vomiting. However, were I to be involved in giving anesthesia in which narcotics aren't needed, peritoneal insufflation isn't needed, etc., then I would probably avoid the use of nitrous oxide. The deficit in this is that one then needs more of another anesthetic. So one has to be concerned with a prolonged wake-up time because most of the other anesthetics have longer half-lives in the body than does nitrous oxide. The modern addition of propofol, soon to come, and alfentanyl, along with isoflurane and perhaps a new inhalation anesthetic soon to be released, may in fact make this latter concern less of a problem.

The other interesting point raised by the study is something that is probably obvious to all, that is, the presence of postoperative nausea and vomiting prolongs recovery room stay and increases the expense of caring for postoperative patients.—M.F. Roizen, M.D.

Nitrous Oxide and Day-Case Laparoscopy: Effects on Nausea, Vomiting and Return to Normal Activity
Sengupta P, Plantevin OM (St Thomas' Hosp, London)
Br J Anaesth 60:570–573, 1988   6–35

Postoperative Morbidity and Administration of
Analgesic and Antiemetic Drugs Before Discharge
(Number of Patients per Group)

		Nitrous oxide	No nitrous oxide
Nausea	Severe	5	3
	Moderate	7	7
	Mild	5	4
	Total	17	14
	Nil	16	17
Vomiting	> 2	0	0
	× 2	5	1
	× 1	6	3
	Total	11	4
	0	22	27
Abdominal pain	Severe	4	7
	Moderate	21	12
	Mild	6	10
	Total	31	29
	Nil	2	2
Analgesia	I.m.	2	2
	Oral	27	19
	Nil	4	10
Anti-emetic		13	10
Awareness		0	1

(Courtesy of Sengupta P, Plantevin OM: *Br J Anaesth* 60:570–573, 1988.)

Nitrous oxide has appeared to reduce the frequency of postoperative nausea and vomiting after laparoscopy. But a significantly reduced incidence of postoperative vomiting occurred when nitrous oxide was omitted from the anesthetic technique. The effect of nitrous oxide on nausea and vomiting and subsequent return to normal activity after day-case laparoscopy was studied.

Eighty unpremedicated adults were randomly assigned to receive a mixture of nitrous oxide and oxygen with enflurane or oxygen with enflurane as part of a standard anesthetic technique for day-case laparoscopy. Postoperative morbidity, particularly nausea and vomiting, and ability to resume normal activity were evaluated over 48 hours. Supplementary administration of propofol during the procedure was required significantly more often in the absence of nitrous oxide. No significant difference was found in the incidence of vomiting before discharge when nitrous oxide was omitted (table). The incidence and severity of nausea during the 48-hour period after surgery were similar in both groups. No difference was noted in analgesic or antiemetic requirements before discharge, and the time taken to resume normal activity was comparable.

Nitrous oxide may be avoided in day-case laparoscopy without affecting postoperative morbidity, particularly nausea and vomiting, or time taken to return to normal activities. There was no significant difference in the incidence of vomiting before discharge when nitrous oxide was omitted from the anesthetic procedure.

▶ Although this article states that nitrous oxide has no effect on nausea and vomiting, the data do not show that to be so. In fact, nitrous oxide was associated with vomiting in 11 of 33 patients who received 33% nitrous oxide as opposed to 4 of 31 patients who did not. This study was just too small to show this difference of 33% versus 12.9% to be statistically different. The difference between vomiting in the 2 groups was over 100%, yet the study sample size was so small as to not show a significant difference when, in fact, it may have existed. This study points up a problem that editors have and that I think needs to be stated in all papers: the probability that the study will find a result if it exists. If this study were enlarged by another 140 patients, such a difference would have been significant at the .05 level.—M.F. Roizen, M.D.

What Is the Potential for Moving Adult Surgery to the Ambulatory Setting?
Roos NP (Univ of Manitoba)
Can Med Assoc J 138:809–816, May 1, 1988   6–36

In 1985, outpatient surgery accounted for about 18% of all surgery performed in the United States. A previously published study suggested that the proportion of outpatient surgery could be increased to between 50% and 60%. Available data indicate that the cost of outpatient surgery is about 30% lower than that of inpatient surgery. Moreover, about 80% of surveyed patients prefer ambulatory surgery to inpatient care for minor procedures. To estimate how much inpatient surgery could be moved to an outpatient setting, the patterns of outpatient surgery performed in the 8 largest hospitals in Manitoba between April 1983 and March 1984 were analyzed.

A surgical procedure was included for analysis only if it was not performed more than 86% of the time as an inpatient or outpatient procedure, with the exception of tooth extraction, which also was included even though it is performed as an outpatient procedure in 89% of the patients in Manitoba. Inpatients discharged within 3 days after admission were considered potential candidates for outpatient surgery. Only patients aged 20 years or older were included in this analysis.

Of 19,286 surgical procedures that could have been performed on either an inpatient or an outpatient basis, 73% were actually performed on an outpatient basis. Analysis of the data indicated that as many as 5,256 inpatient days, or 17.5 inpatient beds per day could have been saved. There were large differences among the 8 hospitals, and among surgeons within each hospital, with regard to the rates of outpatient surgery performed, even after the data were adjusted for patient characteristics and differences in case mix. Surgeons aged 40–54 years and those aged 65 years or older were least likely to perform surgery in an outpatient setting.

Hospitals attempting to rationalize bed use should examine the admitting practices of all physicians whose practices differ considerably from those of their colleagues and should perhaps issue rules about which procedures must be performed on an ambulatory basis.

▶ This article from Winnipeg, Manitoba, looked carefully at how many bed days could be saved by performing as outpatient surgery all that was done on an inpatient basis but had the potential of being done on an outpatient basis. The authors looked at the 19,000 or so surgical procedures that could have been performed on either an inpatient or an outpatient basis between April of 1983 and March of 1984. They judged those based on the fact that similar operations had been done on an inpatient or an outpatient basis elsewhere, using figures in regard to co-morbidity and patient diseases that would not necessitate hospitalization. They estimated that they could improve the percentage done as outpatients from 73% of the 19,000 to approximately 80%, were the maximum for each procedure to be done in any of the hospitals. That would have saved approximately 5,256 inpatient days or roughly 17.5 patient days per day for the 8 hospitals. For hospitals that are pretty full, this makes a major savings and allows them not to build more inpatient beds, as would be the case in the Manitoba hospitals, run by The National Health Service.

However, this is a small number of bed days to save when one considers the cost of increasing the ambulatory surgery services. Because these were divided over 8 different hospitals, one would ask, "How much would one have to increase the number of ambulatory surgery facilities in each of these hospitals, or would one have to increase them at all?" It is obviously a complex decision based on the marginal use of those facilities; that is, how much they are used versus the current crowding in hospitals. The general impression is that most of the surgery that can be moved to the ambulatory surgery suite has been moved.

Another point made in the paper is that the goal was not just cost savings, although it is found that outpatient surgery costs only about 70% of that of inpatient surgery, but that the quality of care actually is thought to improve in the outpatient setting. No good data exist on the latter, and one wonders whether that is true. Clearly for anesthesiologists, the arranging of an outpatient schedule, seeing the patients preoperatively, and having time to evaluate them and think about them requires the initiation of an outpatient preoperative clinic. This has been done in many places but at a reasonably high cost for the benefit.— M.F. Roizen, M.D.

Local Versus General Anesthesia for Laparoscopic Sterilization: A Randomized Study
Peterson HB, Hulka JF, Spielman FJ, Lee S, Marchbanks PA (Univ of North Carolina at Chapel Hill; Ctrs for Disease Control, Atlanta)
Obstet Gynecol 70:903–908, December 1987   6–37

Some authors suggest that local anesthesia is a safe and appropriate alternative to general anesthesia for laparoscopic sterilization, yet randomized studies comparing these techniques have yet to prove it. To better characterize the relative safety and acceptability of these techniques for laparoscopic sterilization, 100 women undergoing bipolar electrocoagulation or spring clip application for tubal ligation were randomly assigned to receive either local or general anesthesia. Both groups weregiven diazepam, 5 mg; fentanyl, 100 μg; and glycopyrrolate, 0.2 mg, for analgesia. For local anesthesia, 10 ml of 2% 2-chloroprocaine was used for periumbilical analgesia and 20 ml of 0.5% bupivacaine was administered to anesthetize the peritoneal surface of the fallopian tubes. For general anesthesia, thiopental and succinylcholine were used for induction. Anesthesia was maintained with nitrous oxide, oxygen, and potent inhalation agents.

Of the 53 women assigned to local anesthesia, 4 had their procedures completed using another technique because of technical problems probably related to obesity. However, in 13 other obese women sterilization was completed with local anesthesia. Women undergoing local anesthesia had slightly less anesthesia time (30 vs. 36 minutes) and less time in the recovery room (65 vs. 78 minutes). Women undergoing general anesthesia were 2.3 times and 1.5 times more likely to have systolic and diastolic hypertension, respectively; 3.2 times more likely to have hypotension; and 5.7 times more likely to have tachycardia. No life-threatening complications of anesthesia occurred in either group. Patient movement (e.g., bucking movement on emergence from anesthesia) was reported to be a problem in 5 women undergoing general anesthesia, but it did not occur in women having local anesthesia. Eighty percent of women in both groups expressed satisfaction with the anesthetic technique used.

These findings suggest that local anesthesia is a safe and acceptable alternative to general anesthesia for laparoscopic sterilization. Because of the hazards of general anesthesia, local anesthesia may be preferable for some properly selected patients.

▶ Considering the doses of local anesthetics administered to the awake patients, it is inappropriate to conclude that this approach is a "safer" approach than general anesthesia. Furthermore, despite an 80% satisfaction rate in both groups, it must be recognized that there was nothing for comparison. It is conceivable that a theoretical patient who was exposed to both techniques would have strongly favored one over the other.—R.K. Stoelting, M.D.

Myalgia in Outpatient Surgery: Comparison of Atracurium and Succinylcholine
Trépanier CA, Brousseau C, Lacerte L (Hôpital de l'Enfant-Jésus, Université Laval, Québec)
Can J Anaesth 35:255–259, 1988   6–38

Muscle pain is the most frequently reported complication of outpatient surgery. Such pain, often severe enough to require bed rest and an analgesic, occurs as an aftereffect of succinylcholine, a commonly used muscle relaxant. Atracurium, a nondepolarizing agent, was evaluated as an alternative to succinylcholine.

Twenty-six patients were given succinylcholine and 34 received atracurium during same-day surgery requiring tracheal intubation. Results in these groups were compared with those in 24 patients whose procedures did not call for intubation or a muscle relaxant.

Patients receiving succinylcholine had a significantly higher rate of myalgia; 76 reported muscle pain, whereas only 23% of those who were given atracurium experienced this complication. Of the patients who took neither muscle relaxant, 21% had myalgia.

Although previous studies have given widely varying reports on the incidence of myalgia, the results indicate that the complication is common in outpatient surgery. That those receiving no muscle relaxant complained of postsurgical muscle pain indicates that there are other causes of this pain. When a muscle relaxant is required, atracurium is far less likely than succinylcholine to cause complications.

▶ After the long debate about succinylcholine and muscle pains, it should be recognized that such pains occur even when muscle relaxants are not given.— R.D. Miller, M.D.

Neonatal Anesthesia

Blood Pressure Response of Neonates to Tracheal Intubation

Charlton AJ, Greenhough SG (St Mary's Hosp, Manchester, England)
Anaesthesia 43:744–746, 1988   6–39

Two recent editorials on neonatal anesthesia suggested that the traditional practice of "awake intubation" of neonates be abandoned because this practice may provoke harmful hypertension, which could predispose to intraventricular hemorrhage. Although the fluctuating pattern of blood pressure seen in sick premature babies whose lungs are ventilated without muscle relaxation has indeed been linked with intraventricular hemorrhage, this blood pressure response has never been linked to tracheal intubation or anesthetic practices. Because a hypertensive response to awake intubation has never been documented, blood pressure and pulse rate changes were investigated in response to tracheal intubation in neonates and infants receiving for anesthetic.

The study was performed with 45 term neonates aged 1–24 days and 15 infants aged 32–93 days, including 12 born at a gestation of 33 weeks or less. The latter 15 infants and 15 of the 45 neonates were intubated when awake, 15 were intubated after halothane inhalation, and 15, after administration of thiopental plus a muscle relaxant. Blood pressures and pulse rates were measured by oscillotonometry immediately before and after intubation. A resting blood pressure was obtained for 21 neonates and 9 older infants at induction of anesthesia.

None of the neonates showed a hypertensive response to intubation, and blood pressures of the 15 neonates who were intubated awake did not differ from those of infants who were intubated under halothane or thiopental plus muscle relaxants. However, the 15 older infants showed a significant increase in systolic and diastolic pressure after intubation, and their systolic pressures were significantly higher than those of the 3 neonatal groups. There was no difference between the resting pulse rates and blood pressures recorded for 9 infants and those recorded for 21 neonates.

A hypertensive response to tracheal intubation is absent at birth but may be present at 1 to 3 months of age. Although awake intubation is believed to be unpleasant but not painful for a neonate, it need not be avoided for fear of a hypertensive response.

▶ I think this study is great, not because it is a good clinical study that gives an answer to a question but because the authors took a statement drawn from unrelated work, designed a study, and refuted the allegation. And, in this instance, neonates are different from somewhat older infants. I am sure other groups will evaluate this problem in their practices, and it will be interesting to see their findings in future YEAR BOOKS OF ANESTHESIA.—G.W. Ostheimer, M.D.

Effects of Fentanyl on Baroreceptor Reflex Control of Heart Rate in Newborn Infants

Murat I, Levron J-C, Berg A, Saint-Maurice C (Hôpital Saint-Vincent-de-Paul, Paris; Janssen Labs, Aubervilliers, France)
Anesthesiology 68:717–722, May 1988   6–40

Previous investigations have demonstrated that intravenously administered and inhalational anesthetics depress the baroreflex-mediated heart rate response in adults. A recent study suggested that the baroreflex control of heart rate is already present in term neonates and that halothane anesthesia depresses the pressor baroresponse more in newborn infants than it does in adults. Because only the pressor baroresponse, but not the depressor baroresponse, was measured in that stusdy, the pressor and the depressor baroresponses were measured in newborn infants before and after administration of fentanyl.

Baroreceptor responses were studied in 10 neonates who were being mechanically ventilated. Four of these infants were born prematurely; but all infants were in stable condition at the time of the study. The pressor response was tested using phenylephrine, and the depressor response was tested using nitroglycerin. Changes in heart rate were plotted against changes in systolic arterial pressure. Baroreflex sensitivity was estimated as the slope of the relationship between arterial pressure and heart period, for which the arterial pressure was the manipulated parameter. After obtaining both pressor and depressor baroresponses, fentanyl, 10 μg/kg, was injected intravenously over 1 minute. Pressor and depressor baroresponses were then again obtained, using the same dosages of phenylephrine and nitroglycerin.

No significant changes in systolic arterial pressure, heart rate, and blood gas values were observed after fentanyl injection compared with control values. However, fentanyl produced significant depression of the baroreflex control of heart rate, with the pressor baroreflex slope declining 48% and the depressor baroreflex slope declining 42% from control values. That the baroreflex control of heart rate is markedly depressed during fentanyl anesthesia may impair the ability of neonates to compensate for rapid changes in systolic arterial pressure.

These results confirm the presence of baroreflex control of heart rate in term neonates and show that fentanyl significantly depresses baroreflex control of heart rate.

▶ The methodology used in this study may be applied to the other narcotics and inhalational anesthetics used in pediatric surgery.—G.W. Ostheimer, M.D.

Paediatric Anaesthetists' Perceptions of Neonatal and Infant Pain
Purcell-Jones G, Dormon F, Sumner E (St Thomas' Hosp, London; Hammersmith Hosp, London; The Hosp for Sick Children, London)
Pain 33:181–187, May 1988   6–41

Because there is much controversy over the use of analgesic drugs in the postoperative management of young and very young infants, all members of the Association of Paediatric Anaesthetists in England and Ireland were queried by mail for their opinions on the perception of pain, its assessment, and their use of opioids and regional anesthesia in newborns and infants younger than age 1 year. Sixty of the 66 members returned their completed questionnaires.

All respondents believed that infants aged 1–12 months are able to perceive pain. Eight-five percent of the respondents believed that newborns between 1 week and 1 month of age can perceive pain, and 80% thought that newborns younger than 1 week can perceive pain. Although most believed that infants can perceive pain, their practices with regard to the use of opioid analgesia or regional and local anesthesia varied widely. However, most respondents never or rarely prescribed opioid analgesia after minor procedures in neonates younger than 1 month of age, whereas more than half usually or always prescribed opioids after major operations for infants older than 1 month of age.

A ranking of clinical signs considered by some as indicators of pain showed no single sign to be more useful than any other. The decision to give analgesia was often made on the very subjective observations of the nursing staff. The results of this analysis underscore the urgent need for practical, reliable, and valid indices of infant and neonatal pain.

Newborn Pain Cries and Vagal Tone: Parallel Changes in Response to Circumcision
Porter FL, Porges SW, Marshall RE (Washington Univ; Univ of Maryland; Case Western Reserve Univ)
Child Dev 59:495–505, April 1988   6–42

Clinical research has confirmed that the cry of the seriously ill newborn is higher and more variable in pitch than the cry of the healthy infant. Previous studies have indicated that the vagal tone of chronically stressed infants is significantly reduced compared with that of normal infants. A neural model of cry production was proposed suggesting that decreased vagal tone among infants at risk may be related to increases in cry pitch.

The relationship between cry acoustics and vagal tone was examined in 32 normal, healthy infants aged 24–48 hours undergoing routine unanesthetized circumcision. Vocalizations, heart rate, and respiratory waveforms were recorded before, during, and after surgery. Recordings were also obtained in 17 controls. Vagal tone was measured by the amplitude of respiratory sinus arrhythmia taken from heart data.

Vagal tone was significantly reduced during circumcision. Reductions in vagal tone were parallel to significant increases in the pitch of the infants' cries. Individual differences in vagal tone measurement before circumcision were predictive of physiologic and acoustic reactivity to subsequent stress.

The findings support the relationship between cry characteristics and vagal tone and demonstrate that decreased vagal tone results in higher-pitched cries. Preoperative measurement of vagal tone might be used to identify infants at greatest risk for adverse reaction to surgery.

▶ Do neonates feel pain? There is increasing and, one would say almost insurmountable, evidence that the neonate feels pain. However, one cannot codify the exact stages in development when the neonate begins to perceive pain and develops adversive responses. Premature babies appear to have pain when invasive procedures are performed in the neonatal intensive care unit. Although we cannot definitively answer at what stage in development the human perceives and integrates a painful stimulus and then responds, it is generally accepted by pediatric anesthesiologists and, hopefully, is becoming more accepted by the general community of anesthesiologists that these babies feel pain. One of the problems in assessing pain in the newborn is that there is no "visual analog scale" that can be applied to the neonate. Their inability to communicate on an understandable level retards investigation in this area. In the Purcell-Jones et al. study (Abstract 6–41), the decision to give analgesia made on subjective observations of the nursing staff was the most pertinent point made for the administration of some form of pain medication. In the Porter et al. study (Abstract 6–42), the investigators used a physiologic observation, i.e., differences in vagal tone, to predict reactivity to the stress of circumcision.

As the advertisement says, "You've come a long way, baby," and so has the anesthesia community. We need to accept that neonates perceive noxious stimuli and formulate a response. However, we may not be able to interpret the response of the baby as an aversive reaction to a painful stimulus. That is a problem that a number of pediatric anesthesiologists interested in pain must assess, and perhaps they will come up with a workable, admittedly subjective system for evaluating the neonate's response to pain. Certainly the withholding of analgesia, except for acute resuscitative procedures, from the neonate is barbaric. Judicious administration of analgesics and anesthetics has been shown to decrease the stress response in preterm and term newborns undergoing surgery. This area of pain evaluation and management should be a fertile field of endeavor in the immediate future.— G.W. Ostheimer, M.D.

Local Anesthesia for Neonatal Circumcision: Effects on Distress and Cortisol Response
Stang HJ, Gunnar MR, Snellman L, Condon LM, Kestenbaum R (Group Health Inc, White Bear Lake, Minn; Univ of Minnesota at Minneapolis St Paul)
JAMA 259:1507–1511, Mar 11, 1988   6–43

Routine circumcision of the newborn is typically performed without anesthesia despite indications that newborns do experience pain. Favorable results have been reported for local anesthesia with the dorsal penile nerve block (DPNB), but few physicians have adopted this technique. A controlled double-blind study was undertaken to determine whether DPNB using lidocaine hydrochloride without epinephrine would reduce behavioral distress and adrenocortical responses to routine neonatal circumcision.

Sixty patients were randomized in equal numbers to undergo circumcision with lidocaine, saline, or no injection. Behavioral state was recorded during the injection and circumcision periods and during a postcircumcision nursery observation period. Blood samples were analyzed for plasma cortisol data.

There were no significant differences in percentage of time spent crying among the groups except during circumcision. Infants receiving injections did not cry more during the injection period than did those not injected. Newborns in the DPNB group cried significantly less during the circumcision period than did those in the other groups. Dorsal penile nerve block with lidocaine attenuated the adrenocortical response to circumcision as compared with the response in the other groups.

Dorsal penile nerve block is safe and effective in reducing distress and modifying the adrenocortical stress response in infants undergoing circumcision. The injection itself apparently does not add to stress reactions.

▶ As previously discussed, the newborn perceives pain, and this has been largely ignored in the history of mankind. Certainly, local infiltration or dorsal penile nerve block appears to be more humane for circumcision than no medication. However, is it safer? Circumcision has been performed for centuries without any significant problems to the health and welfare of the newborn except for complications of the surgery itself. Although I believe that local anesthesia for circumcision is more humane, I am concerned about its application in this group of patients by people untrained in the use of local anesthetics. I am not advocating that anesthesiologist spend their time doing dorsal penile nerve blocks or local infiltration for circumcisions. However, I am urging the establishment of strict rules to be followed for either dorsal penile nerve block or local infiltration. The occurrence of an enlarging hematoma from perforation of 1 of the penile vessels.

Central nervous system toxic reactions and cardiovascular depression are some of the problems that could result from the unintentional excessive injection of local anesthetic. If we as physicians remember the adage "to do no harm" then we can evaluate whether local anesthesia is applicable in every case of circumcision or whether it needs to be applied in a selective manner.—G.W. Ostheimer, M.D.

Does Halothane Anaesthesia Decrease the Metabolic and Endocrine Stress Responses of Newborn Infants Undergoing Operation?
Anand KJS, Sippell WG, Schofield NM, Aynsley-Green A (Harvard Univ; Univ of Kiel, West Germany; John Radcliffe Hosp, Oxford, England; Royal Victoria Infirmary, Newcastle upon Tyne, England)
Br Med J 296:668–672, Mar 5, 1988   6–44

It has been suggested that complications reported with halothane anesthesia may have been the effects of unnecessarily high concentrations. A randomized controlled trial was undertaken to investigate whether stress responses in neonates anesthetized with halothane differed from those in neonates receiving nitrous oxide and curare anesthesia.

Thirty-six neonates scheduled for surgery were randomized to 2 groups: 1 group received anesthesia with nitrous oxide and curare alone; in the other group, halothane was added. Concentrations of metabolites and hormones were measured preoperatively and postoperatively and at 6, 12, and 24 hours after surgery.

Neonates receiving halothane anesthesia had a decreased hormonal response to operation. There were significant differences between the 2 groups in the changes in norepinephrine, epinephrine, and cortisol concentrations, and in the ratio of insulin to glucagon concentration. Changes in blood concentrations of glucose and total ketone bodies, as well as plasma concentrations of nonesterified fatty acids, also were decreased in the group receiving halothane. Neonates in the group receiving unsupplemented nitrous oxide had significantly greater increases in the urinary ratio of 3-methylhistidine to creatine concentration. Their clinical condition was also less stable during and after surgery.

Newborn infants have substantial metabolic and endocrine stress responses to surgery. Effective analgesia and potent anesthesia with halothane or other anesthetic agents should be administered to infants undergoing invasive procedures unless specifically contraindicated.

▶ There is increasing evidence that the neonate perceives pain and demonstrates adverse metabolic responses to surgery if inadequate analgesia/anesthesia is administered. Hopefully, the community of practicing anesthesiologists is receiving this message.—G.W. Ostheimer, M.D.

Pediatric Anesthesia

Perioperative Management of Conjoined Twins
Diaz JH, Furman EB (Tulane Univ; Univ of Washington)
Anesthesiology 67:965–973, December 1987   6–45

On the basis of their most prominent site of connection, conjoined twins are classified as thoracopagus, xiphopagus, omphalopagus, ischiopagus, pygopagus, or craniopagus. Thoracopagus twins, which are joined at the sternum, diaphragm, and upper abdominal wall, are the most common, with a frequency of 40% of all conjoined births. Craniopagus twins, which are joined at the cranial vault and dural venous sinuses, are the rarest, with a frequency of 2% of all conjoined births.

Early prenatal diagnosis of many types of conjoined twins is now possible, allowing early midtrimester termination of such pregnancies when the prognosis is poor, or careful planning for delivery if separation appears possible. Preoperative management of conjoined twins should be unhurried to allow growth and to gather a multidisciplinary separation team. Preoperative evaluation should include a variety of diagnostic studies to define the extent of organ sharing and to demonstrate coexisting congenital anomalies. Conjoined twins with little or no cardiac sharing may be surgically separated immediately after delivery.

Intraoperative anesthetic management of conjoined twins requires a dual team of 1 or 2 anesthesiologists for each twin, plus an additional anesthesiologist who acts as team coordinator. Intra-anesthetic monitoring of conjoined twins must be at least as extensive as that used during routine infant anesthesia. Endotracheal intubation is recommended for intraoperative airway management, as spontaneous ventilation is not recommended because of anesthetic-induced depression of alveolar ventilation. However, endotracheal intubation may be difficult in thoracoabdominally conjoined twins.

At completion of the operation, critically ill newly separated infants require controlled ventilation, followed by a trial of spontaneous breathing with a T-piece and continuous positive airway pressure before tracheal extubation is considered. Tight skin closures may restrict spontaneous ventilation and prolong the need for postoperative controlled ventilation.

Successful intraoperative management of conjoined twins undergoing surgical separation requires timing, teamwork, and an appreciation of the risks involved.

▶ An interesting article that speaks for itself.— R.D. Miller, M.D.

A Single-Blind Study of Pulse Oximetry in Children
Cote CJ, Goldstein EA, Coté MA, Hagin DC, Ryan JF (Harvard Univ; Massachusetts Gen Hosp, Boston; Shriners Burn Inst, Boston)
Anesthesiology 68:184–188, February 1988   6–46

A prospective study was designed to determined the value of pulse oximetry in monitoring oxygen saturation in 152 pediatric surgical patients. The oximeter was applied to a finger or toe before or shortly after anesthetic induction. For 76 patients, the oximeter data and alarms were available to the anesthesia team.

In 17% of patients, the oxygen saturation was 85% or below for longer than 30 seconds, indicating a partial oxygen pressure of about 52 mmHg. Significantly more of these major events occurred when oximeter data were unavailable. Major events were most frequent in children aged 2 years and younger and those weighing less than 10 kg. Four cases of airway obstruction, 3 of laryngospasm, and 3 of hypoventilation were diagnosed, using the oximeter, before diagnosis by the anesthesia team.

Oxygen saturation was maintained at a higher level when oximeter data were known. Cyanosis was not always apparent when the oximeter indicated saturation less than 72%. Vital signs were of little help in diagnosing desaturation. Even experienced anesthesiologists sometimes failed to detect major desaturation clinically. Moderate desaturation occurred less often before transport to the recovery room when oximetry data were available.

Pulse oximetry is a useful adjunct in caring for pediatric surgery patients. Many major hypoxic events will be detected before they are clinically apparent; as a result, oximeters are likely to save many lives and the cost is quite low. Oximetry is a reliable and noninvasive procedure.

▶ This report is not an "outcome" study, but it comes as close as one probably can while still maintaining ethical standards of human research. Although no adverse consequences were reported, because the observer notified the anesthesia team members when oxygen saturation fell below 85%, we can conclude reasonably that, in similar cases in which oxygen saturation is not monitored, potential consequences of unrecognized hypoxemia may be devastating. I don't believe we need any more clear-cut information to be convinced that pulse oximetry (and also expired carbon dioxide monitoring) are not only advisable but also essential to the safe practice of anesthesiology. Dr. David A. Davis of Duke University summed up our current status best when he stated, "It is our view that while the medical sector is concentrating on protecting the circulation, the insurance industry is paying for brain damage" (*Int Anesthesiol Clin* 22:31–42, 1984).—R.R. Kirby, M.D.

Pre-induction of Anesthesia in Pediatric Patients With Nasally Administered Sufentanil
Henderson JM, Brodsky DA, Fisher DM, Brett CM; Hertzka RE (Univ of California, San Francisco)
Anesthesiology 68:671–675, May 1988   6–47

Preinduction of anesthesia in pediatric patients can counter fears of painful procedures and separation from the parents. Nasally administered sufentanil was tried as a replacement for fentanyl in preinducing anesthesia in 80 patients aged 6 months to 7 years. Doses of 1.5, 3.0, and 4.5 μg/kg were compared with a saline placebo.

Patients given sufentanil were more likely to separate willingly from their parents and were more often calm at this time. Ventilatory compliance was reduced in many sufentanil-treated patients, but induction proceeded normally and muscle relaxants were not required. The peak end-tidal halothane concentration was lower in patients given sufentanil. Vomiting after operation was more prevalent among patients given the highest dose of sufentanil.

Nasally administered sufentanil is a useful adjunct to anesthetic induction in pediatric patients. The nasal route is less traumatic than intramuscular injection and more acceptable to older children than rectal administration. Children separate more readily from their parents, and the postoperative course is less unpleasant.

▶ This study demonstrates our continued and heightened interest in new delivery systems for medications. The reader is referred to the accompanying editorial by Dr. Stanley on "New routes of Administration and New Delivery Systems of Anesthetics" (*Anesthesiology* 68:665–668, May 1988). In this very timely editorial, Dr. Stanley reviews different systems available to provide drugs transdermal or transmucosal, encapsulated systems, and a variety of programmable and implantable drug delivery devices.

The advantages of these new routes of administration are increased convenience and safety, improved bioavailability and continuous drug administration without the peaks and valleys of intramuscular administration, thereby providing more effective drug action at reduced dosage and frequency of administration. In preliminary work, there appear to be fewer side effects and possibly decreased cost. This study documents the attempt at opiate administration via the nasal mucous membranes with a less threatening pediatric delivery system in contrast to rectal, intramuscular, or intravenous administration. Future studies should look at a mechanism to titrate the drug administered to a desired end point rather than administering a fixed dosage. Dr. Stanley also speculates on the possibility of administering ketamine, midazolam, or alfentanil in various ways as a rapid onset premedicant or a short-lasting induction agent.

The "down side" of these new drug delivery systems is that the potential for abuse of these drugs may be increased without rigid controls. The other problem occurs when nonskilled anesthetists attempt to administer these potent drugs with new systems in an unsafe setting. Notwithstanding the opportunities for abuse by recreational drug users or for inappropriate utilization by unskilled medical personnel, I agree with Dr. Stanley that new drug delivery systems will open up the ability to make analgesia/anesthesia safer and less traumatic to our patients in the future.—G.W. Ostheimer, M.D.

Sodium Citrate in Paediatric Outpatients
Henderson JM, Spence DG, Clarke WN, Bonn GG, Noel LP (Children's Hospital of Eastern Ontario, Ottawa)
Can J Anaesth 34:560–562, 1987   6–48

Aspiration of foreign material into lungs during anesthesia is rare but can be fatal. Aspiration during anesthesia appears to more common in children than in adults. Almost all children are seen at surgery with a gastric content pH of less than 2.5, whereas only 24% to 75% of adults have a pH this low. As the pH of gastric fluid instilled in the trachea drops below 2.5, the degree of lung damage increases. The efficacy of sodium citrate in raising the gastric content pH preoperatively was studied in 52 outpatients, American Society of Anesthesiologists classification I, aged 7 months to 14 years.

The children were scheduled for ophthalmologic procedures. By random assignment, 25 were given sodium citrate, 0.4 ml/kg, prepared in a 0.3 M solution and 20 received no antacid. Anesthesia was induced either intravenously or with inhalation agents and the gastric pH was measured.

In 23 of the 25 patients who received sodium citrate, the gastric pH value was higher than 2.5. In the control group, only 2 children had a gastric pH higher than 2.5. One child refused to take the medication.

Sodium citrate was readily accepted by this group of children. It should be considered for reducing gastric acidity and thereby aid in decreasing postaspiration morbidity and mortality.

▶ Readers will note that the use of medications to raise gastric pH, thereby lowering gastric acidity, and to decrease gastric volume has been one of the interests of your editor over the years. This study demonstrates the efficacy of sodium citrate in decreasing gastric acidity in pediatric patients even though sodium citrate is not very palatable. One would hope that pharmaceutical companies would address the issue of taste when concocting antacids as they do for cough syrups and other medicinals that can be purchased over the counter.— G.W. Ostheimer, M.D.

The Position of the Larynx in Children and Its Relationship to the Ease of Intubation
Westhorpe RN (Royal Children's Hosp, Melbourne)
Anaesth Intens Care 15:384–388, November 1987   6–49

In a child the larynx is narrower and shorter than in an adult, and the epiglottis is relatively longer and more U-shaped. To define how the structures of the upper airway change position in relation to the cervical spine during growth and how these changes in position relate to effective laryngoscopy and intubation, measurements were obtained on a series of lateral radiographs of the skulls and cervical spines in 30 children aged 1 day to 12 years. Films of another 20 infants, aged 1 day to 3 years, and films of 4 adults also were used to obtain measurements to determine the growth-related changes in position of the tip of the epiglottis, the hyoid, the glottis, and the inferior margin of the cricoid cartilage.

During the first 2 years of life, there is a marked descent of the mea-

R. N. WESTHORPE

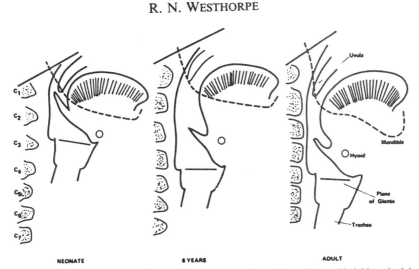

NEONATE   **6 YEARS**   **ADULT**

Fig 6–6.—Relative positions of upper airway structures in newborn, 6-year-old child, and adult. (Courtesy of Westhorpe RN: *Anaesth Intens Care* 15:384–388, November 1987.)

sured structures relative to the cervical spine. They then remain relatively static in position until puberty, when the laryngeal structures descend further (Fig 6–6). In infants the best view is obtained at laryngoscopy with the atlanto-occipital joint fully extended and the head and shoulders on a flat surface. In adults, the best view is obtained with the atlanto-occipital joint fully extended and the head lying on a low pillow.

Because the position of the larynx in relation to the cervical vertebrae is important in ascertaining the degree of difficulty in intubation, it is useful to obtain a lateral radiograph of the neck before undertaking an intubation that might pose problems.

▶ The author states that it is useful to obtain a lateral radiograph of the neck before undertaking an intubation that might pose problems. However, in an emergency, it is often impossible to obtain a diagnostic x-ray film of the neck before proceeding with an emergency operation. Therefore, other means of assessing the difficulty of intubation must be considered. If one can visualize the uvula and the posterior oropharynx on inspection of the mouth, it should be a relatively straightforward intubation. However, the inability to visualize the uvula or the posterior oropharynx should place one on alert for a difficult intubation. One should then consider fiberoptic laryngoscopy.

When faced with a difficult intubation, it is mandatory to have an extra person available to apply cricoid pressure if necessary or to help in manipulation of the head or neck in order to help the laryngoscopist accomplish intubation. If one is forewarned by his own observations to consider a difficult laryngoscopy and intubation then he will be forearmed with the appropriate instrumentation and assistance to accomplish this procedure.—G.W. Ostheimer, M.D.

Hypoxia in Children Following General Anaesthesia

Tomkins DP, Gaukroger PB, Bentley MW (Adelaide Children's Hosp, North Adelaide, Australia)
Anaesth Intens Care 16:177–181, May 1988   6–50

Healthy adults undergoing routine elective surgery under general anesthesia often experience transient postoperative hypoxemia. Therefore, it has become common practice to administer supplementary oxygen in the recovery room. Because children often tolerate masks or nasal catheters poorly, the postoperative use of supplementary oxygen in children is much less common. With the introduction of the pulse oximeter, oxygen saturation can now be measured noninvasively.

A study was done to determine whether general anesthesia also causes postoperative hypoxemia in 152 otherwise healthy children aged 2 days to 19 years. Oxygen saturation was measured continuously with a pulse oximeter for the first 30 minutes after anesthesia, starting immediately on arrival in the recovery room. Any patient whose oxygen saturation fell below 80% was given supplementary oxygen for several minutes.

While breathing room air, 36 of the 152 patients had postoperative oxygen saturation below 90% and 15 patients had it drop below 85%. Ten of these 15 patients appeared clinically normal, and hypoxemia would not have been detected without pulse oximetry. Thus clinical signs were correlated poorly with oxygen desaturation. All patients had their lowest oxygen saturation during the first 5 minutes in the recovery room.

There was no significant correlation with age, weight, procedure, time to awakening, or use of opiates. However, intubation, use of muscle relaxants, intravenous anesthesia induction, and anesthesia duration of more than 1 hour all were associated with an increased incidence of hypoxemia.

All children who undergo general anesthesia should be given postoperative supplementary oxygen during transport to the recovery room and for at least the first 10 minutes in the recovery room.

Postoperative Arterial Oxygen Saturation in the Pediatric Population During Transportation

Kataria BK, Harnik EV, Mitchard R, Kim Y, Admed S (Georgetown Univ)
Anesth Analg 67:280–282, March 1988   6–51

Both adults and children are often hypoxic upon arrival in the recovery room. In a previous study of hypoxia during transfer from the operating room to the recovery room, it was found that 35% of the adult study patients were hypoxic and 12% were severely hypoxic. Because changes in oxygen saturation during postoperative transport have not been well studied in children, a noninvasive pulse oximeter was used to monitor oxygen desaturation during transfer to the recovery room in 60 healthy children aged 1 month to 14 years after they had elective outpatient surgery of various durations. Anesthesia was induced by inhalation in 20 infants aged 0–12 months and by mask plus intravenously administered thiopental or rectal Brevital in 40 children aged 13 months and older. Anesthesia was maintained with oxygen, nitrous oxide, and halothane. Atropine and neostigmine were used to reverse muscle relaxation. Immediately after extubation or removal of the mask, all children were given 100% oxygen for 3 minutes. Oxygen saturation was measured throughout transfer to the recovery room, but only the lowest data point was recorded for each patient.

Although all patients had 100% oxygen saturation before being transferred, desaturation occurred rapidly during transfer to the recovery room. Mean oxygen saturation during transfer ranged from 88% in the youngest infants to 92% in the older infants to 93% in children aged 13 months and older. Thus oxygen desaturation was most pronounced in the youngest infants. Differences in oxygen desaturation between age groups appeared to be attributable mainly to differences in the pulmonary physiology of very young infants.

To avoid potential hypoxia in very young infants after elective outpatient surgery, rapid transport to the recovery room or administration of supplemental oxygen is recommended.

▶ These studies (Abstracts 6–50 and 6–51) document that clinical hypoxemia may not be detected in the postoperative pediatric patient without pulse oximetry. I believe that the findings in these studies were a foredrawn conclusion given the information that has been obtained in a number of recent adult studies. However, these studies needed to be done to establish that clinical hypoxemia can develop in the pediatric patient during the immediate postoperative period and may go undetected. What is most impressive in the Tomkins et al. study (Abstract 6–50) is that, of the 15 pediatric patients with oxygen saturations of less than 85%, 10 appeared clinically normal and the hypoxemia would not have been detected without pulse oximetry. Therefore, the clinical findings of hypoxemia, that is, cyanosis, tachycardia, and alteration in blood pressure, have a very poor correlation with the patient's actual state of oxygenation.

Common sense dictates that certain anesthetic manipulations should key the anesthesiologist to the use of supplemental oxygen in transporting patients from the operating room to the recovery room. These manipulations include intubation, use of muscle relaxants, and duration of anesthesia longer than 1 hour. Interestingly, intravenous induction also led to clinical hypoxemia during the postoperative period in the Tomkins et al. study. It is appropriate that the authors recommend that all children undergoing general anesthesia should be given postoperative supplemental oxygen during transport to the recovery room and during the initial stay in the recovery room. Perhaps our postanesthetic records should be evaluations not only of pulse, blood pressure, respiratory rate, and temperature, but also of oxygen saturation.

Equipment manufacturers are developing monitors that measure blood pressure, pulse, and oxygen saturation, are transportable, and are applicable to the pediatric patient as well as the adult patient. The problems of the occlusion of arterial flow during the monitoring of the blood pressure triggering the alarm on the pulse oximeter is being overcome by instituting a delay mechanism. Bulky transducers must be diminished or eliminated. However, this first generation of combined monitors is a step in the right direction.—G.W. Ostheimer, M.D.

Outpatient Treatment of Upper Extremity Injuries in Childhood Using Intravenous Regional Anaesthesia
Olney BW, Lugg PC, Turner PL, Eyres RL, Cole WG (Royal Children's Hosp, Melbourne)
J Pediatr Orthop 8:576–579, August 1988   6–52

In 1983 a program was initiated that involved treating children in need of closed reduction of upper limb injuries under intravenous regional anesthesia in the emergency department. The results of a prospective study done to assess the safety and effectiveness of this program were reviewed.

Four hundred upper extremity fractures and dislocations in 398 children aged 3–16 years were treated while they were under intravenous regional anesthesia. The nature of the injury and the likelihood that a child would be cooperative during the procedure were the only selection criteria for using this form of anesthesia. Children with fractures that might require open reduction or the use of an image intensifier were admitted for operation under general anesthesia. The quality of the anesthetic was rated as good when there was no or only mild discomfort with direct pressure over the fracture site, fair when there was moderate pain, and poor if the child had severe pain or if the reduction could not be completed.

Anatomical reductions were achieved in 278 injuries, and acceptable reductions, in 113 others. Only 9 (2.3%) patients had unacceptable reductions and required further treatment under general anesthesia. The quality of anesthesia was rated as good in 362 procedures, fair in 14, and poor in 25. However, an anatomical or acceptable reduction was still achieved in 21 of the 25 anesthesias rated as poor.

In 15 patients serum lidocaine levels were measured at different times during the course of anesthesia until 10 minutes after the cuff was released. The serum lidocaine levels in the patient with the highest concentration and in 2 others for whom measurements were available for up to 20–30 minutes after cuff release showed that peak lidocaine levels can occur at different times after cuff release. Because the peak level may not occur until up to 15 minutes after cuff release, patients should be monitored closely during this period. There was only 1 anesthetic complication, this in a 9-year-old girl who experienced myoclonic muscle twitching 25–30 minutes after cuff release. She was admitted for observation, but the twitching was resolved and she was released the next day.

Intravenous regional anesthesia is a safe and effective outpatient procedure for treating selected upper extremity fractures and dislocations in children.

▶ Intravenous regional anesthesia can be used safely in children receiving outpatient surgery, provided there is adequate postoperative observation. The only anesthetic sequela reported in this study is that of a 9-year-old girl who experienced myoclonic muscle twitching 25 to 30 minutes after the release of the cuff. The authors make an excellent recommendation that children receiving intravenous regional anesthesia should be observed for at least 1 hour before they return home with their parents or a responsible adult. I am in complete agreement that intravenous regional anesthesia should be administered only by an anesthesiologist or surgeon who is familiar with its use and possible side effects and subsequently has the patient recover under observation.—G.W. Ostheimer, M.D.

Obstetrical Anesthesia: General Considerations

Recurrent Herpes Simplex Virus Labialis and the Use of Epidural Morphine in Obstetric Patients
Crone L-AL, Conly JM, Clark KM, Crichlow AC, Wardell GC, Zbitnew A, Rea LM, Cronk SL, Anderson CM, Tan LK, Albritton WL (Univ of Saskatchewan)
Anesth Analg 67:318–323, 1988
6–53

In 1985 a possible increase in the frequency of recurrent herpes simplex virus labialis (HSVL) was seen in obstetric patients given epidural doses of morphine for postoperative analgesia after cesarean section at 1 institution. A retrospective study of 291 patients and a prospective study of 729 consecutive patients were begun to analyze this clinical observation.

Thirteen (9.7%) of 134 patients receiving epidural doses of morphine had recurrent oral herpes simplex lesions. Only 1 (0.6%) of 157 patients not receiving the drug had this condition. Opioids in epidural form were administered to 146 of the latter patients. Recurrent HSVL lesions developed in 13 of the 140 given morphine epidurally, for an incidence of 9.3%, but in only 6 of the 583 not given opioids epidurally, for an incidence of 1%. Three of 13 patients with HSVL received both epidural doses of morphine and fentanyl and 10 received only the epidural dose of morphine. Because of the small numbers of patients given only fentanyl, no relationship between HSVL reactivation and epidurally administered fentanyl could be confirmed. The association of recurrent HSVL and the use of morphine epidurally was significant, suggesting that cesarean section was not a confounding factor.

Epidural doses of morphine, a hitherto undescribed triggering agent, apparently were associated with reactivation of HSVL in obstetric patients during the postpartum period.

▶ Well, your editor is not convinced. The difficulty I have with the findings in this study are simply that morphine has been given to patients undergoing cesarean section from the very beginning of the use of cesarean section and, in many cases, very large doses of parenteral morphine have been administered that would produce the same central nervous system concentration as seen with administration of epidural morphine. Heretofore, we have not seen an increase in HSVL in this or any other particular surgical group that has received parenteral morphine.

In our institution, where fentanyl is the most common drug utilized for postoperative pain relief in the obstetric patient, we are not aware of an increase in HSVL. Your editor looks forward to a large prospective study to see whether the authors' initial observations can be substantiated.—G.W. Ostheimer, M.D.

Neuromuscular Transmission Studies in Preeclamptic Women Receiving Magnesium Sulfate

Ramanathan J, Sibai BM, Pillai R, Angel JJ (Univ of Tennessee)
Am J Obstet Gynecol 158:40–46, January 1988   6–54

Intravenous administration of magnesium sulfate is commonly used to prevent convulsions in preeclamptic women. Both animal studies and case reports have documented the occurrence of neuromuscular blockade with consequent potentiation of muscle relaxants during magnesium sulfate administration. However, this neuromuscular transmission defect has not yet been studied in preeclamptic women. A study was done to assess neuromuscular transmission in preeclamptic women while they were receiving magnesium sulfate intravenously to prevent convulsions. The degree of neuromuscular transmission defect was correlated with serum magnesium and calcium concentrations.

The study was done in 14 preeclamptic women who were receiving magnesium sulfate while undergoing induction of labor, 6 preeclamptic women who received magnesium sulfate in the postpartum period, and 10 normotensive controls who were undergoing induction of labor. All patients underwent electromyographic evaluation by standard techniques after measurement of the velocity of motor nerve conduction in the ulnar nerve. Subjects with abnormal nerve conduction were excluded from the study. The patients in the 3 groups were similar in age, height, weight, gravidity, parity, and gestational age.

Preeclamptic patients showed abnormal responses during magnesium sulfate administration that were characterized by an initial low-amplitude muscle action potential followed by a progressive increase in the amplitudes of successive responses. There was a significant correlation in preeclamptic women between the degree of neuromuscular transmission defect and the increase in serum magnesium levels, the decrease in serum calcium levels, and the magnesium-calcium ratio. The highest correlation was between the degree of neuromuscular deficit and the magnesium-calcium ratio during labor (Fig 6–7). All normotensive controls had normal responses to electromyographic testing during magnesium sulfate administration.

The results of this study confirm that neuromuscular transmission in preeclamptic women during magnesium sulfate administration is defective and that the intensity of the transmission defect is correlated significantly with increased serum magnesium levels and decreased serum calcium levels.

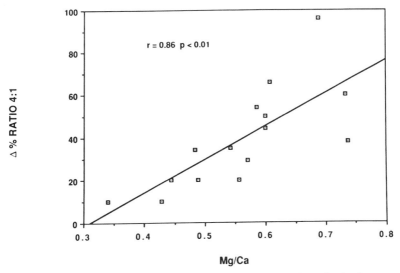

Fig 6–7.—Correlation between degree of neuromuscular transmission defect and ratio of serum concentrations of magnesium and calcium ($r = .86$, $P < .01$). (Courtesy of Ramanathan J, Sibai BM, Pillai R, et al: *Am J Obstet Gynecol* 158:40–46, January 1988.)

▶ This excellent study documents the defect in neuromuscular transmission in patients who receive magnesium sulfate before the administration of muscle relaxants.—R.R. Miller, M.D.

Incidentally Detected Thrombocytopenia in Healthy Mothers and Their Infants

Burrows RF, Kelton JG (McMaster Univ; Canadian Red Cross Transfusion Service, Hamilton, Ontario)
N Engl J Med 319:142–145, July 21, 1988   6–55

The use of automated blood counters for handling routine admission blood samples has led to the identification of thrombocytopenia in numerous asymptomatic pregnant women that would have otherwise gone unnoticed. Some physicians equate a finding of maternal thrombocytopenia with a diagnosis of idiopathic thrombocytopenic purpura, which can affect both mother and child, and recommend delivery by cesarean section for all pregnant women with idiopathic thrombocytopenia. Because the clinical outcome for a mother with unexpected thrombocytopenia and her newborn infant has not yet been determined, a prospective 1-year study was carried out among all women admitted to give birth in the obstetric unit at McMaster University.

Platelet counts were performed on blood samples collected before birth from 2,263 mothers and on neonatal cord blood from 1,350 infants. Thrombocytopenia was defined as a platelet count of less than 150 × 10^9/L. Only 112 asymptomatic women had mild thrombocytopenia ranging from 97 to 150 × 10⁹/L, yielding an 8.3% incidence rate of thromb-ocytopenia. The mild thrombocytopenia had no measurable clinical effect on any of these 112 asymptomatic mothers, and none had excessive bleeding at delivery. The rate of thrombocytopenia for all infants was 4.1 percent, but only 2 infants had a platelet count of less than 50 × 10⁹/L. The frequency of thrombocytopenia among infants born of mothers with mild thrombocytopenia did not differ from that among infants born of mothers with normal platelet counts.

Mild thrombocytopenia among normal pregnant women at term is fairly common and does not seem to affect either the mothers or their infants. To perform cesarean section, merely on a finding of thrombocy-topenia in these mothers, is therefore not justified.

Epidural Anesthesia in Pregnant Patients With Low Platelet Counts
Rolbin SH, Abbott D, Musclow E, Papsin F, Lie LM, Freedman J (Mount Sinai Hosp; St Michael's Hosp, Toronto; Univ of Toronto)
Obstet Gynecol 71:918–920, June 1988   6–56

There is still controversy over the clinical significance of the relatively high incidence of unexplained thrombocytopenia in asymptomatic preg-nant women who are about to give birth. Because a finding of thrombo-cytopenia may affect the choice of anesthetic for use in regional anesthe-sia, platelet counts were performed on blood samples obtained from 686 normal, healthy persons who met the Canadian Red Cross criteria as blood donors and from 2,204 randomly selected, asymptomatic obstetric patients. Women with preexisting conditions usually associated with thrombocytopenia were excluded.

The overall incidence of thrombocytopenia among the 686 controls was 1%. There were 1,621 periparturient women among the 2,204 ob-stetric patients, 104 of whom had unexplained transient thrombocytope-nia, yielding an overall incidence of 6.4%, which was considerably higher than the 1% incidence among the controls. Seventy-four of the 104 thrombocytopenic patients had platelet counts of less than 136 × 10⁹/L.

Sixty-one women with periparturient thrombocytopenia received epi-dural anesthesia; 37 of these received it by the continuous method, whereas the other 24 had a single injection through the epidural needle (table). Epidural anesthesia was refused on the basis of a low platelet count to only 1 patient. None of the women with unexplained thrombo-cytopenia had neurologic complications. In most women the platelet count returned to normal levels within 1 week of delivery. In only 4 women did unexplained thrombocytopenia persist for more than 6 months.

Epidural anesthesia is safe in otherwise healthy pregnant women who became mildly thrombocytopenic when they are about to give birth.

▶ Is there a clinical corollary from these studies for the practicing anesthesiol-ogist? Many obstetric anesthesiologists consider a platelet count of 100,000 to determine whether the parturient should receive a regional anesthetic. How-

Platelet Count Distribution in Patients With
Periparturient Thrombocytopenia

Platelet range	No. of patients	Continuous epidural	Single shot	Total receiving epidural anesthesia
50–74 $\times$ 10^9/L	4	2	0	2
75–99 $\times$ 10^9/L	3	1	0	1
100–125 $\times$ 10^9/L	34	13	4	17
126–150$\times$ 10^9/L	63	21	20	41
Total patients	104	37	24	61

(Courtesy of Rolbin SH, Abbott D, Musclow E, et al: *Obstet Gynecol* 71:918–920, June 1988.)

ever, the literature is replete with studies that demonstrate that a platelet count of greater than 100,000 does not guarantee function and a platelet count of fewer than 100,000 does not guarantee dysfunction. Rolbin et al. (Abstract 6–56) report 104 patients with unexplained transient peripartum thrombocytopenia that was discovered over a 9-month period. Sixty one of the 104 parturients received epidural anesthesia without sequelae. Rolbin et al. defined peripartum thrombocytopenia as a platelet count of fewer than 150,000. However, if we review their patients with a platelet count of fewer than 100,000, there were 7 patients of which 3 received continuous lumbar epidural analgesia without sequelae. Certainly this number of patients is too small to definitively say that we can liberalize our cutoff point for the administration of regional anesthesia. Debate has raged for years on what the cutoff for giving epidural anesthesia is in relation to the number of platelets. However, the number of platelets is not directly related to their function.

The reader is referred to an article by Kelton and associates (*Obstet Gynecol* 65:107–109, 1985) for a review of platelet numbers vs. platelet function in the patient with preeclampsia. It would appear that the generally accepted 100,000 platelets/μl is a good rule of thumb when considering the parturient for an epidural anesthetic. A few patients have fewer than 100,000 platelets/μl, and we obviously have given anesthesia without problems to patients that have fewer than 100,000 platelets/μl of which we were unaware.

Should we consider obtaining a bleeding time on all the patients that have borderline platelet counts? Even with the development of a reasonably reproducible bleeding time technique, its utilization as a sine qua non for the administration of epidural anesthesia is open to question. Certainly, in many institutions, a bleeding time is available from the hematologic laboratory only between 8 A.M. and 5 P.M. Thereafter, it is performed by the intern or resident. Whereas the hematologic technician will do an excellent job that will be reproducible, the physician in training may not pay specific attention to details. The results may be spurious, which directly affect the patient's care. Others have stated that the activated clotting time is an adequate indicator of platelet function and, as such, is used in major cardiovascular cases. However, there is insufficient data at the present time to state that this is the appropriate test for the obstetric patient.

What are we left with as a diagnostic tool to help us ascertain whether to administer a regional anesthetic in patients with marginal platelet counts? Historically, there have been very few epidural or subarachnoid hematomas secondary to epidural or spinal anesthesia in women of childbearing age. One should not proceed with impunity to utilize regional anesthesia in the patient with a borderline platelet count. Adverse occurrences are very rare; however, I think we need to remember the admonition to all anesthesiologists, and that is "to do no harm." A conservative approach would mandate that a patient having a platelet count of 100,000 be further evaluated clinically and hematologically if possible, before the administration of a major regional anesthetic. The anesthesiologist must weigh the pros and cons of administering a block with a platelet count of less than 100,000. Your editor takes a conservative approach with these patients and must be convinced that the administration of a major regional anesthetic in a patient with fewer than 100,000 platelets but with a normal bleeding time is therapeutically in the best interests of the patient. If the reasons to administer regional anesthetic overwhelmingly point to a therapeutic advantage to be gained for the parturient, then it is the responsibility of the individual anesthesiologist to make a decision based on the facts of the matter.

I don't believe there is a difference between administering spinal or epidural anesthesia in a patient with a low but stable platelet count. The typical scenario is that the resident feels that, although the patient's hematologic status is stable, the utilization of a small needle, i.e., 25 or 26 gauge, for the administration of spinal anesthesia will be preferable to the larger needle used for administering the epidural anesthetic. The reader knows what obviously happens. The dural puncture will be bloody and will have to be repeated multiple times before clear fluid is finally obtained, and there goes the rationale for doing a spinal anesthetic with a small needle instead of using a large epidural needle and catheter.

One must always remember that women have had their babies from the beginning of time with a variety of medications for pain relief and that epidural analgesia is an elective procedure that should be administered in the best interest of the patient for delivery. Conversely, general anesthesia can be administered for cesarean delivery if necessary. After weighing the positives and negatives of this approach, one's final decision must always be based on safety for the parturient and the fetus that is about to be born.—G.W. Ostheimer, M.D.

Cardiac Output During Labour

Robson SC, Dunlop W, Boys RJ, Hunter S (Univ of Newcastle Upon Tyne, Freeman Hosp, Newcastle Upon Tyne, England)
Br Med J 295:1169–1172, Nov 7, 1987   6–57

Two thirds of maternal deaths from heart disease occur during or shortly after labor, but the changes in cardiac output at these times are uncertain. To determine the changes in cardiac output during labor and early puerperium, serial measurements of cardiac output and mean arterial pressure were performed in 15 women during the first stage of labor and 1 and 24 hours after delivery. Cardiac output was measured by Doppler and cross-sectional echocardiography at the pulmonary valve, assuming there was no change in pulmonary artery area throughout labor.

Basal cardiac output, as measured between uterine contractions, was increased from a prelabor mean of 6.99 L/minute to 7.88 L/minute at 8 cm of cervical dilatation or greater as a result of an increase in stroke volume. Mean arterial pressure also was increased during this period. During contractions cardiac output was increased further to a mean 10.57 L/minute as a result of an increase in stroke volume and heart rate. The increment in cardiac output became progressively greater as labor advanced. Basal cardiac output was increased by 12% toward the end of labor. Mean arterial pressure was increased further during uterine contractions. One hour after delivery heart rate and cardiac output returned to prelabor values, although mean arterial pressure and stroke volume remained elevated. By 24 hours after delivery all hemodynamic variables had returned to prelabor values.

Hemodynamic changes of this magnitude are of considerable clinical relevance in managing women in labor who have complicated cardiovascular functions.

▶ This is the first study on cardiac output by Doppler and cross-sectional echocardiography. It is refreshing to know that new sophisticated technology has reconfirmed the trends in stroke volume, heart rate, and cardiac output described in previous studies. Hopefully, investigators will reevaluate other physiologic changes in the parturient and either reconfirm or cause a reassessment of previous studies.—G.W. Ostheimer, M.D.

Does Labor Affect the Variability of Maternal Heart Rate During Induction of Epidural Anesthesia?
Chestnut DH, Owen CL, Brown CK, Vandewalker GE, Weiner CP (Univ of Iowa)
Anesthesiology 68:622–625, April 1988   6–58

Several studies have suggested that an increase in maternal heart rate (MHR) is indicative of unintentional intravascular injection of local anesthetic. However, fluctuations in MHR may be related to the cyclic pain of labor. The variability of MHR during induction of epidural anesthesia in women in active labor was compared with MHR in women undergoing elective cesarean section.

The heart rate patterns of 10 women who requested epidural anesthesia during active labor and 10 women electing to receive epidural anesthesia for cesarean section were evaluated. Maternal heart rate was evaluated 10 minutes before and 5 minutes after injection of a test dose of anesthetic; MHR was estimated every 5 seconds during the 15-minute test period.

Successful epidural block was achieved in all patients; therefore, catheters were presumed to have been placed extravascularly within the epidural space. Five women in the labor group, compared with none in the cesarean group, had at least 1 MHR acceleration of at least 25 beats per minute for at least 15 seconds; 2 had 6 accelerations; 1 had 5; 1 had 3; and 1 had 1. Random variance in MHR did not differ significantly between the groups; however, variance associated with 3–5-minute cycles of MHR was significantly greater for the labor group.

Increase in MHR variability during labor appears to be related to cyclic uterine contractions, rather than the lack of preanesthetic medication, pregnancy itself, or intravascular injection.

▶ A wise professor once told me that you are never a prophet in your own church. By this he meant that one can preach a standard of practice and use it successfully, but it takes another investigator or prophet, to get the message across to the reading or listening population. In our Manual of Obstetric Anesthesia it is stated in the section on test-doses for vaginal and cesarean delivery that "All our injections have become test-doses." Following this practice over the last 8 years and after some 40,000 regional anesthetics, we have had 2 transient central nervous system toxic reactions in pregnant women at the Brigham and Women's Hospital with no sequelae. There have been central nervous system manifestations observed after unintentional intravascular injection, and when epinephrine was being administered for cesarean delivery, an increase in pulse or blood pressure has been demonstrated, but not in all cases. We recently found that in a patient on metoprolol there can be an increase in blood pressure without a concomitant increase in heart rate upon the unintentional intravascular injection of an epinephrine-containing solution. Therefore, I am in complete agreement with the authors that every dose given during the initiation or maintenance of epidural analgesia for labor and delivery should be, in effect, a test-dose. And we further agree that the use of epinephrine-containing local anesthetics would be appropriate for cesarean delivery, for which larger amounts of local anesthetic are administered over a short period of time. As is always the case, close attention to the patient is essential for the safe practice of regional analgesia or anesthesia in obstetrics.—G.W. Ostheimer, M.D.

Epidural Analgesia Implies a High Forceps Rate: Can This Be Reduced?
Richmond DH, MacDonald JH, Ryan T (Univ of Liverpool; Mill Road Maternity Hosp, Liverpool, England)
J Obstet Gynaecol 9:24–28, July 1988   6–59

The second stage of labor is considered to be the time when the fetus is at greatest risk from hypoxia and possible trauma from instrumental delivery. Previous studies have reported that epidural analgesia increases the duration of the second stage of labor, leading to a rise in the instrumental delivery rate, particularly rotational delivery. The obstetric outcomes for the 476 patients in labor who received an epidural anesthetic during a 6-month study period were retrospectively reviewed.

Of these 476 patients, 341 (71.6%) had spontaneous vaginal delivery, 110 (23.1%) had occipitoanterior forceps delivery, and 25 (5.3%) had rotational forceps delivery, for a total forceps delivery rate of 28.4%.

None of these patients achieved the second stage and then proceeded to emergency cesarean section. Fifty-nine of the 476 patients had a second stage of at least 3 hours, 33 (55.9%) of whom had a forceps delivery, including 8 (13.5%) rotational deliveries. Three patients delivered infants with low 1-minute Apgar scores. Oxytocin was used to augment labor in 52.8% of the patients, 4 of whom received stimulation within 45 minutes of delivery.

Although the overall forceps delivery rate of 28.4% was low compared with other reported series, the forceps delivery rate increased to well over 50% among women with a second stage of labor lasting for more than 3 hours. Based on these findings, patients in the second stage of labor who have an epidural analgesic in situ, particularly primigravidae, should be examined on an hourly basis. If delivery does not seem imminent, oxytocin to augment labor should be considered, as the results of this retrospective review suggest that a second stage of labor of less than 3 hours may reduce the rate of forceps delivery.

► I agree that epidural analgesia will slightly prolong the first and second stages of labor. Many misinformed obstetricians use this fact to suggest that epidural analgesia should be allowed to wear off in the second stage of labor. On behalf of the parturient, I feel that this is cruel, unusual, and barbaric treatment. In more than 20 years of providing pain relief for laboring women, I have never heard a woman request that her epidural be allowed to completely wear off so that she could have *pain* in order to push more effectively. That concept is a figment of some obstetricians' imaginations. Oxytocin augmentation of uterine contractions will help facilitate the second stage of delivery of labor and delivery of the fetus. Judicious use of fetal scalp capillary pHs, in addition to continuous fetal monitoring, will maintain safety for the fetus. I strongly believe in aggressive obstetric management of the parturient's labor and delivery.— G.W. Ostheimer, M.D.

A Comparative Study of Continuous and Intermittent Epidural Analgesia for Labour and Delivery

Smedstad KG, Morison DH (McMaster Univ)
Can J Anaesth 35:234–241, 1988   6–60

The disadvantage of epidural analgesia administered by intermittent "top-up" doses of local anesthetic in labor and delivery is that analgesia is often allowed to wear off in busy obstetric units, which results in the loss of pain relief. The introduction of safe, accurate mechanical infusion pumps has led to the increased use of continuous epidural analgesia in labor and delivery. The intermittent and continuous routes of administration of epidural anesthesia were compared in 60 healthy primigravid females aged 18–35 years. They were randomly assigned to receive either continuous or intermittent epidural anesthesia. Each patient received an initial injection of 12 ml of 0.25% bupivacaine in divided doses for 10 minutes. One group then received 8 ml of 0.25% bupivacaine per hour using an IVAC 700 Infusion Pump, whereas the other group received 8 ml of 0.25% bupivacaine on an as-needed basis determined by the nurse. Sensory and motor blocks were checked at hourly intervals. Each patient scored her pain on a Visual Analogue Scale on 5 occasions during and after parturition.

Both groups were well matched for age, height, weight, gestation, and length of labor. Patients in both groups had high pain scores before epidural anesthesia was started and significant pain relief after receiving epidural analgesia. Although the patients in the continuous infusion group received significantly more bupivacaine than those in the intermittent administration group, bupivacaine serum levels were lower in the group that received the continuous infusion. However, with such a small number of babies in the study, these concentrations were not considered significant. A number of variables were not controlled or recorded. The incidence of missed segments, degrees of motor block, height of sensory block, length of labor, and fetal outcome were also similar for both groups. Parturients in both groups expressed satisfaction with their pain relief for both labor and delivery.

Epidural anesthesia by continuous infusion pump is as effective in providing satisfactory pain relief as an intermittent top-up regimen.

▶ Continuous epidural analgesia (CEA) has been touted as providing excellent pain relief utilizing a smaller amount of local anesthetic. Clearly the reverse is true in this case, in which more local anesthetic was used. I have used intermittent injection technique for continuous lumbar epidural analgesia for many years and recently have added the utilization of continuous infusions to my practice. Pharmacologically, it stands to reason that continuous infusion of local anesthetic will have the same problems as intermittent technique, that is, unintentional intravascular injection and unintentional subarachnoid administration. The major advantage of CEA is that the local anesthetic concentration can be diminished even more by the addition of a small amount of narcotics. One of the issues to be addressed is the comparison between intermittent and continuous infusions of local anesthetic versus local anesthetic/narcotic mixtures to see whether the amount of local anesthetic can be substantially reduced. Another issue is the question of whether "loading" with narcotic on the initial injection facilitates the continuation of analgesia by the infusion of a dilute anesthetic mixture with narcotic. We continue to make advances to provide pain relief for the parturient during labor and delivery, and we seek the safest method of accomplishing this without jeopardizing the fetus/newborn.—G.W. Ostheimer, M.D.

A Comparative Study of Patient Controlled Epidural Analgesia (PCEA) and Continuous Infusion Epidural Analgesia (CIEA) During Labour
Gambling DR, Yu P, Cole C, McMorland GH, Palmer L (Univ of British Columbia)
Can J Anaesth 35:249–254, 1988   6–61

Patient-controlled analgesia, via the intravenous route, provides optimal postoperative analgesia with less analgesic requirement when compared with more conventional dosing regimes. This method is now used during labor and for postcesarean section analgesia. A randomized, single-blinded, placebo-controlled study was done to compare the level of analgesia provided by continuous infusion epidural analgesia with that of patient-controlled epidural infusions (PCEA) in 25 healthy, nulliparous parturients who were in labor at term. All patients had requested epidural analgesia for labor and delivery.

Fourteen patients were given a background infusion of bupivacaine 0.125% in 4 ml/hour doses with further 4 ml of aliquots by PCEA as required, and 11 patients received continuous infusion of bupivacaine 0.125% in 12 ml/hour doses. Both groups of patients were well matched for age, height, weight, duration and outcome of labor, birth weight, and neonatal Apgar scores. The quality of analgesia was assessed using a visual linear analog scale.

Patients in the PCEA group made more demands for pain relief per hour, as they had to titrate their own analgesia, but overall they required significantly less bupivacaine during labor than did the patients in the group receiving continuous infusion epidural anesthesia. Whereas both groups were satisfied with the anesthesia and pain relief obtained with epidural analgesia, patients in the PCEA group expressed appreciation for being able to control their own pain relief, which rendered them less dependent on the medical staff.

Patient-controlled epidural analgesia is a safe and effective technique of providing optimal analgesia during labor. It allows the patient greater control over her pain relief and requires less local anesthetic than more conventional methods.

▶ We have now seen patient-controlled analgesia used during the postoperative period, in the labor and delivery units, and now for continuous epidural analgesia. There are a number of issues that still need to be addressed with patient-controlled epidural analgesia (PCEA). First and foremost is the question of safety. The pumps must be unable to give an overdose of local anesthetic because of the potential of subarachnoid or intravenous injection. Next, what happens when narcotics are added to either the background solution or the intermittent boluses? And finally, will long-term PCEA present any hazard to the fetus about to be born? Clearly, additional studies are needed to evaluate equipment, drug concentration, and volume (mas) and the maternal and fetal/neonatal effects. Hopefully we will see studies in the immediate future that will assess the use of local anesthetic/narcotic combinations using PCEA.— G.W. Ostheimer, M.D.

Resuscitation in Late Pregnancy
Rees GAD, Willis BA (Univ Hosp of Wales, Cardiff)
Anaesthesia 43:347–349, 1988

Cardiac arrest is rare during late pregnancy, and survival after such an event is unusual unless it occurs during general anesthesia. Several reports of successful resuscitation after immediate cesarean section, which removed aortocaval occlusion, suggest that conventional cardiopulmonary resuscitation in the supine position is unlikely to be successful in obstetric patients at term. An attempt was made to determine whether an effective chest compression force could be applied with the patient inclined to prevent aortocaval compression by the gravid uterus.

To assess the efficacy of resuscitation with the patient at various angles of inclination, a calibrated force transducer was fitted on a plane that could be inclined between 0 and 90 degrees. The transducer was placed at the height of a patient's chest during resuscitation on the ground. Resuscitative force was measured in 8 physician-volunteers at each angle of inclination. Measurements were taken both with hands overlapping and with hands juxtaposed.

The maximum resuscitative force was decreased with increased angle of inclination of the plane. Data were the same for both hand positions. The compression force at an angle of 27 degrees was 80% of that in the supine position. The Cardiff resuscitation wedge was developed as a result of these data. There is a fixed side piece to maintain the patient on the wedge, and the wedge allows easy access for medical personnel. The device is lightweight and portable.

The resuscitation of a pregnant patient at term is problematic and unlikely to be successful unless aortocaval compression by the gravid uterus is relieved. It is practical to apply chest compression forces with the patient inclined at angles of less than 30 degrees. Personnel should be trained in this method.

Complete Maternal and Fetal Recovery After Prolonged Cardiac Arrest
Selden BS, Burke TJ (Alaska Native Med Ctr, Anchorage)
Ann Emerg Med 17:346–349, April 1988   6–63

Complete maternal and fetal recovery after maternal cardiac arrest in pregnancy is rare, and the few reports available deal mostly with perimortem cesarean section, nearly always without successful resuscitation of the mother. Complete maternal and fetal recovery occurred after prolonged cardiac arrest from a massive lidocaine overdose.

Woman, 27, gravida 5, para 2, at 15 weeks' gestation was seen after a minor automobile accident. She had been drinking and had a history of alcohol abuse. Because of increasing ventricular dysrhythmias found on heart monitoring and the possibility of chest trauma, a cardiac contusion was suspected. Immediately after administration of lidocaine, the patient had a grand mal seizure lasting for 1 minute, after which she was apneic and pulseless, despite a normal sinus rhythm. Cardiopulmonary resuscitation was begun and continued for 22 minutes, including 19 minutes of electromechanical dissociation and asystole. A defibrillation attempt with 360 joules converted the patient to a sinus tachycardia at a rate of

200; blood pressure was 150/100 mm Hg. Normal fetal heart function and fetal motion were confirmed by ultrasound immediately after resuscitation.

It was discovered subsequently that the patient had inadvertently been given 1,000-mg of lidocaine intravenously instead of the intended 100-mg dose. This probably explained her seizure and cardiac arrest after injection of the drug. The patient recovered and was delivered of a healthy and neurologically normal infant at 40 weeks' gestation.

Although this is an unusual case, it illustrates that both mother and child may have a good outcome if optimal resuscitation techniques are used even after periods of cardiopulmonary arrest previously thought to be irreversible.

Cardiopulmonary Resuscitation in Late Pregnancy
Oates S, Williams GL, Rees GAD (Univ Hosp of Wales, Cardiff, England)
Br Med J 297:404–405, Aug 6, 1988   6–64

The most recent study of maternal mortality reported that half of all maternal deaths are the direct result of acute causes. In the third trimester of pregnancy, the uterus compresses the aorta and vena cava, which complicates resuscitation.

Woman, 27, gravida 2, para 1, was admitted at 38 weeks' gestation after having collapsed at home about 10 minutes earlier. Her antenatal history had been uneventful, and she had no history of uterine contractions or ruptured membranes. On admission, the patient was deeply cyanotic and apneic and had fixed, dilated pupils and no pulse. Cardiopulmonary resuscitation was initiated, intubation was performed, and a right internal jugular line was inserted. An electrocardiogram showed asystole. She was tilted to the left lateral position, but resuscitation in this position could not be accomplished.

Five minutes after admission, a lower segment cesarean section was performed while the patient was still on the stretcher, and the infant was delivered within 1 minute. The uterus was atonic, and there was no bleeding during operation. Cardiopulmonary resuscitation was continued throughout. Immediately after delivery, the patient developed ventricular fibrillation that was successfully treated by defibrillation.

The results of laboratory testing were consistent with disseminated intravascular coagulation and showed amniotic squames consistent with amniotic fluid embolism. The patient was treated with packed red blood cells, cryoprecipitate, platelets, and fresh frozen plasma. However, severe bilateral pulmonary edema developed 20 hours after operation, necessitating total support until extubation on day 14 when a trascheostomy was inserted. At 16 months after operation, her physical condition was good with minimal weakness on the right side and she was continent of urine and feces, but her mental state remained severely impaired, her speech was poor, and she required constant attendance. The infant was born with no detectable heart rate, but shortly after intubation spontaneous respiration started. His development was normal at 6, 12, and 16 months.

If a pregnant patient in cardiac arrest does not respond after 5 minutes of resuscitation, urgent cesarean section is critical to the survival of the mother and the infant.

▶ These papers (Abstracts 6–62 through 6–64) demonstrate that aggressive cardiopulmonary resuscitation can result in a poor to excellent outcome for the parturient who sustains cardiac arrest. Rees and Willis (Abstract 6–62) have developed a wedge to allow the resuscitators to perform closed chest cardiac massage on the parturient. At the same time, there is uterine deviation to decrease aortocaval compression. Selden and Burke (Abstract 6–63) describe an unusual case but demonstrate that a good outcome can result if aggressive cardiopulmonary resuscitative efforts are undertaken. Anesthesiologists responsible for overseeing the provision of obstetric analgesia/anesthesia in the labor and delivery suite should take it upon themselves to review cardiopulmonary resuscitation of the adult and neonate with labor and delivery personnel on a regular basis. It might be a reasonable thing to stage mock drills on an irregular basis to instill a sense of readiness in obstetric nursing, anesthetic, and pediatric personnel. It is interesting in the second case report that the patient received a massive dose of intravenous lidocaine for cardiac arrhythmias, which is similar to an unintentional intravascular injection of local anesthetic during the administration of epidural anesthesia. Notwithstanding that there are differences between local anesthetics and their effect on the cardiovascular system, this study demonstrates that aggressive resuscitative management can result in a good outcome for both the mother and her fetus.

And finally, Oats and associates (Abstract 6–64) demonstrate that, if initial aggressive cardiopulmonary resuscitation with closed chest cardiac massage, endotracheal intubation, and defibrillation is not immediately successful, emergency cesarean delivery must be accomplished to save the mother and the baby.

A clinical corollary to the above but not to that extreme can be applied to the failed intubation for delivery under general anesthesia. In a number of cases over the years, your editor has found that ventilation of the parturient is much easier once the uterus has been evacuated by cesarean delivery. In the emergency situation in which anesthesia has been induced and intubation cannot be accomplished, I have found that rapid decompression of the abdominal contents has allowed me to effectively ventilate patients who, before delivery, were extremely difficult to ventilate. Obviously, this response has been my experience; everyone must make his or her own judgment in each circumstance.
—G.W. Ostheimer, M.D.

Anesthesia for the Obstetric Patient With Multiple Sclerosis
Bader AM, Hunt CO, Datta S, Naulty JS, Ostheimer GW (Brigham and Women's Hosp, Boston; Harvard Univ)
J Clin Anesth 1:21–24, 1988   6–65

Because the literature contains only limited information on the effects of regional anesthesia on postpartum relapse rates in obstetric patients with multiple sclerosis, a computerized medical records search was performed to identify all patients with multiple sclerosis who had given birth at Brigham and Women's Hospital from 1982 through 1987. The search identified 20 women who had a total of 32 deliveries, including 8 cesarean and 24 vaginal deliveries, after a clinical diagnosis of multiple sclerosis had been established. Eighteen of the 20 women were contacted by mail or by telephone to obtain information on relapses experienced during the first 3 months postpartum. The anesthetic records were reviewed for anesthetic technique used and type and amount of anesthetic drugs administered during delivery. Relapse was defined as any worsening in a patient's neurologic condition, regardless of neurologic location.

Nine of the 32 pregnancies were associated with postpartum relapse, 2 in the cesarean delivery group and 7 in the vaginal delivery group. The incidence of relapse among women who received epidural anesthesia for vaginal delivery was not significantly higher than that among women who received anesthesia using local infiltration or pudendal block. Three women who received bupivacaine in concentrations higher than 0.25% and 2 women who were given 2% lidocaine experienced postpartum relapse.

Although these numbers were too small for meaningful statistical analysis, the findings suggest that the concentration of the anesthetic agent used may influence relapse rates. In view of various other factors such as infection, hyperpyrexia, and emotional stress being known to adversely influence the clinical course of multiple sclerosis, the results of this study cannot be considered evidence that patients who undergo epidural anesthesia have a higher incidence of relapse in the postpartum period than those who do not receive regional anesthesia. Therefore, obstetric patients with multiple sclerosis should not be denied the advantages of epidural anesthesia during labor and delivery.

▶ The world of obstetric anesthesia was saddened recently with the passing of J. ("Jeff") Selwyn Crawford who for many years was considered the leading obstetric anesthetist in the United Kingdom. I had the privilege to visit with Dr. Crawford in the mid-1970s, and at that time, we discussed the administration of epidural analgesia/anesthesia for patients with neurologic disease. We both shared the opinion that there was no reason to deny epidural analgesia to the parturient with a chronic neurologic process, and we doubted whether it made any significant difference in the patient with an acute neurologic process. However, we realized that in our current medicolegal situation someone would look upon the administration of an epidural or a spinal anesthetic in the patient with acute neurologic symptoms as a deviation from good medical practice.

Subsequently, Drs. Warren and Datta and I reported a patient with multiple sclerosis who received lumbar epidural anesthesia (*Anesth Analg* 61:1022– 1023, 1982). A short time thereafter, Dr. Crawford commented in the same journal (62:617–621, 1983) on epidural analgesia for patients with chronic neurologic disease.

In an effort to bring some reason to whether or not to administer an epidural anesthetic to a patient with neurologic disease, specifically, multiple sclerosis,

Dr. Bader and our group reviewed the patients in our newly formed institution, the Brigham and Women's Hospital, by a computerized medical records search for the years 1982–1987 and found the information that has been summarized in the paper. Clearly we feel strongly that the obstetric patient with multiple sclerosis or, in fact, any chronic neurologic disease should not be denied the advantages of epidural analgesia/anesthesia for delivery. The utilization of spinal anesthesia is less clear because the drug is placed directly in the cerebrospinal fluid and may have a more direct impact at higher concentrations on the central nervous tissue. We believe that the risks and benefits must be explained to the parturient so that she can make an informed decision in consultation with her anesthesiologist. One would hope that other institutions with large obstetric services will be able to accumulate more data on situations such as this and publish them so that "old wives" tales about when or when not to use various forms of analgesia/anesthesia can be dispelled.—G.W. Ostheimer, M.D.

Risk of Multiple Sclerosis Exacerbation During Pregnancy and Breast-Feeding

Nelson LM, Franklin GM, Jones MC, the Multiple Sclerosis Study Group (Univ of Colorado Health Sciences Ctr, Denver)
JAMA 259:3441–3443, June 17, 1988   6–66

Previous studies have confirmed that women with multiple sclerosis (MS) are at increased risk of exacerbations of the disease during the postpartum period. To determine whether breast-feeding alters this risks, a study was done with 435 females aged 18–55 years with clinically confirmed MS. All were interviewed with regard to pregnancy and breast-feeding history. Of these 435 mothers, 111 (26%) had given birth to 1 or more children after the onset of MS. Findings in 191 pregnancies were analyzed.

Ninety-six (50%) of the 191 mothers breast-fed their infants. The average duration of breast-feeding was 6.3 months. Thirty-six (37.5%) of the breast-feeding mothers and 29 (30.5%) of the non-breast-feeding mothers experienced postpartum exacerbations of MS. The difference was statistically not significant. The mean time to exacerbation in the breast-feeding group was 3.0 months, and in the non-breast-feeding group, 3.1 months. These findings indicate that breast-feeding does not hasten or delay exacerbations of MS in the postpartum period. Most MS exacerbations in the breast-feeding group occurred before or during the same month as cessation of breast-feeding. Exacerbations were more than 3 times as likely to occur during the 9-month postpartum period as during the pregnancy itself, with the highest risk occurring in the 3-month period immediately after childbirth. The postpartum exacerbation rate reported in this study was 34%, which was comparable to that reported in other studies.

Although exacerbation of MS during pregnancy and the postpartum period both may be related to hormonal effects on the immune system, the hormonal effects of breast-feeding do not seem to similarly affect the risk of MS exacerbation.

▶ The following letter to the editor and reply (*JAMA* 260:2838, Nov 18, 1988) have been submitted as a comment to this article.

To The Editor
We would like to respond to the article by Nelson et al. (1) entitled "Risk of Multiple Sclerosis Exacerbation During Pregnancy and Breast-feeding" in the June 17, 1988, issue of *JAMA.*

An area of major concern to obstetric anesthesiologists is the potential for exacerbation of the symptoms of multiple sclerosis after delivery. Although a correlation between the use of regional anesthesia (epidural and spinal) for labor and delivery has been suggested, no study thus far has demonstrated conclusively the role that regional anesthesia may play in an exacerbation of the disease.

In reviewing the records of all parturients with multiple sclerosis who received regional anesthesia for labor from 1982 through 1987, data at the Brigham and Women's Hospital, Boston, suggest that the choice of anesthetic may indeed affect the course of the disease (2). This remains a controversial area in the practice of anesthesiology, and, unfortunately, there is no clear answer to give the parturient who asks, "Will an epidural cause my multiple sclerosis to worsen?"

Therefore, we were disappointed to note that the study by Nelson et al. failed to mention whether regional anesthesia was used in any of their patients. If some of the patients did receive epidural analgesia while others did not, this adds a variable that must be taken into consideration before the authors can make a positive or negative statement regarding the correlation of exacerbation of multiple sclerosis and breast-feeding itself.

David J. Birnbach, MD
St Luke's-Roosevelt Hospital
New York
Angela Bader, MD
Gerard W. Ostheimer, MD
Brigham and Women's Hospital
Harvard Medical School
Boston

References

1. Nelson LM, Franklin GM, Jones MC, et al: Risk of multiple sclerosis exacerbation during pregnancy and breast-feeding. *JAMA* 1988; 259:3441–3443.
2. Bader AM, Hunt CO, Datta S, et al: Anesthesia for the obstetric patient with multiple sclerosis. *J Clin Anesth*, in press.

In Reply
The effect of spinal anesthesia on exacerbation risk in the postpartum period is one of several obstetrical concerns in multiple sclerosis that deserve rigorous study. Our study did not allow us to address this issue because the data was collected in the context of a larger study in which detailed information regarding labor and delivery was not sought.

As Dr Birnbach and colleagues point out, the studies published to date have not provided strong evidence that spinal anesthesia is a risk factor for disease exacerbations. Most of the published studies on this issue have been small case series that are limited in their generalizability. The most widely cited study of the effect of anesthesia in multiple sclerosis found that one of three women studied who received spinal anesthesia during delivery experienced an exacerbation in the postpartum period (1). This percentage (33%) is almost identical to the postpartum exacerbation rate (34%) obtained in our study for a large unselected group of women with multiple sclerosis. There have been single case reports of disease exacerbations after spinal (2) or epidural (3) anesthesia, but given that one third of all women with multiple sclerosis will have exacerbations in the postpartum period, the occasional case report of an exacerbation in a woman who received spinal anesthesia is not surprising. Dr Birnbach and colleagues cite an article in press that suggests that choice of anesthetic may affect the course of the disease. Even if spinal analgesia is a risk factor for exacerbation in the postpartum period, the major results of our study would be influenced only to the extent that women who breast-feed differ from women who do not breast-feed with regard to their tendency to receive spinal anesthesia.

While we acknowledge that spinal analgesia might have a transient effect on exacerbation risk, we remain convinced that the immunologic changes of pregnancy are largely responsible for the suppression of disease relapses during pregnancy and the "rebound" exacerbations that occur during the postpartum period. Other immunologic disorders (ie, rheumatoid arthritis, systemic lupus erythematosus, and myasthenia gravis) also are characterized by disease suppression during pregnancy and an increased risk of postpartum relapses, which suggest that immunologic phenomena rather than spinal anesthesia is responsible for relapses of immune-mediated disorders in the postpartum period. Pregnancy-related suppression of immune-mediated disorders also is supported by animal studies. Pregnancy has been demonstrated to prevent or inhibit an animal model of demyelinating disease (i.e., experimental autoimmune encephalomyelitis) (4).

It is encouraging that clinicians from a variety of disciplines have interest in the reproductive issues of women with multiple sclerosis. Future studies are warranted that investigate the myriad of factors (immunologic, endocrinologic, and obstetric) surrounding pregnancy and childbirth that could influence the risk of exacerbation.

Lorene M. Nelson, MS
Gary M. Franklin, MD, MPH
Monica C. Jones
Rocky Mountain Multiple Sclerosis Center
University of Colorado Health Sciences Center
Denver

References

1. Bamford C, Sibley W, Laguna J: Anesthesia in multiple sclerosis. *Can J Neurol Sci* 1978; 5:41–44.
2. Keschner M: The effects of injuries and illness on the course of multiple sclerosis: Research publications. *Assoc Nerv Ment Dis* 1950; 28:533–547.

3. Warren TM, Datta S, Ostheimer GW: Lumbar epidural anesthesia in a patient with multiple sclerosis. *Anesth Analg* 1982; 61:1022–1023.
4. Evron S, Brenner T, Abramsky O: Suppressive effect of pregnancy on the development of experimental allergic encephalomyelitis in rabbits. *Am J Reprod Immunol* 1984; 5:109–113.

Combined Epidural Sufentanil and Bupivacaine for Labor Analgesia
Phillips GH (Texas Tech Univ Health Sciences Ctr Lubbock, Tex)
Reg Anesth 12:165–168, October–December 1987   6–67

Epidural administration of local anesthetic during labor usually controls pain well, but unwanted side effects can occur. More dilute local anesthetic solutions might avoid motor block but might also fail to provide analgesia of the same quality as higher concentrations. Combining epidural opioids and local anesthetic solutions may minimize the disadvantages of each agent alone and maximize the benefits. A study was done to determine whether sufentanil, 2 μg/ml, added to epidurally administered bupivacaine, 0.125%, would provide analgesia during labor of a quality comparable to that of bupivacaine, 0.25%.

Fifty patients in labor at term were randomly divided into 2 groups of 25. The first group received epidurally administered bupivacaine, 0.25%, and the second received epidurally administered bupivacaine, 0.125%, with sufentanil, 2 μg/ml. The time to onset and quality of analgesia were comparable in both groups. No motor block was detected among women in the second group, whereas 10 patients in the first group had a mild or moderate degree of motor block. The total dose and the dose rate per hour of bupivacaine were significantly lower in the second group than in the first. Nine patients in the second group complained of mild pruritis. No other significant side effects were encountered.

These findings demonstrate that epidurally administered bupivacaine, 0.125%, combined with sufentanil, 2 μg/ml, can be substituted safely for bupivacaine, 0.25%, for labor analgesia. Patient benefits were minimal motor block and decreased risk of drug toxicity.

▶ Your editor has no problem with the findings of this study; however, I would like to raise the question of how much epidural narcotic is necessary to augment the local anesthetic block in providing effective pain relief. Depending upon the equivalency one applies, 2 μg of sufentanil is equal to 10–20 μg of fentanyl. Whereas the physicochemical characteristics are somewhat different, the higher lipid solubility is the predominant factor governing the dosage of sufentanil. The rapid absorption of this opioid from the epidural space into blood vessels and across the dura into the cerebrospinal fluid and then onto the cord and its opiate receptors required a higher concentration of drug than is necessary with fentanyl. Clearly the effects produced with sufentanil in combination with the local anesthetic in this study can be produced by adding 1–2 μg offentanyl instead to the same concentration of local anesthetic. Therefore the higher dose equivalents of sufentanil required because of the physicochemical characteristics of the drug result in a higher incidence of side effects denoted by an incidence of 45% for pruritus in the bupivacaine and sufentanil group.

In choosing the appropriate narcotic to add to the local anesthetic, one must be cognizant of its physicochemical characteristics, potency, and propensity to produce a side effect in the healthy parturient. Other investigators are looking at various combinations of local anesthetics and lipid soluble opioids with and without epinephrine as a means of providing the best possible analgesia for the patient in labor with little or no motor blockade and, at the same time, keeping the bothersome but not life-threatening side effects to a minimum.—G.W. Ostheimer, M.D.

FURTHER READING

The following articles are recommended to the reader.

1. Doll DC, Ringenberg QS, Yarbro JW: Management of cancer during pregnancy. *Arch Intern Med* 148:2058–2064, September 1988.
2. Field DR, Gates EA, Creasy RK, et al: Maternal brain death during pregnancy: Medical and ethical issues. *JAMA* 260:816–822, Aug 12 1988.
3. Schrier RW: Pathogenesis of sodium and water retention in high-output and low-output cardiac failure, nephrotic syndrome, cirrhosis, and pregnancy: Part I. *N Engl J Med* 319:1065–1072, Oct 20, 1988.
4. Schrier RW: Pathogenesis of sodium and water retention in high-output and low-output cardiac failure, nephrotic syndrome, cirrhosis, and pregnancy: Part II. *N Engl J Med* 319:1127–1134, Oct 27, 1988.

Obstetrical Anesthesia: Fetal Outcome

Survival After Cardiopulmonary Resuscitation in Babies of Very Low Birth Weight: Is CPR Futile Therapy?
Lantos JD, Miles SH, Silverstein MD, Stocking CB (Univ of Chicago)
N Engl J Med 318:91–95, Jan 14, 1988   6–68

Babies of very low birth weight (less than 1,500 gm) account for 50% of all neonatal deaths, even though they represent only 1.15% of all live births in the United States. The relation between mortality and birth weight is shown in Figure 6–8.

True cardiac arrest is relatively rare in neonates. Cardiopulmonary resuscitation (CPR) in the neonatal intensive care unit involves mechanical ventilation and administration of intravenous inotropic agents to neonates with intractable bradycardia and hypotension. Previous studies on survival of neonates after CPR showed an overall rate of 14%, with 7% of babies still alive 1 year after discharge. The outcome of CPR in infants of very low birth weight was studied retrospectively in 158 such infants admitted to a neonatal intensive care unit in 1985. The average birth weight was 1,031 gm and the average gestational age was 28 weeks.

Forty-nine (31%) of 144 viable infants received CPR. All had epinephrine treatment and mechanical ventilation as part of their resuscitation.

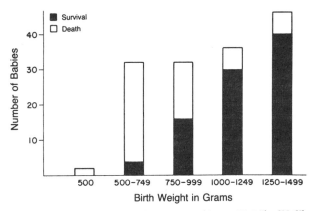

Fig 6–8.—Outcome according to birth weight. (Courtesy of Lantos JD, Miles SH, SIlverstein MD, et al: *N Engl J Med* 318:91–95, Jan 14, 1988.)

Other interventions included atropine, vasopressor infusions, chest compressions, and emergency intubation. The need for CPR was associated with low birth weight, low Apgar scores, birth asphyxia, pulmonary interstitial emphysema, hyaline membrane disease, and severe intraventricular hemorrhage.

Only 4 (8%) of 49 infants who required CPR survived, compared to 83 of 95 (87%) infants who did not require CPR. None of the 38 infants who received CPR during the first 72 hours of life survived, but 4 of 11 who received CPR after the first 72 hours did. Three of these had residual neurologic deficits.

The poor outcome of CPR in the neonatal intensive care unit may reflect both the seriousness of underlying conditions that affect infants of very low birth weight and the aggressiveness of care that these infants receive before initiation of CPR. According to federal legislation passed in 1984, treatment is not legally required if "the provision of such treatment would be virtually futile in terms of the survival of the infant and . . . would be inhumane."

Because survival rates after CPR in infants of very low birth weight are worse than those reported in older children, CPR may be considered a nonvalidated therapy in very-low-birth-weight infants, particularly during the first 72 hours of life. It should not be instituted automatically in very-low-birth-weight infants as though it were a validated treatment, but it can be offered as potentailly life-saving, but experimental, therapy administered upon parents' informed consent.

▶ There is no question that underlying disease may make optimal CPR futile. This report documents the futility of CPR performed in the first 72 hours of life when birth weight is less than 1,500 gm. Such information will facilitate prospective decisions that are most likely to benefit parents and society.—R.K. Stoelting, M.D.

**Effects of Intrapartum Intravenous Infusion of 5% Dextrose or Hartmann's
Solution on Maternal and Cord Blood Glucose**
Loong EPL, Lao TTH, Chin RKH (The Chinese Univ of Hong Kong, Prince of
Wales Hosp, Hong Kong)
Acta Obstet Gynecol Scand 66:241–243, 1987   6–69

Dextrose and Hartmann's solutions are commonly used during labor.
Because glucose homeostasis is essential to the fetus and the expectant
mother, a study was done to assess the effects of intrapartum infusion of
5% dextrose or Hartmann's solution on maternal and cord blood glucose
levels.

Sixteen patients received infusions of 5% dextrose solution, used as a
vehicle for oxytocin; 16 others received Hartmann's solution before epidurally administered analgesia; the 16 controls received no fluids intravenously before delivery. None of the patients had experienced significant
complications during pregnancy. At delivery, the umbilical cord was
clamped and blood samples were taken from the umbilical vein. Maternal blood samples were collected at delivery or soon after from the ante-
cubital vein of the contralateral arm. The 3 groups were comparable in
maternal age, parity, gestation at delivery, and birth weight.

The mean maternal blood glucose concentration was higher than the
mean cord blood concentration for all 3 groups. The difference was statistically significant in the dextrose and the control groups, but not in the
Hartmann group. The mean maternal blood glucose concentration in the
Hartmann group was significantly lower than that in the dextrose and control groups. However, cord blood glucose concentrations did not differ significantly between the 3 groups. The volume of Hartmann's solution administered was significantly greater than that of 5% dextrose solution, but
none of the patients received more than 1.2 L of either solution.

These results indicate that maternal infusion of 5% dextrose or Hartmann's solution in routine intrapartum management does not adversely
affect fetal blood glucose levels.

**Euglycemic Hydration With Dextrose 1% in Lactated Ringer's Solution
During Epidural Anesthesia for Cesarean Section**
Peng ATC, Shamsi HH, Blancato LS, Shulman SM, Chervenak FA, Castro JL (St
Luke's–Roosevelt Hosp Ctr, New York; Columbia Univ)
Reg Anesth 12:184–187, October–December 1987   6–70

Rapid intravenous loading with a crystalloid solution before epidural
anesthesia for cesarean section is an accepted method of preventing maternal hypotension. However, massive maternal glucose administration
from using glucose or dextrose in the infusate can lead to maternal hyperglycemia, which can be deterimental to the infant. Total absence of
glucose is also undesirable. The effects of 3 glucose concentrations administered intravenously to precesarean patients on neonatal umbilical
glucose levels were investigated.

Thirty women undergoing elective cesarean section were randomly assigned to 1 of 3 groups of 10. Group A received Ringer's lactate, 1,000 ml; group B received dextrose 1% in Ringer's lactate, 1,000 ml; and group C received dextrose 5% in Ringer's lactate, 1,000 ml. Umbilical artery glucose levels were 46.8 ± 13.8 mg/dl in group A; 79.1 ± 19 mg/dl in group B; and 207.1 ± 45.9 mg/dl in group C. Two neonates in group C in whom umbilical artery glucose was very high later developed hypoglycemic seizures. In contrast, dextrose 1% in Ringer's lactate infusion resulted in euglycemic levels.

The use of dextrose 1% in Ringer's lactate, 1,000 ml, for rapid loading is a simple technique for euglycemia hydration. This solution appears to be optimal in maintaining maternal and fetal euglycemia before delivery.

► The study by Loong (Abstract 6–69) reemphasizes that the intrapartum administration of small amounts of glucose to the laboring parturients does not have a negative effect on the neonate whereas rapid infusion of large amounts of glucose will cause maternal hyperglycemia and secondary fetal hyperglycemia, which after delivery may develop into neonatal hypoglycemia and, possibly, acidosis. Peng and associates (Abstract 6–70) demonstrate that using small amounts of dextrose, i.e., 1% dextrose in lactated Ringer's, does not have this effect after rapid intravenous loading before cesarean section. Unfortunately, I am not aware that 1% dextrose in lactated Ringer's solution is commercially available. Hopefully, further investigations will demonstrate whether these preliminary findings are significant enough to warrant the commercial development of such a solution.—G.W. Ostheimer, M.D.

The Relationships Among the Fetal Biophysical Profile, Umbilical Cord pH, and Apgar Scores
Vintzileos AM, Gaffney SE, Salinger LM, Kontopoulos VG, Campbell WA, Nochimson DJ (Univ of Connecticut, Farmington)
Am J Obstet Gynecol 157:627–631, September 1987   6–71

The fetal biophysical profile is the most accurate single antepartum test for fetal compromise, partly because of the combination of acute and chronic markers of fetal condition. The relationship among the profile, umbilical cord blood pH, and Apgar scores were examined in a prospective series of 124 pregnant patients at 26–43 weeks' gestation who underwent section delivery of single infants. The patients had intact membranes and were not in labor. Infants with congenital anomalies were excluded.

The mean gestational age was 34 weeks. The fetal biophysical profile score was 8 or higher for 82% of patients. When a criterion of umbilical cord arterial pH less than 7.20 was used to diagnose fetal acidosis, the fetal biophysical profile score was 90% sensitive and 96% specific. The positive and negative predictive values were 82% and 98%, respectively. By using the combination of a nonreactive nonstress test and absent fetal breathing, the test was 100% sensitive and 92% specific, but its positive predictive value was only 71%. The profile was more sensitive than the 1- and 5-minute Apgar scores in detecting fetal acidosis.

The fetal biophysical profile is significantly related to fetal acid-base status at the time of testing. A nonstress test or assessment of fetal breathing is preferred, as is a determination of the amniotic fluid volume. In more than 6,500 cases studied in 4 years no fetal deaths of structurally normal fetuses have occurred within a week of a reassuring biophysical assessment.

▶ We know that the Apgar score is a poor predictor of outcome for the new-born. For some unexplained reason, obstetricians have been reluctant to use the scalp capillary blood pH as a further assessment of abnormal fetal heart rate patterns during labor. The fetal biophysical profile offers a noninvasive way to assess the fetus before and during labor that may help the clinician evaluate the fetal condition. In this study, the authors demonstrate a strong relationship between the fetal biophysical profile and the fetal acid-base status at the time of delivery. Although the authors are known as strong proponents of the use of the fetal biophysical profile, the evidence appears to be mounting that ultrasonic fetal evaluation is a tool that should be in the armamentarium of the practicing obstetrician.— G.W. Ostheimer, M.D.

Perinatal Brain Damage: Predictive Value of Metabolic Acidosis and the Apgar Score
Ruth VJ, Raivio KO (Univ of Helsinki)
Br Med J 297:24–27, July 2, 1988   6–72

Perinatal asphyxia is an important cause of morbidity and mortality in the newborn infant and of neurologic disability in later life. The incidence of asphyxia and its role in outcome are difficult to assess because no reliable diagnostic criteria have as yet been identified. The Apgar score has a poor sensitivity for predicting neurologic damage because of asphyxia. Measurement of the blood pH in the umbilical artery is now routinely used to assess asphyxia and fetal distress. Whether acidosis at birth and the 5-minute Apgar score have predictive value for perinatal brain damage was studied during a 2-month period in 982 infants.

Arterial acid-base values were determined for 964 of these infants, and lactate concentrations were measured in 931. Of these infants, 111 (12%) had acidosis, 70 (7%) had a high base deficit, 83 (9%) had high lactate concentrations, and 32 (3%) had low 5-minute Apgar scores. Twelve (11%) of the 111 infants with acidosis had low Apgar scores, and 12 (41%) of the 29 infants with low Apgar scores had acidosis.

After 1 year of follow-up, 35 of the 982 study infants could not be traced, 22 had an adverse outcome unrelated to asphyxia, and 883 (95%) showed normal development. The remaining 42 infants had an adverse outcome, probably caused by asphyxia. Four of the 42 infants had died, 28 showed slightly abnormal development, and 10 showed clearly abnormal development.

The sensitivity of perinatal acidosis for an adverse outcome was 21%, and the positive predictive value was 8%. High lactate concentration had a sensitivity of 12% and a predictive value of 5%. A low 5-minute Apgar score had a sensitivity of 12% and a predictive value of 19%. Metabolic acidosis determined in blood from the umbilical artery at birth is a poor predictor of perinatal brain damage.

▶ We know from the American cooperative perinatal project of 1959–1966 that the Apgar score at 5 minutes after birth is a poor predictor of neurologic damage due to asphyxia. Investigators have searched for a better means to predict the development of perinatal brain damage and have looked at a variety of markers, including metabolic acidosis. This study demonstrates that we still do have an accurate predictor of perinatal brain damage from the perinatal period. The fetus and newborn are resistant to the development of neurologic damage in many instances. However, this resistance must not be counted upon to protect the newly born. Every newborn deserves aggressive cardiopulmonary resuscitation by trained personnel unless there is overwhelming evidence of the presence of lethal congenital abnormalities.—G.W. Ostheimer, M.D.

Intrapartum Asphyxia: A Rare Cause of Cerebral Palsy
Blair E, Stanley FJ (Univ of Western Australia, Queen Elizabeth II Med Ctr, Nedlands, Australia)
J Pediatr 112:515–519, April 1988   6–73

Several studies have questioned the association between cerebral palsy (CP) and birth asphyxia. To investigate this relationship, data on perinatal events in 183 children with spastic CP were compared with those on such events in 549 control children matched for year of birth (between 1975 and 1980) and closely for birth weight. All were born in Western Australia. The likelihood that birth asphyxia caused the perinatal brain damage was assessed by 2 independent observers who used defined criteria.

There was a significant relationship between birth asphyxia and spastic CP (relative risk, 2.84; 95% confidence interval, 1.85–4.37). This was strongest in infants who weighed more than 1,500 gm at birth. However, the overall population-attributable risk proportion, which is an estimate of the expected reduction in spastic CP if all perinatal signs that are associated with asphyxia are eliminated, was 14.1%. Furthermore, it was estimated that in only 8.2% of all children with spastic CP was intrapartum asphyxia the possible cause of their brain damage.

Intrapartum events and obstetric mismanagement probably contribute less to overall CP rates than was previously thought. It appears that CP is not a good measure of intrapartum care as currently practiced.

▶ The title of this paper, "Intrapartum Asphyxia: A Rare Cause of Cerebral Palsy," is somewhat misleading. Clearly there is a significant relationship between birth asphyxia and spastic cerebral palsy, and it is strongest in infants heavier than 1,500 gm at birth. However, the majority of patients with spastic CP did not have any evidence of intrapartum or perinatal asphyxia resulting in brain damage, which has been documented in a number of other recent studies. Thus cerebral palsy can not be used as evidence for intrapartum asphyxia, and other causes (genetics, neurologic abnormalities, etc.) must be considered.— G.W. Ostheimer, M.D.

Motor and Cognitive Deficits After Intrapartum Asphyxia in the Mature Fetus
Low JA, Galbraith RS, Muir DW, Killen HL, Pater EA, Karchmar EJ (Queens Univ, Kingston, Ont)
Am J Obstet Gynecol 158:356–361, February 1988   6–74

The theory of a continuum of casualty with regard to fetal asphyxia postulates that a small amount of asphyxia causes little damage and a larger amount causes more severe damage. The range of major and minor motor or cognitive deficits was assessed at 1 year of age in 37 mature children who had experienced an intrapartum fetal asphyxial insult; the findings were compared with those in 76 children who had no evidence of fetal asphyxia at delivery. The criterion of intrapartum fetal asphyxia was evidence of metabolic acidosis at delivery, as expressed by an umbilical artery buffer base of less than 34 mmole/L.

The incidence of major deficits (14%) and minor deficits (27%) in infants with asphyxia was significantly greater than that in controls. Major deficits were characteristic of cerebral palsy, accompanied in some cases by mental retardation. Minor deficits were characteristically motor developmental delays with apparently satisfactory cognitive development. A distinct number of these children were unable to roll over from the supine to the prone position, suggesting a deficiency of shoulder girdle or truncal motor function. The severity of metabolic acidosis was correlated with the presence of deficits at 1 year of age, and was most striking when the umbilical artery buffer base was no more than 20 mmole/L. There was a trend toward an increased incidence of fetal growth retardation in children with deficits.

These results provide evidence for a continuum of casualty with regard to morbidity as a result of intrapartum fetal asphyxia.

▶ The findings in this study clearly take issue with those of the previous study (Abstract 6–73) in that these investigators did find that the severity of metabolic acidosis demonstrated in umbilical artery blood was correlated with the presence of motor and cognitive deficits in these children at 1 year of age. The authors suggest a continuum of morbidity related to increasing fetal asphyxia. Whether the analysis of umbilical arterial blood for metabolic derangement will predict the future development of abnormalities in the newborn is still open to conjecture. Clearly our efforts should be directed toward preventing intrauterine and intrapartum birth asphyxia from whatever cause. Since we are unable to predict the duration of hypoxia in almost all cases in which asphyxia is present at birth, it behooves the listener to remember when faced with the depressed newborn that aggressive cardiopulmonary resuscitation can often make the difference between a child that will develop neurologic abnormalities and one that may not.—G.W. Ostheimer, M.D.

Umbilical Cord Acid Base Changes Associated With Perinatal Cardiac Failure
Brar HS, Wong MK, Kirschbaum TH, Paul RH (Univ of Southern California)
Am J Obstet Gynecol 158:511–518, March 1988   6–75

Electronic fetal heart rate monitoring is widely used in the management of obstetric patients. Acceleration of fetal heart patterns during labor is commonly associated with fetal well-being. In 2 patients intrapartum fetal heart rate monitoring failed to detect fetal distress.

Case 1.—Woman, 24, primigravida, presented in labor with 1-cm dilation and the fetus in a breech position. Fetal heart rate monitoring documented a baseline fetal heart rate of 140 to 145 beats per minute with average variability and uterine contractions every 3 to 6 minutes. As labor progressed, the fetal heart rate tracing demonstrated occasional accelerations over the baseline heart rate. Four hours after admission, oxytocin infusion was started because of inadequate contractions. The fetal heart rate remained unchanged with periodic accelerations until 10 hours after admission, when a variable deceleration of fetal heart rate to 95 beats per minute was noted. A direct fetal electrocardiogram revealed a momentary fetal heart rate of 140–145 beats per minute, followed by an abrupt drop to 30–40 beats per minute. Fetal bradycardia did not resolve with oxygen administration. Cesarean section was performed, and a 2,500-gm infant was delivered within 13 minutes after onset of bradycardia. Neonatal resuscitation failed to save the infant, which was pronounced dead 20 minutes after birth. Umbilical cord blood gas analysis revealed moderate predominantly metabolic acidosis. Postmortem examination showed cardiac dilation and moderate to severe chronic cardiac failure.
Case 2.—Woman, 25, primigravida, presented in labor at 42.5 weeks' gestation with a history of leaking amniotic fluid for 2 days and a temperature of 101.2 F. The baseline fetal heart rate was 110–120 beats per minute with decreased to absent variability and repetitive late decelerations. The scalp pH was 6.7. A 3,280-gm infant was delivered by emergency cesarean section but died 16 hours after birth. Neonatal echocardiography revealed large dilated left and right ventricles. Postmortem examination confirmed cardiac dilatation and hypertrophy consistent with cardiac failure. Umbilical cord values were indicative of mixed metabolic and respiratory acidosis.

In both infants, there was a wide difference in values between umbilical arterial and venous blood, with umbilical venous blood values approaching those of maternal uterine venous blood. Such findings appear to be associated with perinatal cardiac failure. Both umbilical venous and arterial blood samples should be obtained to assess fetal acid-base status.

▶ I thought that the umbilical arterial and venous blood were always sampled at the time of delivery. Apparently that is not so in many institutions, and therefore the recommendation of the authors that both vessels be sampled at the time of delivery is sound advice for every obstetric unit to heed. Hopefully, obstetricians will attempt to obtain a long portion of the umbilical cord in order to make umbilical arterial sampling easier—G.W. Ostheimer, M.D.

Cesarean Section-Related Maternal Mortality in Massachusetts, 1954–1985
Sachs BP, Yeh J, Acker D, Driscoll S, Brown DAJ, Jewett JF (Harvard Univ; Brigham and Women's Hosp, Boston)
Obstet Gynecol 71:385–388, March 1988   6–76

The cesarean section rate has increased markedly in this country during the past 2 decades, and presently nearly 1 in 4 infants is born by cesarean section. Maternal mortality data were analyzed in Massachusetts for the period 1954–1985. The number of deaths directly due to cesarean section per 100,000 live births did not change significantly during this period. The section delivery rate rose from about 5% in 1954 to 23.4% in 1984. Half the deaths directly due to section delivery were considered preventable. In 1976–1984, the rate of deaths directly related to section delivery was 5.8 per 100,000 sections, compared with 10.8 deaths per 100,000 vaginal deliveries.

This survey, which excluded deaths due to ectopic pregnancy and septic abortion, showed a low risk of maternal death from cesarean section. The risk can probably be further reduced, but the morbidity associated with section delivery justifies efforts to lower the cesarean section rate. The risk of maternal morbidity from cesarean section remains much higher than that associated with vaginal delivery.

▶ Unfortunately studies of this nature are becoming more difficult to perform because of the threat of medical malpractice. Dr. John F. Jewett, Chairman of the Committee on Maternal Welfare of the Massachusetts Medical Society had extraordinary cooperation from clinicians and institutions in the state during his tenure because the stated purpose of the committee was to educate rather than to discipline physicians and institutions. In many cases, notification of a maternal death was made by the obstetrician, the institution at which it occurred, or both. Simultaneously, information was also provided by the state department of health.

In 1963, the Commonwealth of Massachusetts enacted legislation to help prevent the misuse, in cases of litigation, of information pertaining to the Committee's proceedings. The Committee, after its investigation, would determine whether the death was preventable, and if so, an assessment of probable responsibility was made regarding the physicians involved, the patient, the hospital, or a combination thereof. The Committee's report was then shared with the physicians involved. On occasion, very informative cases were presented, for their educational value, in the *New England Journal of Medicine*. Dr. Jewett's incisive and often acerbic analysis was extremely instructive, with the objective being education and, hopefully, prevention of similar future occurrences. Interestingly, the leading cause of death was pulmonary embolism, as was recently demonstrated in several other studies. Unfortunately, anesthesia contributed to a number of deaths in this study.

Finally, the risk of maternal death attributable to cesarean delivery is very low in Massachusetts commpared with prior studies in other states and countries. As with any operative procedure there is a certain mortality, and this obviously could be decreased by reducing the overall rate of operative deliveries. With the present medicolegal climate, in which to perform a cesarean delivery is to do all you can for the mother and her fetus, one must wonder whether a reduction in cesarean deliveries will occur.—G.W. Ostheimer, M.D.

Anesthesia-Related Maternal Mortality in Michigan, 1972 to 1984
Endler GC, Mariona FG, Sokol RJ, Stevenson LB (Wayne State Univ; Hutzel Hosp, Detroit; Harper/Grace Hosp, Detroit)
Am J Obstet Gynecol 159:187–193, July 1988   6–77

Maternal mortality in the United States and other industrialized nations has declined during recent decades, but anesthesia-related maternal mortality has decreased to a lesser degree. Data on maternal deaths occurring from 1972 through 1984 in the state of Michigan were reviewed to identify all of those in which anesthesia was either the primary cause or a contributory factor.

Fifteen maternal deaths occurred in which anesthesia was the primary cause of death, accounting for 6.9% of direct maternal deaths, or 0.82/100,000 live births; in 4 maternal deaths anesthesia was considered a contributory factor. Causes of deaths attributable to anesthesia included pulmonary complications in 1 patient, cardiac complications in 9, central nervous system complications in 2, and reactions to spinal or lumbar puncture in 3 patients (table).

Fourteen of the 15 patients had 1 or more of several complicating factors known to increase the risk of anesthesia. Twelve (80%) patients were obese, 5 morbidly so, i.e., twice their normal weight. Anesthesia was administered to 12 (80%) patients under emergent conditions, including 11 who required cesarean section. Eight (53%) patients were hypertensive. Only 1 patient had none of the above-cited risk factors; she died of a reaction to epidural anesthesia. Thirteen deaths occurred in black patients and 2 deaths occurred in white patients, resulting in an anesthesia-related maternal mortality rate 30 times higher in black patients compared with white patients. The reason for the increased mortality among black patients could not be identified clearly, but the darker complexion of black patients may have masked the onset of cyanosis. Complications of regional anesthesia were the main cause of death during the early part of the study period,

Causes of Deaths Attributable to Anesthesia

ICD-9-CM Code	Complications	No. of deaths	Subtotal
668.0	Pulmonary complications		1
	Inhalation of stomach content	1	
668.1	Cardiac complications		9
	Cardiac arrest	6	
	Cardiac arrest resulting from aberrant placement of endotracheal tube	2	
	Cardiac arrest resulting from failure to place endotracheal tube	1	
668.2	Central nervous system complications		2
	Cerebral anoxia	2	
349.0	Reactions to spinal or lumbar puncture	3	3
Total			15

(Courtesy of Endler GC, Mariona FG, Sokol RJ, et al: *Am J Obstet Gynecol* 159:187–193, July 1988.)

whereas the inability to accomplish endotracheal intubation was the principal cause of death in more recent years.

Among the many specific steps that can be taken to improve the safety of anesthesia, several appear particularly pertinent, including the assignment of well-rested anesthesia personnel to the obstetric unit during off-hours and provision of around-the-clock coverage by anesthesiologists who have an interest and experience in obstetric anesthesia.

▶ Michigan is another one of the states that has done an excellent job of assessing maternal mortality. I can only echo the conclusions of the authors that adequately trained and rested anesthesia personnel must be assigned to the obstetric unit and hospitals must provide around-the-clock coverage by anesthesiologists who have an interest, experience, and expertise in obstetric anesthesia.—G.W. Ostheimer, M.D.

Obstetrical Anesthesia: Cesarean Delivery

Neonatal Status in Relation to Incision Intervals, Obstetric Factors, and Anesthesia at Cesarean Delivery

Andersen HF, Auster GH, Marx GF, Merkatz IR (Albert Einstein College of Medicine, New York)
Am J Perinatol 4:279–283, October 1987   6–78

The interval between uterine incision and delivery is thought to be critical to the immediate condition of the newborn infant delivered by cesarean section. Although it was believed previously that long intervals between anesthesia induction and delivery resulted in a depressed, anesthetized infant, later studies suggested that the time interval from uterine incision to delivery is a more critical parameter. However, the many obstetric factors other than anesthesia that may influence neonatal outcome were not taken into account in those earlier studies.

Stepwise multiple linear regression analysis was used to identify the relative contributions of the interval from skin incision to delivery, the interval from uterine incision to delivery, and other obstetric and anesthetic factors to the newborn infant's birth weight, Apgar scores, and umbilical cord blood gas volume. The study population included 204 evaluable patients delivered by cesarean section.

Labor complications, infant birth weight, surgical technique, and type of anesthesia significantly influenced Apgar scores and umbilical cord blood gas volumes, whereas skin incision and uterine incision to delivery intervals did not significantly affect either Apgar scores or umbilical cord blood gases.

Careful evaluation of maternal status before cesarean delivery, optimal anesthetic management, and gentle, atraumatic surgical technique are the most important factors affecting immediate neonatal status at cesarean delivery.

▶ The authors suggest that careful attention to maternal status and optimal treatment of maternal complications before cesarean delivery are the most important factors in the immediate neonatal status at the time of delivery. Subsequently they go on to discuss some of the obstetric problems that can occur and that would lead to newborn depression, such as an inadequate uterine incision to deliver the fetus. As one of the authors of one of the papers to which they referred in their introduction, I can state that a relationship existed between neonatal depression and prolonged uterine incision-to-delivery intervals in healthy mothers and newborns. Andersen and associates have failed to take into account the consideration under which different studies were performed. Our conclusion that increased uterine incision-to-delivery intervals produced a tendency toward acidosis was, and we believe still is, true for a healthy population. Certainly, if we consider all patients, or just high-risk patients, then other compounding variables enter the equation. We appreciate that our initial work, along with Dr. Jeff Crawford's work, has spurred on these investigators to look at the obstetric and anesthesia practices in their institution. Hopefully, other institutions will follow suit to demonstrate the variables that affect neonatal outcome in their practices.— G.W. Ostheimer, M.D.

Bupivacaine Disposition in Mother, Fetus, and Neonate After Spinal Anesthesia for Cesarean Section
Kuhnert BR, Zuspan KJ, Kuhnert PM, Syracuse CD, Brown DE (Cleveland Metropolitan Gen Hosp, Cleveland; Case Western Reserve Univ)
Anesth Analg 66:407–412, May 1987   6–79

Nationally, spinal anesthesia is the preferred regional anesthetic method for cesarean section. Maternal blood levels have been assumed to be low or undetectable. However, detectable levels of lidocaine in maternal and fetal plasma at delivery after subarachnoid injection have been found. The disposition of bupivacaine, more highly protein bound than lidocaine, and its metabolite in maternal, fetal, and neonatal plasma and in neonatal urine after spinal anesthesia for elective cesarean section was determined.

Six pregnant women and their infants were studied. Maternal plasma levels were 59 ± 32 ng/ml, only about 5% of those found in a previous study of epidural anesthesia. Mean plasma umbilical venous bupivacaine levels were 20.2 ± 21 ng/ml, or 7% of those found after epidural anesthesia. Mean umbilical venous/maternal venous bupivacaine ratios were 0.34 ± 0.12, and mean umbilical arterial/umbilical ratios were 0.81 ± 0.3. No bupivacaine could be detected in neonatal plasma 24 hours after delivery. For at least 36 hours after delivery, neonatal urine had measurable levels of both bupivacaine and its inactive metabolite.

Bupivacaine crosses the placenta and reaches the fetus, but only in very small amounts. Transplacental passage occurs despite injection of small doses of a highly protein-bound drug into the subarachnoid space.

▶ A nicely done study that continues the authors' work to delineate the metabolism of local anesthetics in the parturient and newborn. The only thing missing from this study is the neurobehavioral evaluation of the newborn. Previous studies have demonstrated no known neurobehavioral effects from these concentrations of bupivacaine in patients receiving epidural anesthesia; however, it would have been nice to have that correlation in this group of patients.—G.W. Ostheimer, M.D.

Epidural Anesthesia With Fentanyl and Lidocaine for Cesarean Section: Maternal Effects and Neonatal Outcome

Preston PG, Rosen MA, Hughes SC, Glosten B, Ross BK, Daniels D, Shnider SM, Daily PA (Univ of California, San Francisco)
Anesthesiology 68:938–943, June 1988   6–80

Epidurally administered lidocaine is widely used for local anesthesia during cesarean delivery. However, some patients still experience discomfort with 2% lidocaine and require supplemental medication. Clinical studies have shown that the addition of fentanyl to lidocaine administered epidurally after delivery of the neonate improves maternal comfort during the latter part of cesarean section. A randomized, double-blind study was carried out to determine the effects on maternal comfort and on the newborn infant when fentanyl is added to 2% lidocaine at the onset of epidural blockade.

The study population consisted of 30 healthy women who were undergoing elective cesarean section. At the start of the procedure, 15 women received epidural anesthesia with 2% lidocaine and saline, whereas the other 15 patients received 2% epidural lidocaine with fentanyl anesthesia. Intraoperative pain was treated with supplemental epidural administration of 2% lidocaine. Analgesics and sedatives were administered intravenously if relief was still not obtained. Each patient was asked to rate her surgical pain on a 4-point pain scale at predetermined intervals.

Patients who were administered fentanyl and lidocaine epidurally experienced a significant decrease in moderate and severe pain during the operation compared with control patients. Pain relief lasted from incision to peritoneal closure. Additional requirements for supplemental intraoperative medication were significantly reduced in the epidural fentanyl group. There was no difference in the condition of the neonates after delivery by cesarean section with either epidurally administered lidocaine alone or with fentanyl plus lidocaine.

Maternal epidural fentanyl administration at the onset of epidural anesthesia for elective cesarean section augments the analgesic effectiveness of 2% lidocaine without significant maternal or fetal side effects.

▶ Additional work in our institution supports the conclusion of these investigators. Hopefully, future investigations will look at the other lipid soluble opiates, sufentanil and alfentanil, for possible use in this manner.—G.W. Ostheimer, M.D.

Influence of Epinephrine on the Spread of 0.75% Bupivacaine in Epidural Anesthesia for Cesarean Section
Carvalho JCA, Mathias RS, Senra WG, Cremonesi E (Univ of São Paulo, Brazil)
Reg Anesth 13:91–93, April–June 1988   6–81

The quality and duration of epidural anesthesia after the addition of epinephrine to the anesthetic solution have been widely studied, but the impact of epinephrine on the extent of epidural blockade has not previously been evaluated. This study was carried out before the FDA's issued warnings against the use of 0.75% bupivacaine solutions in obstetrics.

The study population comprised 406 term pregnant women who underwent elective cesarean section under epidural anesthesia. One hundred twenty-nine patients were injected epidurally with 20 ml of a 0.75% bupivacaine solution, 97 patients received a 0.75% bupivacaine solution to which epinephrine 1:400,000 had been added, and 180 patients were given a bupivacaine solution containing epinephrine 1:200,000. The level of sensory blockade was determined by pinprick at 10-minute intervals along each midclavicular line until peak cephalad spread was obtained, usually 30–60 minutes after epidural injection. The total number of blocked segments and the number of blocked segments above the puncture site were recorded for each patient. Multivariate analysis of variance was used to correct the data for age, height, weight, body mass index, and gestational age, as these factors are known to influence the spread of anesthetic solution.

The total number of blocked segments and the number of blocked segments above the puncture site were greatest in the group that received bupivacaine with epinephrine 1:200,000 solution. The total number of blocked segments and the number of blocked segments above the puncture site in the other 2 groups were similar.

The addition of epinephrine 1:200,000 to 0.75% bupivacaine solution used for epidural anesthesia in term pregnant patients undergoing elective cesarean section resulted in greater extension of the sensory blockade. The addition of epinephrine 1:400,000 to bupivacaine solution did not affect the spread of epidural blockade in this particular study population. It is suggested that the reduction of local anesthetic absorption could account for these results.

▶ The effect of epinephrine on local anesthetics administered into the epidural space has been a subject of investigation and discussion over many years. In this study, the authors demonstrate that epinephrine, perhaps by decreasing the absorption of the local anesthetic, allows more molecules to act on nervous tissue and provides analgesia/anesthesia. The clinical importance of this study lies in the demonstration that 1:200,000 epinephrine potentiates the effect of local anesthesia, whereas higher dilutions of epinephrine appear to have no effect.—G.W. Ostheimer, M.D.

Maternal Hemodynamic Responses to Epinephrine-Containing Local Anesthetics in Mild Pre-eclampsia

Dror A, Abboud TK, Moore J, Swart F, Mosaad P, Davis H, Gangolly J, Mantilla M, Makar A, Zaki N (Los Angeles County–Univ of Southern California Med Ctr, Los Angeles)
Reg Anesth 13:107–111, July–September 1988   6–82

Epinephrine is often omitted from anesthetic solutions used for epidurally administered anesthesia in preeclamptic patients for fear of excessive hypertension and possible adverse effects on uterine activity and uterine blood flow. Because actual occurrence of hypertension in preeclamptic patients has never been documented, a double-blind, randomized study was conducted to assess maternal hemodynamic responses to epinephrine during epidural anesthesia for labor and delivery.

Thirty mildly preeclamptic patients were studied, including 16 who received 1.5% lidocaine with 1:200,000 epinephrine added, and 14 who received plain 1.5% lidocaine. All patients had ruptured membranes. Monitored parameters included maternal blood pressures and heart rates, fetal heart rates, duration of analgesia, and neonatal outcome. There was no significant difference between the groups with regard to maternal age, weight, height, parity, infant's gestational age, and birth weight.

None of the patients in either group became hypertensive. The mean systolic and diastolic arterial blood pressure was decreased significantly below baseline values for the epinephrine group 5 minutes after administration of the anesthetic and remained decreased up to 60 minutes. No such decreases were observed in the lidocaine-only group. The duration of anesthesia in the epinephrine group was significantly longer than that in the lidocaine-only group. None of the neonates in either group had any abnormal heart rate patterns attributable to the anesthetic, and all had Apgar scores of 9 or more at 5 minutes.

It appears that mildly preeclamptic patients are not likely to experience hypertension when small amounts of epinephrine are added to the anesthetic solution used in epidural anesthesia.

▶ Contrary to most obstetric anesthesiologists, I have used lidocaine with epinephrine for cesarean delivery in the mildly preeclamptic patient for several years. I am in agreement with Heller and Goodman (*Anesthesiology* 65:224–226, 1986) and the authors that the mildly preeclamptic patient can receive epidural analgesia/anesthesia with epinephrine-containing local anesthetics without adverse effect on the mother or the fetus.—G.W. Ostheimer, M.D.

Ventricular Tachyarrhythmias During Cesarean Section After Ritodrine Therapy: Interaction With Anesthetics
Shin YK, Kim YD (Georgetown Univ)
South Med J 81:528–530, April 1988   6–83

The β-adrenergic agonist ritodrine hydrochloride is presently the only drug approved by the FDA for use as tocolytic therapy. However, ritodrine can cause serious cardiovascular complications, including cardiac arrhythmias. Ventricular tachycardia and subsequent cardiac arrest developed in a patient after ritodrine infusion to arrest preterm labor.

Primigravida, 22, admitted for preterm labor at 31 weeks' gestation, was scheduled for emergency cesarean section because of failure to stop labor despite maximal ritodrine therapy intravenously. The patient had also been admitted 3 days earlier because of preterm labor, which was controlled with ritodrine. In the operating room she was given a rapid intravenous infusion of lactated Ringer's solution, and a lumbar epidural block using ephedrine was initiated. The patient was apprehensive before operation and as surgery began she continued to be so. Her infant was delivered approximately 30 minutes after discontinuation of ritodrine infusion. About 5 minutes after the delivery, the patient's systolic pressure suddenly dropped to 80 mm Hg and shortly thereafter she went into ventricular tachycardia and fibrillation. Cardiopulmonary resuscitation including external cardiac compression, endotracheal intubation, intermittent positive pressure ventilation with 100% oxygen, and sodium bicarbonate intravenously was initiated. External direct current counter shocks successfully restored the heart to sinus rhythm. After closure of the abdomen, the patient was taken to the intensive care unit where she was soon extubated. Her postoperative course was uneventful, and the patient was discharged without sequelae on the tenth postoperative day.

This case report illustrates that patients receiving ritodrine for preterm labor may be at risk for interactions between the residual β-mimetic effects of ritodrine and the effects of anesthetics during cesarean section, even after ritodrine administration has been discontinued. Anesthesia induction should be delayed whenever possible following ritodrine administration. The cautious use of carefully titrated doses of ephedrine is strongly advised.

▶ Although it is true that patients receiving ritodrine for inhibition of preterm labor may be at risk for interactions between the residual β-mimetic effects of ritodrine and the effects of anesthetics during vaginal delivery or cesarean section, in this case the interaction was between the residual effects of ritodrine and ephedrine. However, the possibility of an air embolus was not considered by the authors and clearly could be a possibility because of the time frame in which the hypotensive episode occurred. The corollary to this case report is that immediately discovered cardiovascular collapse treated aggressively with appropriate cardiopulmonary resuscitation will result in an excellent outcome for the parturient. Drug interactions are a major problem in obstetric anesthesia, and the occasional obstetric anesthesiologist needs to be reminded of the possibility of their occurrence.—G.W. Ostheimer, M.D.

Incidence of Hypotension Associated With Epidural Anesthesia Using Alkalinized and Nonalkalinized Lidocaine for Cesarean Section
Parnass SM, Curran MJA, Becker GL (Michael Reese Hosp, Chicago)
Anesth Analg 66:1148–1150, November 1987   6–84

Because of its more gradual and predictable onset of action, epidural anesthesia is often preferred to spinal anesthesia for cesarean section. A major disadvantage is the marked decrease in cardiac output and blood pressure resulting from rapid onset of a high sympathetic block and decrease in venous return. The onset of epidural anesthesia is accelerated significantly by the use of alkalinized lidocaine. Women having elective cesarean section were studied to determine whether epidural alkalinized lidocaine is also associated with a higher incidence of hypotension than is epidural nonalkalinized lidocaine.

Twenty-one full-term unpremedicated women in American Society of Anesthesiologists classifications I and II were studied. By random assignment, 10 patients were given lidocaine with epinephrine plus $NaHCO_3$ and 11 patients were given lidocaine with epinephrine alone. Women in the first group had significantly greater decreases in systolic blood pressure (32% from baseline values) than those in the second group had (19%). Women in the first group also had a greater rate (9% per minute) of systolic blood pressure decline to those minimum values than did those in the second group (3% per minute). These differences were observed despite that patients given lidocaine with epinephrine plus $NaHCO_3$ received no less ephedrine and no more additional anesthetic than the control group.

Systolic hypotension was significantly greater, both in magnitude and rate of development, during epidural blockade for cesarean section when lidocaine and epinephrine alkalinized with bicarbonate were used to obtain more rapid onset of anesthesia. Caution was recommended in the use of this preparation as a bolus injection.

The Incidence and Neonatal Effects of Maternal Hypotension During Epidural Anesthesia for Cesarean Section

Brizgys RV, Dailey PA, Shnider SM, Kotelko DM, Levinson G (Univ of California, San Francisco)
Anesthesiology 67:782–786, November 1987   6–85

Cesarean sections often are done with epidural anesthesia. Maternal hypotension, leading to metabolic abnormalities in umbilical cord blood, is a major side effect of epidural anesthesia. A large group of laboring and nonlaboring women undergoing repeat or primary cesarean section during epidural anesthesia was studied to determine whether a specific prophylactic and therapeutic regimen could decrease the incidence of maternal hypotension.

In a 4-year period, 583 parturients having delivery by cesarean section during epidural anesthesia were divided into 5 groups. Group 1 consisted of 183 women undergoing repeat cesarean section without labor; 39 nonlaboring women undergoing planned primary cesarean section formed group 2, and 88 laboring women without fetal distress undergoing repeat cesarean section comprised group 3; group 4 included 229 laboring women with no fetal distress undergoing primary cesarean section, and group 5 comprised 44 laboring women with mild-to-moderate fetal distress undergoing primary cesarean section. To prevent hypotension before delivery, all patients were given a rapid intravenous infusion of 1L of lactated Ringer's solution before epidural anesthesia.

The overall incidence of maternal hypotension was 29%; of those women, 92% were given ephedrine intravenously to normalize blood pressure. Women in groups 1 and 2 had a significantly higher incidence of hypotension than women in the other 3 groups: 36% vs. 24% (Fig 6–9). However, transient maternal hypotension did not affect the clinical condition of the neonates. When the mean umbilical blood acid-base val-

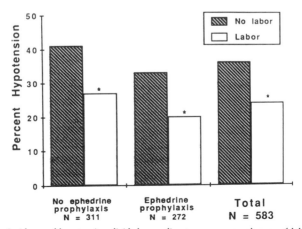

Fig 6–9.—Incidence of hypotension divided according to presence or absence of labor and use of prophylactic ephedrine. * Significant difference between nonlaboring and laboring mothers. (Courtesy of Brizgys RV, Dailey PA, Shnider SM, et al: *Anesthesiology* 67:782–786, November 1987.)

ues of infants of all normotensive mothers were compared, infants of women in group 5 were found to have significantly lower values for umbilical arterial base excess and umbilical venous pH, PO_2, and base excess than infants of women in the other groups. Infants from groups 3 and 5 had significantly lower umbilical arterial pH and significantly higher umbilical venous PCO_2 values compared with the other groups. Hypotension occurred in 26% of the women treated prophylactically with ephedrine and 32% of those not treated. Laboring mothers treated prophylactically had a 20% incidence of hypotension, and nonlaboring mothers had a 33% incidence.

Epidural anesthesia is a safe technique for cesarean section; maternal hypotension need not adversely affect fetal outcome. The higher incidence of maternal hypotension among nonlaboring mothers indicates that they are possibly at greater risk for complications with epidural anesthesia.

▶ The findings of Parnass et al. (Abstract 6–84) that epidural anesthesia with alkalinized lidocaine for cesarean delivery results in maternal hypotension because of rapid onset of sympathetic blockade are similar to the findings of Dr. Shnider's group at the University of California, San Francisco, a number of years ago, which were that the rapid onset of sympathetic blockade with 2-chloroprocaine produced maternal hypotension and a tendency toward acidosis in the newborn. Dr. Brizgys et al. (Abstract 6–85) reviewed their experience at the University of California, San Francisco, in regard to maternal hypotension at cesarean delivery and found that the administration of 1 L of crystalloid solution prior to epidural block for cesarean delivery may be inadequate hydration, particularly for the nonlaboring mother. In addition, the early administration of intravenous ephedrine to treat hypotension helps maintain normal blood pressure and has no adverse affect on the fetus.

It has been our practice at the Brigham and Women's Hospital to administer at least 1,500 ml of crystalloid solution before the initiation of spinal anesthesia and at least 2,000 ml of crystalloid to the patient receiving epidural anesthesia for cesarean delivery by the time of delivery. Although we have diminished the number of patients with hypotension, we believe firmly in the administration of intravenous ephedrine if there is any hypotension whatsoever. By this approach we demonstrated excellent maternal and neonatal outcomes (Datta et al: *Anesthesiology* 56:68–70, 1982).

However if the reader thinks we have solved all the problems related to cesarean delivery by the use of appproximately 2 L of crystalloid by delivery and the liberal use of intravenous ephedrine, let me remind you that there are patients who get extreme tachycardia from the use of intravenous ephedrine even after receiving 2–3 L of crystalloid. These patients often manifest signs (chest pain, anxiety, and shortness of breath) that are comparable to angina in the older person, probably from extreme myocardial stress. Therefore, is ephedrine the best drug for the parturient (and her baby) at cesarean delivery? A number of investigators are now looking at the utilization of phenylephrine in place of ephedrine at cesarean delivery. Let me remind the reader that phenylephrine was *not* evaluated in the Ralston et al. study (*Anesthesiology* 40:354,

1974). α-Adrenergic drugs, metaraminol and methoxamine, were evaluated, and their effects were attributed to phenylephrine because of their pharmacologic similarities. Indeed the vasopressor of choice for the sick cardiac parturient and the routine surgical patient is intravenous phenylephrine. Several investigators are comparing phenylephrine and ephedrine at this time, and readers will be updated on the studies concerning these drugs in future YEAR BOOKS.— G.W. Ostheimer, M.D.

Neonatal Neurobehavior After Epidural Anesthesia for Cesarean Section: A Comparison of Bupivacaine and Chloroprocaine
Kuhnert BR, Kennard MJ, Linn PL (Case Western Reserve Univ)
Anesth Analg 67:64–68, January 1988   6–86

There have been conflicting reports as to whether bupivacaine has adverse neurobehavioral effects when used for cesarean section. Studies with the Brazelton Neonatal Neurobehavioral Assessment Scale indicate that significant neonatal effects do occur; however, the Scanlon scale and the Neurologic and Adaptive Capacity Scoring System have failed to demonstrate adverse effects. Brazelton Scale scores were compared in 55 infants after elective section delivery using epidural anesthesia. Twenty-nine mothers received 0.5% or 0.75% bupivacaine and 26 received 3% chloroprocaine.

Orientation behavior was significantly better in the bupivacaine group, even after adjusting for parity, age, and the time from anesthetic injection to delivery. Infants in the bupivacaine group tended to do better than those whose mothers received chloroprocaine in most neurobehavioral tests. Scores for motor and autonomic function and orientation improved with advancing age in both groups.

Performance on the Brazelton Scale is better after epidural anesthesia with bupivacaine than with chloroprocaine. Chloroprocaine may not be innocuous to the infant, although the reason for this is not clear.

▶ This comparison of bupivacaine and chloroprocaine epidural anesthesia for cesarean delivery using the Brazelton Neonatal Neurobehavioral Assessment Scale is a welcome addition to the obstetric anesthesia literature. There has been a great deal of controversy regarding these 2 drugs in relation to their effects on neonatal neurobehavior. Claims have been pressed for chloroprocaine as the best local anesthetic for obstetric anesthesia because the drug is rapidly metabolized and therefore would have little pharmacologic effect on the fetus/ newborn. On the other hand, bupivacaine, a highly lipid soluble local anesthetic, traverses the placenta in small amounts but can be easily stored in the fatty tissues and organs of the neonate/newborn. Subsequent release of the drug could produce long-term neurobehavioral effects.

Although this is clearly a well-done study by an outstanding group in perinatal pharmacology, I doubt that this report will change clinical practice in obstetric anesthesia. Those institutions that are using the amide local anesthetics lidocaine and bupivacaine will continue to do so, whereas those institutions that rely on chloroprocaine will not change their utilization of the drug. With the increasing use of local anesthetics combined with narcotics by intermittent or continuous infusion for vaginal delivery, the dosage of drugs is so low that serum levels are negligible.

Having been part of neurobehavioral investigations from the inception of the concept in obstetric anesthesia, I feel comfortable making a few overall evaluations of the studies to date. In the early phases of the investigations, the exposure of the fetus/neonate to large amounts of amide local anesthetics demonstrated neurobehavioral changes, particularly with mepivacaine, which had an extremely long half-life in the newborn. Maintenance of uteroplacental perfusion is paramount to decreasing neurobehavioral effects because hypotension has been linked to altered neurobehavioral responses. At cesarean delivery, a uterine incision-to-delivery interval of greater than 3 minutes can lead to progressive fetal hypoxia and acidosis, which can by itself produce neurobehavioral changes regardless of the anesthetic technique used.

In conclusion, we have come a long way with the neurobehavioral assessments of obstetric analgesia and anesthesia for labor and vaginal or cesarean delivery. Maintenance of uteroplacental perfusion seems to be of paramount importance in diminishing neurobehavioral changes. However, the utilization of mepivacaine and now, possibly, chloroprocaine, must be questioned. In our institution, bupivacaine is the primary drug used for labor analgesia; lidocaine is the primary drug used for cesarean delivery whereas chloroprocaine is used when indicated for cesarean delivery of an elective or emergent nature. The obstetric anesthesia community should be indebted to all the contributors for their evaluations of obstetric anesthesia by neurobehavioral techniques, as these inquiries have led to the safer application of techniques and drugs for vaginal or cesarean delivery.— G.W. Ostheimer, M.D.

Combined Intrathecal Morphine and Bupivacaine for Cesarean Section
Abouleish E, Rawal N, Fallon K, Hernandez D (Univ of Texas, Houston)
Anesth Analg 67:370–374, April 1988   6–87

The addition of morphine to hyperbaric spinal bupivacaine would seem to provide several advantages in analgesia during cesarean section. A double-blind, randomized prospective study of 34 patients undergoing cesarean section was conducted to test this hypothesis.

Seventeen patients in the study group received morphine sulfate added to hyperbaric bupivacaine just before the intrathecal injection; 17 controls received saline instead of morphine. Clinicians monitored intraoperative and postoperative arterial blood pressures, graded the state of consciousness, and determined the narcotic requirement during total hospital stay.

Eighty-two percent of patients who received morphine did not require analgesic supplementation to spinal anesthesia during surgery; 41% of patients without morphine did require supplementation. Postoperatively, patients receiving morphine did not request additional analgesia for 27 hours compared with control patients who required analgesia after 2 hours. Neonates had no adverse effects from the morphine.

The addition of morphine, 0.2 mg, to hyperbaric spinal bupivacaine for cesarean section is a safe and effective method of reducing intraoperative pain and providing prolonged postoperative analgesia.

▶ The subarachnoid administration of morphine (or fentanyl) is directly accomplishing what has already been achieved by epidural opioid administration but with a markedly decreased dose. The listener can expect to hear about the addition of a wide variety of opioids to spinal bupivacaine and lidocaine in the near future. It will be interesting to see whether there will be a difference between epidural and subarachnoid administration in the incidence of side effects, most notably pruritus, nausea, and vomiting.—G.W. Ostheimer, M.D.

7 Monitoring

Hypoxemia During Ambulatory Gynecologic Surgery as Evaluated by the Pulse Oximeter
Raemer DB, Warren DL, Morris R, Philip BK, Philip JH (Brigham and Women's Hosp, Boston; Harvard Univ)
J Clin Monit 3:244–248, October 1987   7–1

An adverse outcome is rare after anesthesia in healthy patients undergoing ambulatory gynecologic surgery. Several studies suggest, however, that even patients classified in American Society of Anesthesiologists categories I and II are at risk. The incidence of hypoxemia during general anesthesia administered by experienced anesthetists was determined in 108 female patients undergoing ambulatory gynecologic operation. Pulse oximetry was used to determine arterial oxygenation saturation (SaO_2).

Eleven patients experienced 1 or more hypoxemic episodes. Five of these had severe hypoxemia (SaO_2 less than 85%), and 6 had moderate hypoxemia (SaO_2 less than 90%). Moderate hypoxemia was associated with non-laparoscopic gynecologic operation, obesity, and age older than 35 years, whereas severe hypoxemia was associated with obesity and age older than 35 years. Among operative events, moderate hypoxemia was found only with the lithotomy position, manual ventilation, and during arousal. The anesthetist was aware of the hypoxemia in none of 7 patients who had moderate hypoxemia and in 2 of 7 with severe hypoxemia.

Seven episodes of hypoxemia occurred during resumption of spontaneous ventilation during arousal. Two occurred in obese patients during tracheal intubation without preoxygenation, 1 episode occurred after uneventful extubation, 3 occurred during maintenance of mask anesthesia, and chronic hypoventilation was responsible in 1 patient.

Cost-benefit analysis, based on a cost of $1.35 per patient for monitoring with pulse oximeter, showed that a mortality of 1 in 40,000 among patients who actually become moderately hypoxemic would justify the cost of monitoring SaO_2.

Most hypoxemic episodes result from inadequate management of ventilation during an otherwise uncomplicated anesthesia. Pulse oximetry should be part of routine anesthetic management for ambulatory gynecologic patients.

▶ This is one of the early studies that demonstrated that pulse oximetry was a valuable adjunct to the clinical management of the surgical patient with or without endotracheal intubation. Pulse oximetry, along with capnography, should be the standard of care in circumstances under which general anesthesia is being administered. The pulse oximeter should be applied routinely to the patient undergoing a surgical procedure with major regional anesthesia. It will be interesting to see whether the utilization of these 2 monitors will decrease the number of adverse occurrences in anesthesia and, if so, what effect their prevention will have on the medical malpractice situation. Some states are already decreasing the classification of anesthesiologists and are lowering their medical malpractice premiums if they present evidence of the utilization of pulse oximetry and capnography in their operating suites. Aggressive risk management and prevention appears to be having a beneficial effect in our practices.—G.W. Ostheimer, M.D.

Auditory Alarms During Anesthesia Monitoring
Kestin IG, Miller BR, Lockhart CH (Children's Hosp, Denver; Univ of Colorado)
Anesthesiology 69:106–109, July 1988   7–2

Most monitors used in anesthesia now employ alarm systems that produce a sound signal when a high or low limit is passed. Five such monitors were routinely used in performing elective general, ophthalmic, orthopedic, or dental operations on 50 pediatric patients. Monitoring included ECG, oscillometric blood pressure, oxygen analyzer, pulse oximetry, and inspiratory ventilator pressure.

Three fourths of all alarms that sounded were spurious, and only 3% indicated actual risk. On average, 10 alarms sounded per patient. Most alarms were from the ECG, blood pressure monitor, and pulse oximeter. With the ECG (Fig 7–1) and the saturation alarm on the pulse oximeter, most alarms were spurious. However, most alarms from the blood pressure monitor and the heart rate alarm on the pulse oximeter were recorded as a change above the upper alarm limit.

Heart rate, arterial pressure, and oxygenation are such fundamental aspects of patient status that monitors probably do not require auditory alarms. If an alarm is to be used, one of the new type emitting a sequence of notes to aid localization would be preferable. In contrast, disconnec-

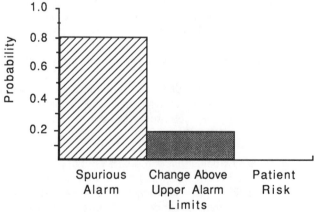

Fig 7–1.—Probability that ECG alarm will be spurious alarm, patient risk, or change above upper alarm limits. (Courtesy of Kestin IG, Miller BR, Lockhart CH: *Anesthesiology* 69:106–109, July 1988.)

tion alarms or inspired oxygen monitors rarely sound, and when they do, extreme hazard is likely to be present.

▶ While there can be no doubt that the availability of various innovative monitoring devices has dramatically increased in the last few years, there is little or no evidence that these devices have actually improved patient outcome. On the other hand, such data are difficult to obtain. While no one can logically argue against the benefit of obtaining as much information as possible, these monitors may have some drawbacks. Certainly this study verifies that, when an alarm sounds, it is often difficult to assess which alarm is sounding and what its significance is. Hopefully, these valuable monitoring devices will have a more coordinated alarm system that will aid in immediately identifying the difficulty.—R.D. Miller, M.D.

Critical Incidents Detected by Pulse Oximetry During Anaesthesia
McKay WPS, Noble WH (Univ of Toronto)
Can J Anaesth 35:265–269, 1988   7–3

The greatest value of the pulse oximeter is in detecting early signs of hypoxemia, but other indications for its use have not been developed. The clinical usefulness of oximetry during anesthesia to determine when and where it shortens the time to detect critical events was assessed.

The Critical Incident Technique was used in 4,797 patients undergoing anesthesia to identify and estimate the frequency of anesthesia-related incidents that might put the patient at risk. Changes that met the criteria included oxygen saturation less than 95% and changes in pulse, blood pressure, or temperature that would be expected to lead to a poor outcome in a given patient. A pulse oximeter signaled the critical incident.

A critical incident occurred with 6% of reported patients. Desaturation was the most common incident (Table 1). Airway and intubation problems were the most common primary causes of desaturation (Table 2). Desaturations were milder but more frequent during the maintenance phase than during induction or emergence. The oximeter was the first indication of a poorly tolerated heart rhythm in 45 patients. The oximeter

TABLE 1.—Physiologic
Change Signaled

Desaturation	151
Heart rhythm change	45
Temperature decrease	7
Blood pressure decrease	4
Blood pressure increase	3

(Courtesy of McKay WPS, Noble WH: *Can J Anaesth* 35:265–269, 1988.)

TABLE 2.—Primary Cause and Most Important Contributing
Cause of Desaturation

Condition	Primary cause (%)	Contributing cause (%)
Upper/lower airway spasm/oedema/ soft tissue obstruction	37 (19)	
Lung disease	29 (15)	22 (11)
Narcosis	26 (14)	
Intubation problem	22 (11)	
Obesity		28 (15)
Other illness		20 (10)

(Courtesy of McKay WPS, Noble WH: *Can J Anaesth* 35:265–269, 1988.)

also first signaled temperature less than 35 C in 7 patients, potentially dangerous blood pressure drop in 4, and severe unexpected hypertension in 3. The false critical incident rate was 2%.

Early detection of critical incidents by pulse oximeter can prevent disastrous results. Hypoxia, which is associated with the most severe outcomes of anesthesia, is poorly detected by other means. A pulse oximeter should be used in addition to other monitors in all anesthesias.

▶ There is no question that the introduction of pulse oximetry has further increased the safety of patients undergoing and recovering from anesthesia. It is academic to debate those instances when use of the pulse oximeter is most useful; every patient deserves this monitor during the intraoperative and early postoperative period.— R.K. Stoelting, M.D.

Central Venous Cannulation Done by House Officers in the Intensive Care Unit: A Prospective Study

Sessler CN, Glauser FL (Med College of Virginia; McGuire VA Med Ctr, Richmond, Va)
South Med J 80:1239–1242, October 1987   7–4

Central venous cannulation (CVC) may be complicated by inadvertent arterial puncture, pneumothorax, hemothorax, and air embolism. It is a procedure often performed by house staff in the intensive care units of teaching hospitals. The success and complications associated with CVC in a teaching hospital were evaluated prospectively.

Consecutive CVC attempts by house staff were assessed in a 14-month period. Cannulation was successful in 172 patients after 231 attempts, for a success rate of 74%. Fourteen complications occurred, for a rate of 6.1%. Five complications required intervention, but none was fatal. The overall success rate was higher with the internal jugular approach and lower with the external jugular approach than for other sites. The success rate of Swan-Ganz catheterization also was higher with the internal jugular than with the subclavian approach. During resuscitation, CVC often was unsuccessful (in 41% of the patients) or complicated (13.6%). Although the success rates were comparable, CVCs performed by experienced house officers were more commonly associated with complications than were CVCs performed by interns, possibly because of patient selection. A trend toward fewer or less severe complications was noted in the course of the month and in the study.

The indications for and techniques of CVC must continually be reappraised. Overall, the internal jugular approach appeared to be more reliable than the external jugular approach in this series.

▶ Central venous catheterization is associated with a significant incidence of complications, a fact often lost sight of now that the procedures used are so commonplace. The surprising fact was that experienced house officers had more problems than interns (10% versus 2%, respectively). The difference may well have been related to patient selection, as suggested. Presumably, the highest incidence of complications would have resulted if attending staff complications had been tallied!—R.R. Kirby, M.D.

A Community-Wide Assessment of the Use of Pulmonary Artery Catheters in Patients With Acute Myocardial Infarction
Gore JM, Goldberg RJ, Spodick DH, Alpert JS, Dalen JE (Univ of Massachusetts, Worcester)
Chest 92:721–727, October 1987   7–5

Trends in the use of pulmonary artery catheters were studied in more than 3,200 patients with acute myocardial infarction. The patients were seen at 16 hospitals in 1975, 1978, 1981, and 1984. Hemodynamic monitoring with a pulmonary artery catheter has increased progressively over time. Most recently, one fifth of patients were monitored. Catheter use was more frequent at teaching hospitals.

In 1984 nearly one third of the patients with congestive heart failure had monitoring by pulmonary artery catheter. Three fourths of those patients in cardiogenic shock were monitored. Monitoring was associated with a longer hospital stay, whether or not acute complications occurred; however, monitoring did not influence the long-term outlook after complicated infarction.

In view of the increasing use of pulmonary artery catheters, risk-benefit studies are needed. Patients with acute infarction who are not likely to benefit from this form of monitoring should be identified.

▶ Pulmonary artery catheterization (and other forms of invasive monitoring) are becoming increasingly controversial. The authors of this study and Dr. Eugene Robin of Stanford University who wrote an accompanying editorial (*Chest* 92:727–731, October 1987) are clearly biased against what they believe to be nonselective use of pulmonary artery catheters. In this regard, I tend to agree with them: uncritical usage has led to abuse, which is obvious in almost any critical care settings and many operating room settings today. In previous writings, Robin has soundly condemned pulmonary artery catheterization (Robin ED: The cult of the Swan-Ganz catheter: Overuse and abuse of pulmonary flow catheters. *Ann Intern Med* 103:445–449, 1985; and Robin ED: Iatroepidemics: A probe to examine systematic preventable errors in (chest) medicine. *Am Rev Respir Dis* 135:1152–1156, 1987). He has suggested that perhaps 5,000 deaths occur in the United States annually as a direct result of catheter insertion and use. Nevertheless, I think Gore and associates and Robin are guilty of overkill in the present article and editorial. One comes away with the impression that pulmonary artery catheters alone were the cause of differing morbidity and mortality in the patients studied and that the disease processes and other variables played little or no role. Keep in mind that this was a retrospective study with *no* control of variables. Hence, to single out the pulmonary artery catheter as the single, or at least prime, offender in bad outcomes is scientifically invalid.

Nevertheless, more care in selection and application of such monitoring clearly is indicated, as is a good, prospective, randomized clinical trial at a multi-institutional level. We shouldn't discard these devices yet, but we should be much more careful in how and when we use them.— R.R. Kirby, M.D.

The Relationship Between Central Venous Pressure and Pulmonary Capillary Wedge Pressure During Aortic Surgery
Ansley DM, Ramsay JG, Whalley DG, Bent JM, Lisbona R, Derbekyan V, Wynands JE (Royal Victoria Hosp, Montreal; McGill Univ)
Can J Anaesth 34:594–600, 1987   7–6

It has been suggested that a preoperative left ventricular ejection fraction greater than 0.5 is predictive of a strong correlation between central venous pressure (CVP) and pulmonary capillary wedge pressure (PCWP) when preload is altered. A study was conducted to determine whether a correlation exists between PCWP and CVP during periods of altered preload and afterload in patients undergoing aortic reconstructive surgery.

Multiple unit gated acquisition angiography scans were used to determine the resting left and right ventricular ejection fractions in 23 patients scheduled to undergo aortic surgery. Both CVP and PCWP were measured with the patient in the prone, 24 degrees head up, and 24 degrees head down table-tilt positions. The correlation between absolute values and changes in PCWP and CVP and the degree to which preoperative knowledge of left ventricular ejection fractions and right ventricular ejection fractions predicted these correlations were examined.

The range of resting left ventricular ejection fraction was from 0.1 to 0.84. Thirteen patients lacked a significant correlation between the absolute values of PCWP and CVP either before or after aortic crossclamp.

There was a small but significant correlation before aortic crossclamp, but not after, when the correlation coefficients from this analysis were compared with left ventricular ejection fraction. There was a significant correlation between a change in PCWP and a change in CVP in all patients at all times both before and after aortic crossclamp; however, low correlation coefficients and wide confidence intervals suggested that estimates of a change in PCWP based on a change in CVP would be unreliable. In a few patients, the direction of change of PCWP was opposed to the change in CVP.

The CVP and PCWP should be independently assessed if the surgeon needs to know the filling pressures of both ventricles during aortic surgery. Preoperative knowledge of the ejection fraction is not a reliable predictor of a correlation between CVP and PCWP.

▶ This information corroborates the findings of Civetta et al. 16 years ago (*Ann Surg* 76:753, 1972) and reinforces the concept of ventricular disparity in this subgroup of patients with significant cardiovascular disease. Hence, pulmonary artery catheterization seems a reasonable and prudent choice for monitoring. What is not clear is whether a knowledge of changes in CVP and PCWP, presumably to be used in choosing therapeutic interventions, anesthetic techniques, etc., results in improved outcome, i.e., reduced morbidity and mortality.—R.R. Kirby, M.D.

Central Mixed and Splanchnic Venous Oxygen Saturation Monitoring
Dahn MS, Lange MP, Jacobs LA (Wayne State Univ)
Intensive Care Med 14:373–378, 1988   7–7

Monitoring of central mixed venous oxygen saturation (SvO_2) is being increasingly used to evaluate critically ill patients, but splanchnic venous oxygen saturation may be markedly depressed in the presence of a normal or high SvO_2. Levels of SvO_2 and hepatic venous oxygen saturation were measured in 7 postoperative and 15 septic patients who required more than 3 days in intensive care. No patient was hypotensive or had a major decrease in cardiac output within 48 hours before the study.

Survival was 40% in the septic group and 71% in nonseptic patients. Septic patients had higher total body oxygen and splanchnic oxygen delivery rates, but the differences were not significant. Central mixed venous and hepatic venous oxygen saturation were somewhat depressed in the injured patients. In the septic group, hepatic venous oxygen saturation averaged only 55.6%, a significant reduction compared with the central mixed venous saturation. Lactate levels were slightly higher in the septic patients.

It may be very helpful to assess organ oxygen transport and utilization by regional venous oxygen saturation monitoring in some seriously ill patients. Data on SvO_2 must be interpreted cautiously in these patients. If a major reduction in venous saturation is sustained, relatively minor events can precipitate splanchnic ischemia, compromise clearance of lactate, and lead to sudden cardiovascular deterioration.

▶ The lack of correlation between Sv_{O_2} and overall cardiovascular performance in septic patients has been demonstrated repeatedly. Perhaps regional venous oxygen saturation monitoring will be of greater value, but can it be done satisfactorily and routinely in a clinical setting? Of more importance, if a low hepatic venous saturation is demonstrated when Sv_{O_2} is normal, what therapeutic response is appropriate? As is the case with all good research, more questions are raised than are answered.—R.R. Kirby, M.D.

8 Special Patient Groups

Patients With Myocardial Ischemia

Perioperative Myocardial Ischemia: Importance of the Preoperative Ischemic Pattern

Knight AA, Hollenberg M, London MJ, Tubau J, Verrier E, Browner W, Mangano DT, SPI Research Group (Univ of California, San Francisco; VA Med Ctr, San Francisco)
Anesthesiology 68:681–688, May 1988
8–1

Previous studies have not related preoperative myocardial ischemia to perioperative ischemia. To evaluate the impact of anesthesia and surgery on preexisting patterns of myocardial ischemia, ischemic patterns throughout the perioperative period in patients undergoing coronary artery bypass grafting (CABG) were studied.

The frequency and severity of ischemic episodes before, during, and after surgery were compared in 50 patients undergoing CABG. Patients were monitored by Holter monitor for 2 days each before and after surgery and also intraoperatively.

Preoperatively, 42% of patients had ischemic episodes of which 87% were clinically silent. Only 18% had perioperative ischemia, and 40% had episodes of postoperative ischemia. The number of ischemic episodes per hour was similar during all periods. There was similarity in the duration of episodes preoperatively and intraoperatively, but ischemic episodes were longer following surgery. Most intraoperative ischemias occurred without significant change in blood pressure or heart rate. Intraoperative ischemia occurred in 7% of patients without preoperative ischemia but in 33% of those with preoperative ischemia; however, neither preoperative nor perioperative ischemia was predictive of postoperative ischemia.

Frequent, usually silent, episodes of myocardial ischemia occur despite antianginal therapy. The intraoperative ischemic pattern is no worse than the preoperative pattern. Because perioperative ischemic patterns appear to recapitulate preoperative patterns, it is relevant to study preoperative ischemia to analyze the effect of anesthesia and surgery on ischemia during CABG.

▶ It seems possible that episodes of silent ischemia are as likely to occur during anesthesia as during the awake state. Failure of these silent episodes to be associated with changes in blood pressure and heart rate further clouds the issue of the significance of these changes. An important question is whether signs of myocardial ischemia detected on the intraoperative electrocardiogram and not associated with hemodynamic changes should be treated. Obviously, the same changes in an awake patient would remain silent and untreated.— R.K. Stoelting, M.D.

Intravenous Diltiazem Worsens Regional Function in Compromised Myocardium
Leone BJ, Philbin DM, Lehot J-J, Wilkins M, Foëx P, Ryder WA (Oxford Univ)
Anesth Analg 67:205–210, March 1988   8–2

The calcium antagonists verapamil, nifedipine, and diltiazem relieve angina and coronary spasm in patients with stable angina pectoris and coronary artery disease. Recent experimental studies in dogs showed that verapamil used in combination with halothane caused regional myocardial dysfunction in the form of continued myocardial postsystolic segment shortening, even though there was no obstruction of coronary inflow.

The effect of intravenously administered diltiazem on regional myocardial function was assessed in a canine model of critical constriction of the left anterior descending coronary artery (LAD) during maintenance anesthesia with fentanyl, nitrous oxide, and halothane.

Maintenance anesthesia caused regional dysfunction, measured as postsystolic shortening in the compromised LAD territory. After intravenous injection of diltiazem, 0.1 mg/kg or 0.2 mg/kg, the heart rate showed no change from baseline, and all of the dogs continued to have sinus rhythm. However, postsystolic segment shortening was substantially depressed, and regional myocardial dysfunction was significantly worse after administration of diltiazem, 0.1 mg. Postsystolic shortening was essentially abolished with diltiazem, 0.2 mg. These changes in regional function were accompanied by decreases in global left ventricular performance.

When given intravenously during anesthesia, diltiazem causes significant depression of regional systolic shortening and substantial worsening of regional dysfunction in myocardium with a compromised blood supply. Although extrapolation to clinical situations is difficult, deleterious effects on myocardium with a compromised blood supply may occur when diltiazem is given intravenously during anesthesia.

▶ These animal data do not support the use of diltiazem in patients with ischemia-induced myocardial dysfunction. It seems unlikely that confirmation in patients will be pursued considering the likely clinical usefulness of this drug therapy.— R.K. Stoelting, M.D.

Does Chronic Treatment With Calcium Entry Blocking Drugs Reduce Perioperative Myocardial Ischemia?
Slogoff S, Keats AS (Texas Heart Inst, Houston)
Anesthesiology 68:676–680, May 1988   8–3

There is a significant relationship between perioperative myocardial is-chemia and the occurrence of postoperative myocardial infarction after coronary artery bypass grafting (CABG). If coronary spasm were respon-sible for the new myocardial ischemia, its incidence could be reduced by administration of calcium entry blocking drugs (CEB).

Four hundred forty-four patients undergoing CABG were divided into 4 groups: 180 patients received neither CEB nor adrenergic β-blocking drugs (BB), 119 patients received CEB only, 74 received both CEB and BB, and 71 received BB only. Perioperative patient characteristics having prognostic significance were compared among the groups.

Almost 47% of patients had new ischemia. Ischemia occurred at ar-rival to the operating room in 55 patients, after induction in 86 patients, and at both times in 67 patients. Sixty-six percent of all ischemia was un-related to extremes of heart rate or blood pressure. Incidence of this type was not reduced in patients receiving CEB, but it did occur less fre-quently in both groups receiving BB. The incidence of ischemia during anesthesia was doubled when peak heart rate reached or exceeded 110 beats per minute. At lower heart rates, the incidence of ischemia during anesthesia was similar among the groups (Fig 8–1). For all types of is-chemia, CEB-treated patients did not differ from those receiving no an-tianginal therapy.

Optimal hemodynamic control will not prevent ischemia in 30% of patients with coronary artery disease. Most tachycardia-related isch-emia can be prevented by preoperative administration of BB, but pre-

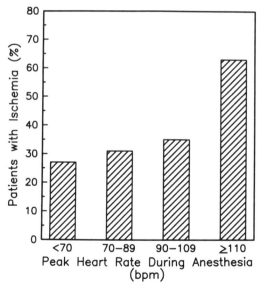

Fig 8–1.—Frequency of ischemia during anesthesia in 4 groups of patients based on peak heart rate achieved during this period. In ascending order, groups included 49, 229, 136, and 30 patients. Ischemic episode did not necessarily occur during period of peak heart rate. Incidence of ischemia sharply in-creases in patients who can increase heart rate in excess of 109 beats per minute (bpm) ($P < .005$ vs. heart rate < 110 bpm). (Courtesy of Slogoff S, Keats AS: *Anesthesiology* 68:676–680, May 1988.)

operative administration of CEB offers no benefit for the control of perioperative ischemia.

▶ Although the authors could not demonstrate a protective effect of calcium entry blockers on the incidence of perioperative myocardial ischemia, there is no suggestion these drugs should be discontinued prior to induction of anesthesia. The 2 clear messages from this study are (1) the unpredictable occurrence of angina pectoris in vulnerable patients and (2) the importance of avoiding increases in heart rate in minimizing this unpredictable occurrence.—R.K. Stoelting, M.D.

Effects of Isoflurane and Halothane on Coronary Vascular Resistance and Collateral Myocardial Blood Flow: Their Capacity to Induce Coronary Steal

Cason BA, Verrier ED, London MJ, Mangano DT, Hickey RF (VA Med Ctr, San Francisco)

Anesthesiology 67:665–675, November 1987   8–4

Isoflurane is a powerful coronary vasodilator. Although it may benefit patients with coronary artery disease, it may also endanger them if it causes an intercoronary redistribution of blood, i.e., coronary steal, away from potentially ischemic areas. Net coronary blood flow does not increase with halothane, so its potential for causing ischemia through coronary steal should be negligible. The potential for coronary steal in both isoflurane and halothane was studied.

Chronic occlusion of the left anterior descending coronary artery was induced in 10 dogs. Eight weeks later, the dogs were anesthetized with fentanyl and pentobarbital, and a stenosis was created on the circumflex coronary artery. Diastolic aortic pressure was held constant while either isoflurane or halothane was administered. Diastolic coronary artery pressure and collateral myocardial blood flow were measured.

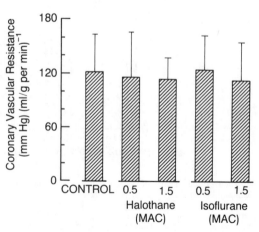

Fig 8–2.—Effects of halothane and isoflurane on coronary vascular resistance. (Courtesy of Cason BA, Verrier ED, London MJ, et al: *Anesthesiology* 67:665–675, November 1987.)

The effects of both halothane and isoflurane on diastolic coronary pressure, coronary vascular resistance (Fig 8–2), and collateral myocardial blood flow were minimal. There was no evidence of coronary steal or ischemia. In canines, neither halothane nor isoflurane is likely to cause myocardial ischemia by coronary steal if diastolic hypotension is avoided.

▶ The original concern that isoflurane could produce coronary artery steal in the presence of coronary artery disease was derived from patients in whom coronary perfusion pressure often decreased substantially. Subsequent complex and invasive animal models seemed to confirm the ability of isoflurane, but not halothane, to reduce coronary vascular resistance and divert coronary blood flow away from potentially ischemic areas of myocardium. Nevertheless, clinical experience, when isoflurane was administered in the presence of acceptable coronary perfusion pressure, consistently failed to demonstrate drug-related myocardial ischemia. The present data are, likewise, reassuring to those of us who feel isoflurane is a safe anesthetic. See the following article (Abstract 8–5) for data on administration to patients with coronary artery disease.—R.K. Stoelting, M.D.

Addition of Nitrous Oxide to Fentanyl Anesthesia Does Not Induce Myocardial Ischemia in Patients With Ischemic Heart Disease
Cahalan MK, Prakash O, Rulf ENR, Cahalan MT, Mayala APG, Lurz FC, Rosseel P, Lachitjaran E, Siphanto K, Gussenhoven EJ, Roelandt JRTC (Univ of California, San Francisco; Erasmus Univ, Rotterdam, the Netherlands)
Anesthesiology 67:925–929, December 1987   8–5

Nitrous oxide is commonly administered to patients with ischemic heart disease, but recent reports suggest that it may induce myocardial ischemia in these patients. Because nitrous oxide is a common adjunct to fentanyl anesthesia before and during coronary artery surgery, its effects on segmental left ventricular function and the ST segment of the ECG during fentanyl anesthesia were studied in 18 patients who required coronary artery bypass grafting. None had valvular or left ventricular dysfunction. The results were compared in a crossover design with those of treatment with an equal concentration of nitrogen.

After endotracheal intubation and 20 minutes of ventilation with 100% oxygen, either 60% nitrous oxide or 60% nitrogen (randomly assigned) was added to the inspired gas mixture of each patient for 10 minutes. This was followed by 10 minutes of 100% oxygen, and then 10 minutes of 60% nitrous oxide or 60% nitrogen, whichever had not been administered previously. Patients were monitored for myocardial ischemia using a standard 12-lead ECG and transesophageal 2-dimensional echocardiography.

In none of the patients did myocardial ischemia develop, i.e., an ST segment change of more than 1 mm, during the study. In addition, none had a new segmental wall motion abnormality during inhalation of either nitrous oxide or nitrogen.

Contrary to previous reports, this study indicates that nitrous oxide does not induce myocardial ischemia when used as an adjunct to fentanyl anesthesia in patients with severe coronary artery disease and normal left ventricular function.

▶ The design of this study is superb for the question asked and for providing data in patients that were previously implied from animal data. Although the use of nitrous oxide is not recommended following cardiopulmonary bypass, the present data suggest that, in contrast to animal studies, this anesthetic does not produce myocardial ischemia in patients with coronary artery disease.—R.K. Stoelting, M.D.

Patients With Hypotension and Taking Diuretics

Diuretics, Serum Potassium, and Ventricular Arrhythmias in the Multiple Risk Factor Intervention Trial

Cohen JD, Neaton JD, Prineas RJ, Daniels KA (Multiple Risk Factor Intervention Trial Research Group)
Am J Cardiol 60:548–554, Sept 1, 1987   8–6

Diuretics were the initial drugs of choice for hypertensive men in the Multiple Risk Factor Intervention Trial. Because patients who have abnormal resting ECGs at the outset are at increased risk of coronary and sudden death, the relation between diuretic treatment and ventricular premature complexes (VPCs) is of concern. Among about 360,000 men aged 35–57 years who were screened, nearly 13,000 without overt coronary artery disease were randomized to special intervention or usual care.

About 2% of participants had VPCs on the baseline resting ECG; these appeared most often in men with ECG abnormalities. In patients given special intervention and also in the usual care group, diuretic use was more frequent in those having VPCs. In addition, the serum potassium was lower, and the use of potassium, more frequent. A decline of 1 mEq/ L in serum potassium levels was associated with a 28% higher risk of VPCs in patients given usual care and with an 18% higher risk in patients given special intervention.

Premature ventricular beats are more frequent in hypertensive men who receive diuretic therapy, whether or not the ECG is abnormal. Hypokalemia may underlie this association. Regardless of the cause, the relation of diuretic use to ventricular arrhythmia requires urgent study.

▶ The issue of potassium has seemed to have been clarified substantially in the previous decade, and its relationship to anesthesia seems to be clearer. This article is derived from a statistical analysis of data from the Multiple Risk Factor Intervention Trial in which patients who were hypertensive were given either special intervention, which involved very aggressive diuretic therapy, counseling on cessation of smoking, and counseling on change in diet, or their usual care, which may or may not have included diuretic therapy. The study became controversial when the special intervention group that was hypertensive actually had a slightly higher risk of coronary artery death and sudden death than did the usual care group. Most people presumed this was caused by the perhaps overly aggressive therapy with diuretics.

In the currently reported statistical analysis of this study, the authors tried to correlate development of ventricular premature beats on follow-up examination with factors responsible for it. In other studies, this has been related to the presence of hypokalemia, the presence of hypomagnesemia, and ECG abnormalities at the start of study. In this study, that is exactly what was found as well; however, the authors did not study the presence of hypomagnesemia and whether that correlated with VPCs. Thus, I'm left with the question, "What should we do with the patient who is on diuretics?" Should we give serum potassium and, if we do, should we start treating before surgery? Data from Slogoff and colleagues and Vitez and colleagues imply that a serum potassium level of more than 2.5 is not associated with the development of more dysrhythmias during the anesthetic period than is a normal serum potassium in the same patients. In addition, data from the Boston collaborative drug study group show that there is either a fatal or life-threatening drug reaction in a little more than 1 in 200 patients who receive potassium in the hospital setting. That is, if you have about 197 patients to whom you give either intravenous, oral, or a combination of the 2 potassium therapies to treat hypokalemia, one of them will either die or have a life-threatening reaction to it. In addition, another 11 or slightly more will have a serious episode of hyperkalemia.

The data presented in this paper and others in the literature, however, indicate that the development of premature ventricular contractions is correlated with an abnormally low serum potassium level and is more prevalent with exercise. Thus, what I do with a patient who is taking diuretics is get a serum potassium level preoperatively and justify in the chart the lack of treatment because of the risk if the potassium value is between 2.5 and 3.5 mEq/L. However, if new ventricular premature contractions develop intraoperatively, I begin treatment. The other approach would be to begin slow oral potassium repletion or discontinue the diuretic and switch to another antihypertensive agent preoperatively in the patient who has ventricular premature beats on preoperative electrocardiogram and has hypokalemia. Perhaps the third approach for patients who are on diuretics is not to measure the serum potassium unless they have premature ventricular contractions on electrocardiogram; then one would measure only the serum potassium and treat the patient if ventricular premature contractions developed.—M.F. Roizen, M.D.

Thiazide Therapy Is Not a Cause of Arrhythmia in Patients With Systemic Hypertension
Papademetriou V, Burris JF, Notargiacomo A, Fletcher RD, Freis ED (Georgetown Univ; VA Med Ctrs, Washington, DC)
Arch Intern Med 148:1272–1276, June 1988　　　　　　　　8–7

Although diuretics have long been considered safe and effective as initial therapy in the treatment of hypertension, several recent reports have raised concern that mild-to-moderate diuretic-induced hypokalemia may aggravate cardiac arrhythmias. However, such an association has never been confirmed.

To assess the effect of diuretic therapy on cardiac arrhythmias, 44 black men with uncomplicated mild-to-moderate systemic hypertension underwent 48-hour electrocardiographic monitoring, measurement of potassium plasma levels, and assessment of renal function before and after 4 weeks of treatment with 100 mg of hydrochlorothiazide per day, taken in 2 divided doses. At baseline, all patients had normal plasma potassium levels and renal function. Twenty-eight patients had evidence of left ventricular hypertrophy by echocardiographic criteria, and 20, by electrocardiographic criteria.

As expected, thiazide therapy significantly decreased body weight and blood pressure compared with baseline values. After thiazide therapy, 27 patients had potassium levels of 3.4 mmole/L or less, whereas the other 17 patients had remained normokalemic. Twelve of the 27 hypokalemic patients had more than minimal ectopy of class 2 to class 5 before thiazide administration, whereas 11 patients had it after thiazide therapy. Similarly, 8 of the 17 normokalemic patients had class 2 to class 5 ectopy before thiazide therapy, and 6 had it after treatment (Table 1). These differences were not statistically significant.

The 28 patients with pretreatment echocardiographic evidence of left ventricular hypertrophy had more premature ventricular contractions per hour and more repetitive beats then the other 16 patients, but the differences were not statistically significant (Table 2). However, the difference in the average grade per hour between these 2 groups was statistically significant. There were no statistically significant differences in arrhythmias between the 20 patients who had pretreatment evidence of left ventricular hypertrophy by electrocardiographic criteria and the other 24 patients who did not.

TABLE 1.—Ventricular Ectopy in Patients With or Without Hypokalemia Receiving Diuretic Therapy

Variable*	Hypokalemia (n=27)		No Hypokalemia (n=17)	
	Baseline	Diuretic	Baseline	Diuretic
BW, kg	92.2±17.5	90.1±17.6†	81.1±14.4	79.8±14.1†
PK, mmol/L (mEq/L)	4.00±0.22	3.08±0.24†	4.20±0.28	3.81±0.28†
PVC/h	16.8±50.7	9.1±22.9	2.6±5.9	5.1±9.2
Total couplets	124	12	5	6
Total VT episodes	2	2	5	1
AGR/h	0.72±0.78	0.59±0.64	0.48±0.54	0.57±0.76

*BW, body weight; PK, plasma potassium; PVC, premature ventricular contractions; VT, ventricular tachycardia; AGR, average grade.
TP < .001, statistics compare values before and after diuretic therapy.
(Courtesy of Papademetriou V, Burris JF, Notargiacomo A, et al: *Arch Intern Med* 148:1272–1276, June 1988.)

TABLE 2.—Ventricular Ectopy in Patients With or
Without LVH Before and After Hydrochlorothiazide*

Variable	LVH (n = 28)		No LVH (n = 16)	
	Baseline	**Diuretic**	**Baseline**	**Diuretic**
LVPWT	1.39 ± 0.14	...	1.03 ± 0.07	...
BW, kg	86.3 ± 14.7	85.4 ± 14.7†	90.0 ± 20.8	88.1 ± 20.6†
PK, mmol/L (mEq/L)	4.06 ± 0.23	3.39 ± 0.45†	4.10 ± 0.32	3.33 ± 0.43†
PVC/h	16.6 ± 49.8	10.1 ± 22.9	2.1 ± 5.0	3.0 ± 5.9
Total couplets	123	15	6	3
Total VT episodes	5	3	2	0
AGR/h	0.79 ± 0.78	0.68 ± 0.74	0.34 ± 0.40‡	0.41 ± 0.54

LVH, left ventricular hypertrophy; *LVPWT*, left ventricular posterior
wall thickness; *BW*, body weight; *PK*, plasma potassium; *PVC*, premature
ventricular contractions; *VT*, ventricular tachycardia; *AGR*, average
grade.
†$P < .001$, compare values before and after diuretic; $P < .05$, compare values between groups at baseline.
(Courtesy of Papademetriou V, Burris JF, Notargiacomo A, et al: *Arch Intern Med* 148:1272–1276, June 1988.)

The findings in this study did not support any correlation between plasma potassium levels and any type of arrhythmias or arrhythmia grade, not even for patients with overt hypokalemia.

▶ This is an important article by a group that has had a major role in hypertension treatment. Freis is the original lead investigator in the Veterans Administration Cooperative Study. In this study, they selected patients who had hypertension, took them off all antihypertensives for a period of time, and then studied them for dysrhythmias on two 24-hour Holter monitors. They then gave each patient a diuretic twice daily for 4 weeks and examined the development both of hypokalemia and of dysrhythmias. Hypokalemia developed in 27 of the 44 patients, or about 60% of the total patient population had serum potassium levels in the hypokalemic range (less than or equal to 3.4 mEq/L). Neither these patients nor the other patients showed any increase (or any decrease) in their dysrhythmic frequency. This time period should have been enough for equilibration to occur and for magnesium deficiency to also occur, were it to occur. Thus, these data are pretty substantial evidence that dysrhythmias will not be a problem or should not be a problem in the average patient.

The authors go on to cite the data on the large variation in day-to-day recording of ventricular abnormalities with Holter monitoring. They state that the most frequently cited investigation using 24-hour ECG monitoring, Holland's study (Holland et al: Diuretic-induced ventricular ectopic activity. *Am J Med* 70:762–768, 1981), failed to take into account the day-to-day variability in dysrhythmic activity. They cite, for instance, that it was biased in favor of patients who initially had few dysrhythmias and thus would show an increase in dysrhythmias because patients with more than 6 premature ventricular beats per hour at baseline (prior to diuretic therapy) were excluded from that study. They feel that bias was introduced by selecting baseline recordings with low levels of aberrant ventricular activity, that is, because of the possibility of day-to-day variability, the likelihood of finding increased dysrhythmias on the second recording would be increased simply because of regression toward the mean rather than because of hypokalemia per se.

In the accompanying editorial for this paper, the reviewer cites that, although we may not have to worry about the dysrhythmic complications of hypokalemia induced by thiazides, other complications such as changes in cholesterol metabolism and disturbances in glucose and insulin metabolism induced by diuretics may still be of concern. Thus, they believe that these authors have not proved that the potassium level should be treated with "benign neglect."

Does this study mean that we don't have to get a serum potassium level preoperatively on patients who chronically take diuretics? I don't believe that question has been answered, but I believe it surely needs to be investigated.—M.F. Roizen, M.D.

Characterization of Antihypertensive Therapy by Whole-Day Blood Pressure Monitoring
Weber MA, Cheung DG, Graettinger WF, Lipson JL (VA Med Ctr, Long Beach, Calif; Univ of California, Irvine)
JAMA 259:3281–3285, June 10, 1988   8–8

Whole-day ambulatory monitoring is used for diagnosing hypertension and gauging response to therapy. Both of these uses were assessed in an antihypertensive trial with the calcium channel blocker diltiazem hydrochloride to determine whether diltiazem is more effective than placebo in lowering blood pressures of patients with mild to moderate hypertension, whether diltiazem has antihypertensive efficacy all day, and whether there are differences in the effects of diltiazem therapy in patients in whom whole-day blood pressure monitoring has confirmed or failed to confirm the clinical diagnosis of hypertension.

Thirty patients with an average age of 58 years had had essential hypertension diagnosed clinically by exclusion of secondary forms of hypertension. Systolic and diastolic blood pressures fell significantly in patients who received diltiazem, whereas no consistent change occurred in those who received placebo. Diltiazem also decreased systolic and diastolic blood pressures evenly throughout the day. The 15 diltiazem-treated patients were divided into those whose clinically diagnosed hypertension was confirmed by pretreatment blood pressure monitoring and those whose blood pressures were not. Diltiazem decreased average whole-day blood pressures by 18/13 mm Hg in the 9 hypertensive patients but only by 0/1 mm Hg in the 6 nonhypertensive patients.

Whole-day blood pressure monitoring strengthens antihypertensive trials by documenting efficacy and duration of treatment. It also enhances the diagnosis of hypertension, thereby identifying patients in whom treatment is justified.

▶ It appears that whole-day blood pressure monitoring may gain wider acceptance, as it differentiates those with "white-coat" hypertension from those who were hypertensive throughout the day. It also leads to effective characterization of the antihypertensive effect of therapy. In this case, the calcium channel blocker diltiazem lowered blood pressure to a more normal range in those who were actually hypertensive and kept it at a normal range in those who had "white-coat" hypertension. Thus it appears that, as with most therapies, something is brought to a normal set point, and this was beautifully demonstrated with the ambulatory whole-day blood pressure monitoring technique. Perhaps this technique can be used to better distinguish those patients who are hypertensive and in whom therapy before surgery may be a benefit from those patients who only have "white-coat" hypertension and in whom postponement of surgery may not lead to a benefit. One would then, of course, have to do a study on those with sustained hypertension to see whether, in fact, antihypertensive therapy before surgery leads to a benefit or not.—M.F. Roizen, M.D.

Patients With Congestive Heart Failure

Relative Efficacy of Vasodilator Therapy in Chronic Congestive Heart Failure: Implications of Randomized Trials
Mulrow CD, Mulrow JP, Linn WD, Aguilar C, Ramirez G (Univ of Texas, San Antonio; Univ of Texas at Austin; Academy of Health Sciences at Fort Sam Houston, San Antonio, Tex)
JAMA 259:3422–3426, June 17, 1988   8–9

The status of vasodilator therapy for patients with chronic heart failure remains uncertain. Data on 28 randomized, placebo-controlled trials involving nearly 2,000 patients were reviewed. All the studies had clinical end points, and treatment lasted for at least 4 weeks. Patients with symptomatic heart failure despite digitalis and diuretic therapy were included. Most were middle-aged men. About half of the patients had coronary disease. Three independent observers assessed the trial results.

The quality of the trials varied substantially. Treatment duration ranged from about 1 month to 2 years. All the vasodilator drugs used, except hydralazine, were associated with functional improvement. However, the only class of drugs exhibiting both improved functional status and lower mortality were the angiotensin converting-enzyme inhibitors. In general, patients given active vasodilator therapy were nearly 5 times more likely than placebo recipients to improve their functional status.

Angiotensin converting-enzyme inhibitors may lower mortality among patients with chronic heart failure, as well as bring about functional improvement. The best time to initiate treatment remains to be determined.

▶ In this analysis, the efficacy of vasodilator therapy for chronic congestive heart failure is evaluated. The addition of vasodilator therapy benefits approximately 200,000 patients yearly in functional status improvements. Only 1 therapy, which was with angiotensin converting-enzyme inhibitors, seemed to appear both to decrease mortality (by 50%) as well as to improve functional status. The age-old warning to anesthesiologists dealing with patients who were at poor risk (that is, don't let the patient get hypotensive or hypoxic) was dealt a death blow by this treatment of congestive heart failure. Bill Hamilton's adage to lower the blood pressure has finally been picked up by cardiologists as well as anesthesiologists. If you look at the contributions of William K. Hamilton to medicine in advocating PEEP for the newborn child as an effective therapy for respiratory disease of the newborn, in helping to uncover the mechanism of oxygen toxicity in adults, and in advocating the use of vasodilators in patients with heart disease, you will see that he has been a stalwart and has led our specialty admirably. One can only hope that anesthesia will have great giants such as him in the next generation, as we have had in the past.—M.F. Roizen, M.D.

Patients With Malignant Hyperthermia

Non-invasive Evaluation of Malignant Hyperthermia Susceptibility With Phosphorous Nuclear Magnetic Resonance Spectroscopy
Olgin J, Argov Z, Rosenberg H, Tuchler M, Chance B (Univ of Pennsylvania, Hahnemann Univ, Philadelphia)
Anesthesiology 68:507–513, April 1988   8–10

Phosphorus nuclear magnetic resonance spectroscopy (^{31}P NMR), a noninvasive method for determining intracellular changes in high energy phosphates, has been successfully used to assess several muscle diseases, primarily metabolic myopathies. This technique was employed in vivo to determine the levels of phosphocreatine, inorganic phosphate, and adenosine triphosphate in the muscles of patients susceptible to malignant hyperthermia (MH) in the hope of distinguishing this population from normal people.

The NMR spectra of the flexor muscles of the forearm of 13 patients considered MH-susceptible on the basis of in vitro caffeine/halothane contracture tests were compared with those from 25 normal volunteers. Levels of phosphocreatine, inorganic phosphate, and adenosine triphosphate during rest, graded exercise, and postexercise recovery were measured. The MH-susceptible persons had significantly higher inorganic phosphate and phosphocreatine values at rest than the normal volunteers had. (Fig 8–3). Also, a significantly slower postexercise recovery rate was noted in the MH-susceptible group. There were no significant differences between the 2 groups in the relationship of work rate to inorganic phosphate/phosphocreatine.

These findings suggest that unchallenged MH-susceptible patients can be distinguished from normal subjects using ^{31}P NMR spectroscopy to measure muscle inorganic phosphate/phosphocreatine at rest. Subjects with inorganic phosphate/phosphocreatine levels higher than 0.175 were shown to be MH-susceptible by contracture tests, whereas normal controls had levels lower than 0.160.

▶ This article shows that there is a way of doing a noninvasive evaluation of malignant hyperthermia using magnetic resonance spectroscopy. There is little overlap between the ratio of inorganic phosphate/phosphocreatine between controls and malignant hyperthermic-positive patients in this study of 13 malig-

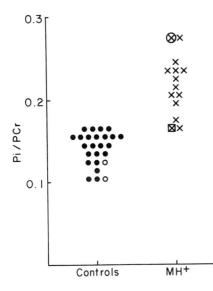

Fig 8–3.—Distribution of resting inorganic phosphate/phosphocreatine values for normal volunteers *(circles)* and malignant hyperthermia-susceptible patients *(x)*. Note that this distribution clearly defines 2 almost distinct populations, and that 2 controls proven nonsusceptible by biopsy (◯) fall within range of normal volunteers. (Courtesy of Olgin J, Argov Z, Rosenberg H, et al: *Anesthesiology* 68:507–513, April 1988.)

nant hyperthermia-susceptible patients diagnosed with caffeine contracture tests and 25 normal controls. I hope that many magnetic resonance spectroscopists learn how to use this technique and that we as a specialty can benefit from this technology.—M.F. Roizen, M.D.

Modified ECT Using Succinylcholine After Remission of Neuroleptic Malignant Syndrome

Devanand DP, Sackeim HA, Finck AD (New York State Psychiatric Inst, New York; Columbia Univ)
Convulsive Ther 3(4):284–290, 1987   8–11

Neuroleptic malignant syndrome and malignant hyperthermia exhibit similar clinical characteristics, such as tachycardia, tachypnea, hyperthermia, autonomic dysfunction, rigidity, and disordered cardiac conduction. Although these disorders appear to have different causes, there is some evidence that they share a primary peripheral etiology. Two patients with histories of neuroleptic malignant syndrome underwent successful treatment with bilateral electroconvulsive therapy (ECT), in which methohexital was used as an anesthetic and succinylcholine was used as a muscle relaxant. This supports the hypothesis that rigidity and intermittent hyperthermia in neuroleptic malignant syndrome may have a central origin, in contrast to malignant hyperthermia, which results from a genetic defect in skeletal muscle.

Both patients had symptoms of rigidity and elevated temperature. Neuroleptic malignant syndrome developed in 1 patient while under treatment with neuroleptic medication. When admitted to hospital, he exhibited extensive delusional behavior. High doses of lorazepam and a trial of clonidine were ineffective, so ECT was instituted. The patient received 11 bilateral treatments along with intravenously administered succinylcholine. The other patient underwent 6 bilateral treatments and the same regimen of succinylcholine.

There were no complications with either patient and no cardiac abnormalities. There was little clinical response in the first patient; however, the second patient had complete remission of symptoms after treatment. Because of poor outpatient compliance, the second patient had 3 subsequent hospitalizations for manic episodes. For each episode, he was treated with ECT and succinylcholine without complications or cardiac arrhythmias.

The results indicate that ECT can be used in conjunction with succinylcholine for treatment of neuroleptic malignant syndrome. This report does not support the view that use of succinylcholine will precipitate malignant hyperthermia; however, it must be remembered that these patients had short exposure to succinylcholine and anesthesia. It appears that muscle rigidity and hyperthermia are centrally caused in neuroleptic malignant syndrome.

▶ The resurgence of interest in electroconvulsive therapy has provided the anesthesiologist with difficult decisions regarding drug interactions and the impact of co-existing medical diseases. An elderly patient with angina pectoris being treated with appropriate cardiac drugs plus antidepressant medication is not an infrequent challenge. It could be an equally unnerving challenge to begin the day faced with a patient with a history of neuroleptic malignant syndrome. In this regard, the safety of using succinylcholine in such a patient would be comforting information.—R.K. Stoelting, M.D.

9 Postoperative Problems

General

Unexpected Focal Neurologic Deficit on Emergence From Anesthesia: A Report of Three Cases

Oliver SB, Cucchiara RF, Warner MA, Muir JJ (Mayo Clinic and Mayo Med School, Rochester, Minn)

Anesthesiology 67:823–826, November 1987   9–1

A patient emerging from anesthesia with a new and unexpected focal neurologic abnormality must be assumed to have had an acute focal injury from ischemia or hemorrhage. Patients with a global cerebral insult from profound hypotension, hypoxia, or cardiac arrest may have diffuse neurologic abnormalities without localizing signs. Three cases illustrate the various etiologies for unexpected focal neurologic deficit on emergence from general anesthesia.

Case 1.—Man, 65, underwent percutaneous ultrasonic lithotripsy after percutaneous placement of a wire into the renal pelvis under local anesthesia. General anesthesia was induced intravenously with 400 mg of thiopental and was maintained with 50% nitrous oxide and 0.5% to 1.5% enflurane in oxygen. Ten minutes postoperatively, dense right hemiplegia was noted. The diagnosis was focal left cerebral hemispheric infarction, probably caused by emboli of cardiac origin.

Case 2.—Woman, 32, underwent pelvic laparoscopy for persistent pelvic pain. General anesthesia was induced intravenously with 500 mg of thiopental and was maintained with 60% nitrous oxide and 0.5% to 1.5% enflurane in oxygen after endotracheal intubation was facilitated intravenously by 100 mg of succinylcholine. Thirty minutes after the procedure, a right hemiparesis and facial paresis were noted. The patient's combination of cardiac arrhythmias during intra-abdominal carbon dioxide insufflation without hypotension or hypoxia and focal neurologic deficit on emergence suggest the diagnosis of paradoxical carbon dioxide embolism.

Case 3.—Woman, 57, underwent a hysterectomy. After anesthesia was induced and the trachea was intubated, ventricular bigeminy lasting about 15 seconds was noted and the arterial blood pressure by cuff increased for 5 minutes from 120/70 mm Hg to 180/90 mm Hg. Anesthesia was maintained with 50% nitrous oxide and 1% to 2% enflurane in oxygen. Two hours postoperatively, the patient was still very lethargic; computed tomographic head scan revealed a large right intracerebral hematoma.

Perioperative neurologic injury is usually caused by ischemia or hemorrhage. Ischemic injury can result from embolic events, thrombosis of damaged arteries, or arterial compression. Patients with atherosclerotic disease of the carotid or vertebral system may have ischemia from emboli or inadequate blood flow through stenotic vessels. Pertinent information in the history of a patient awakening from anesthesia with a new neurologic deficit includes transient ischemic attacks or subarachnoid hemorrhage, medical conditions associated with increased risk of emboli, and type of operative procedure.

▶ This series by Oliver et al. clearly explains the potential mechanisms and reviews the diagnostic algorithm that can be followed should a patient have a focal neurologic deficit after anesthesia. This algorithm begins with a history. I would hope only that the history is simply repetition of history obtained beforehand, as a prior history of neurologic events suggestive of transient ischemic attacks or subarachnoid hemorrhage and of medical conditions that increase the risk for emboli should become known, I would think, before operation, even in busy practices that utilize nurses. Being able to critically evaluate those things that are important to care and adjust to those things may be a factor that differentiates physician-directed from physician-undirected nurse anesthesia. There is no definite evidence of a difference, but I firmly believe that difference in evaluating medical history is a major difference and the reason that physicians spent their time in medical school to broaden their base of knowledge.

The changes in computed tomographic scan that accompany both ischemic and hemorrhagic infarction are reviewed, although perhaps it should be stated that there are cerebral areas that are more likely to be affected during ischemic changes, such as the border zones where there is selective vulnerability. This vulnerability is characteristic of the cerebral cortex, especially in the parietal and occipital areas, mostly in the sulci, and affects preferentially layers 3, 5, and 6 of the gray matter. The Sommer sector of hippocampal gyrus in the temporal lobe is a favorite site for the development of ischemic changes as well, whereas the basal ganglia and diencephalic areas are affected variably by cerebral ischemia of the low blood pressure with normal oxygen content type.

Emphasis in this article is placed also on the finding that 40.3 person years of anesthesia would get an expected stroke rate of only 0.1 episodes, which means that if you were to anesthetize 60,000 people for an average period of 6 hours, you would expect only 0.1 stroke. I find this extremely low for the age group of their population, but I think this paper makes an important contribution to our understanding of stroke and of perioperative neurologic deficit. The authors are to be congratulated for their excellent contribution.— M.F. Roizen, M.D.

Thiamine Status, Vitamin Supplements, and Postoperative Confusion
Day JJ, Bayer AJ, McMahon M, Pathy MSJ, Spragg BP, Rowlands DC (Cardiff Royal Infirmary, Cardiff; Llandough Hosp, Penarth, Wales)
Age Ageing 17:29–34, January 1988   9–2

Vitamin B_1 deficiency is thought to be common among elderly patients with fractured proximal femurs and may significantly affect recovery, especially by contributing to postoperative confusion. A prospective, randomized, controlled study of the effects of a parenteral preparation of vitamins B and C on mental and thiamine status of elderly patients hospitalized after an acute fracture of the proximal femur was done.

Patients aged 60 years or older were included. Twenty-eight were allocated to receive vitamin supplements, of whom 26 received the full course of injections; 32 patients served as controls. The treated patients had significant improvement in thiamine status immediately postoperatively, but by day 14 the thiamine pyrophosphate effect had returned to near baseline values. Controls had a significant increase in thiamine status 2 days after surgery, when 14 of they had thiamine pyrophosphate values indicating borderline or definite thiamine deficiency. Neither thiamine status nor vitamin supplementation influenced mortality, length of hospital stay, or final placement of survivors. There was no significant association between thiamine pyrophosphate effect preoperatively or at any subsequent assessment of mental status of patients in either group.

Vitamin supplementation significantly but transiently improved postoperative thiamine status in elderly patients. However, it had no influence on mental state or outcome during the postoperative period. Thus, the use of parenteral vitamins for postoperative confusion cannot be justified on a routine basis.

▶ This study neatly addresses the conclusion of whether the thiamine status is responsible for postoperative confusion and comes to the conclusion that, in the vast majority of patients, it is not.—M.F. Roizen, M.D.

Analgesia

Epidural Bupivacaine and Morphine Plus Systemic Indomethacin Eliminates Pain but not Systemic Response and Convalescence After Cholecystectomy
Schulze S, Roikjaer O, Hasselstrøm L, Jensen NH, Kehlet H (Herlev Univ, Hvidovre Univ, Copenhagen)
Surgery 103:321–327, March 1988   9–3

Epidurally administered anesthetics have proved less effective in upper abdominal and thoracic surgery than in operations on the lower abdomen or lower extremity. Twenty-four patients undergoing elective cholecystectomy were randomized to receive conventional treatment of postoperative pain with intermittent nicomorphine and acetaminophen or to receive thoracic epidural analgesia. The epidural anesthesia was maintained with plain 0.5% bupivacaine alone for 24 hours, and then 0.25% bupivacaine for another 24 hours. Patients also received morphine, 4 mg, administered epidurally every 8 hours for 4 days, plus indomethacin, 100 mg, administered systemically on the same schedule.

Postoperative pain was less in the epidural group. The increase in rectal temperature was less marked in this group. Epidurally administered anesthesia did not alter the rise in plasma glucose after surgery, or the granulocytosis. Serum transferrin levels decreased more in the epidural group. Hand grip strength was unaffected in both groups.

A combination of epidurally administered bupivacaine and morphine plus systemically administered indomethacin relieves pain after cholecystectomy. Metabolic responses to surgery are not substantially altered, suggesting that factors other than pain must be controlled to lower postoperative morbidity.

▶ This is a fascinating study in which epidural analgesia with local anesthetic, and then morphine when combined with indomethacin, provided substantially more postoperative pain relief than intermittent narcotic and acetaminophen therapy. Although there are minor and, according to the authors, clinically unimportant changes in plasma cortisol, glucose, transferrin, white blood cell counts, temperature peak flow, and fatigue, the differences between the 2 groups in quality of postoperative pain relief is striking. Clearly, factors other than pain must be controlled and modulated in order to reduce postoperative morbidity. In a few select patients, and in an uncontrolled study, I have combined ibuprofen and oral analgesics. I was very impressed by the qualitative improvement in well-being between patients receiving an oral analgesic and those receiving an oral analgesic and the nonsteroidal anti-inflammatory agent. Not only was the quality of pain relief improved, but the overall outlook of the patient was clearly better during convalescence. Certainly more studies need to be done in the area of combining narcotics with nonsteroidal anti-inflammatory agents during which several parameters known to demonstrate adequate postoperative convalescence can be assessed.—G.W. Ostheimer, M.D.

Patient-Controlled Analgesia vs. Conventional Intramuscular Analgesia Following Colon Surgery

Albert JM, Talbott TM (Ferguson Clinic, Grand Rapids, Mich)
Dis Colon Rectum 31:83–86, February 1988   9–4

Conventional techniques of intermittent intramuscular administration of analgesic fall short of meeting the needs of patients after major abdominal surgery. Patient-controlled analgesia (PCA) is a safe and effective method of postoperative pain control. The efficacy and cost of PCA and intramuscular administration of the same narcotic agent for the same type of operation were compared in a prospective, randomized trial in 62 patients aged 38–90 undergoing elective colon surgery. All had partial or total elective colon resection via a vertical midline incision. Thirty-two were assigned to postoperative pain control with PCA-administered morphine and 30 were assigned to intramuscular-administered morphine. The PCA system contained a 60-cc syringe pump filled with morphine, 1 mg/cc, and was set to deliver 1 mg per administration with a programmable lockout period set to 10 minutes. The usual intramuscular morphine orders ranged from 5 to 12 mg every 3 to 4 hours.

The mean dose of morphine in the PCA group during the 72-hour postoperative period was 69.6 mg; the mean dose of morphine in the intramuscular group was 92.2 mg. The difference was statistically significant. The mean cost per patient for injectable narcotics in the PCA group was $109.00, which included the use of the PCA apparatus for 3 days; the mean cost per patient for the intramuscular group was $75.00. There was no statistical difference in the amount of nausea, vomiting, and the level of sedation and analgesia between the 2 study groups. Many patients in the PCA group preferred PCA to intramuscular injections for pain control.

▶ Patient-controlled analgesia has made intermittent intramuscular administration of opioids for postoperative pain relief a historical procedure.—R.K. Stoelting, M.D.

Patient-Controlled Analgesia in Pediatric Surgery
Rodgers BM, Webb CJ, Stergios D, Newman BM (Univ of Virginia)
J Pediatr Surg 23:259–262, March 1988   9–5

Patient-controlled analgesia (PCA) has been studied frequently in adult patients, but no reports of its use in children are available. The safety and efficacy of PCA for relief of postoperative pain in children and adolescents were studied in 15 patients aged 11–18 years undergoing major thoracic or abdominal surgery. Postoperative PCA was available via a microprocessor-operated infusion syringe. Patients and their parents were taught how to use the equipment before surgery.

The mean duration of PCA was 2.6 days. There were no major mechanical difficulties with the equipment. Patient acceptance of PCA was excellent; only 2 patients preferred some other method of analgesia. A nurse assessed pain relief twice daily using a verbal-visual pain scale. The average pain relief was 7.2 on a 10-point scale. Eight patients had previous surgery; 7 reported preferring PCA as a method of pain control. In comparison with patients receiving conventional analgesia, PCA-treated patients used less postoperative analgesia overall but more during the first 24 hours.

Patient-controlled analgesia is safe and effective in pediatric patients. Satisfactory pain relief can be achieved with less analgesia and with less nursing attention. This procedure is recommended for postoperative pediatric patients.

▶ Patient-controlled analgesia is again demonstrated to be an effective means of providing pain relief, even in this study with a small number of pediatric patients. I know a number of unpublished studies that will demonstrate that even younger patients can effectively utilize PCA by themselves or through their responsible parents.

How many of our readers have had pain in the hospital and realized after 1 or 2 requests for medication that they must time their requests from 30 to 90 minutes before the actual need because of the inability of the nursing staff to respond due to understaffing and being overworked? The nursing shortage is not going to improve in the near future, and therefore, inventive ways of providing analgesia will be a necessity for good patient care. Patient-controlled analgesia remains the best attempt to date to utilize parenteral medication for pain relief. Interestingly, in almost all the studies I have reviewed, the patients do not want to totally remove their pain to a pain score of 0. They prefer to have a little discomfort knowing that they can decrease their discomfort when necessary. The ability to control one's own pain relief appears to be the overriding consideration in the acceptance of PCA by our patients.—G.W. Ostheimer, M.D.

Use of Patient-Controlled Analgesia for Management of Acute Pain
White PF (Stanford Univ)
JAMA 259:243–247, Jan 8, 1988

9–6

Previous studies have found that small intravenous doses of opioid analgesics administered on demand to postoperative patients provided improved pain relief with smaller total drug dosages. Because repeated administration of small intravenous bolus doses of opiate compounds is impractical owing to the demands placed on the nursing staff, instruments have been designed that allow patients to self-administer small intravenous doses of opioid drugs when they feel the need for pain relief. Patient-controlled analgesia (PCA) devices have been improved over the years so that it is now possible for a patient to safely self-administer small intravenous bolus doses of an analgesic by depressing a button located at the end of a cord that extends from an infusion pump connected to a timing device. The purpose of the timer is to provide a safeguard against administration of additional doses until a specific time interval has elapsed. This so-called lockout, or delay interval, allows the first dose to exert its maximal pharmacologic effect and prevents overdose.

For PCA therapy to be successful, patients should be given thorough preoperative instructions, so that they understand the concept of this form of therapy. The ideal drug for PCA therapy has not yet been found, but the opiate analgesics are the most widely used parenteral drugs in postoperative analgesia, as these drugs have rapid onset of analgesic action and are highly efficacious in relieving pain. In a carefully controlled randomized study, patients who used PCA required significantly less narcotic medication to achieve comparable postoperative analgesia than did patients who received conventional intramuscular injections for the treatment of acute postoperative pain. Patients especially like the PCA system because it provides them with a certain measure of control over their pain and it removes the anxiety of waiting for an injection when the pain is already severe. Patients who use PCA are usually able to maintain a near optimal state of analgesia with minimal sedation and few side effects. Although the risk of clinically significant respiratory depression in patients receiving PCA therapy is low, some investigators suggest that special precautions, such as the use of apnea monitors, should be taken to minimize the risk of this potentially life-threatening complication.

It appears that PCA is safe and effective in the management of acute pain in postoperative patients. The concept of PCA could well be extended to other patient populations with severe pain.

▶ This is a nice review article of the current status of a very useful technique for managing postoperative pain. This technique and epidural narcotics are revolutionizing approaches to postoperative pain management.—R.D. Miller, M.D.

Epidural Narcotic, and Patient-Controlled Analgesia for Post-cesarean Section Pain Relief
Harrison DM, Sinatra R, Morgese L, Chung JH (Yale Univ)
Anesthesiology 68:454–457, March 1988   9–7

Postoperative pain can be controlled by either intramuscular or epidural administration of narcotics or by patient-controlled analgesia (PCA). These 3 modalities were compared in a randomized prospective study of 60 patients after undergoing cesarean section.

Twenty-two patients in group A received morphine epidurally after surgery; 18 patients in group B received PCA; and 20 patients in group C received morphine intramuscularly. Pain level was graded from mild to severe, and patient satisfaction, presence of pruritus, nausea and vomiting, and respiratory rates were noted.

In group A, 85% of patients reported mild pain, compared with 40% in group B and 45% in group C. Patients in group B did not have significantly lower pain scores than those in group C. Significantly lower pain scores in group A persisted for 16 hours after delivery. Respiratory rates, incidence of nausea and vomiting, and length of hospital stay were comparable in all groups. In group A, 45% of patients required treatment for pruritus, compared with 11% in group B and 6% in group C. Two patients in group A said they would not undergo the therapy again because of the severity of the pruritus. All patients receiving PCA expressed satisfaction with this form of analgesia.

Epidurally administered morphine provides the best pain relief, but with a higher morbidity. A high rate of patient satisfaction and uniform analgesia offered by PCA make this therapy an attractive alternative.

Patient-Controlled Analgesia Following Cesarean Section: A Comparison With Epidural and Intramuscular Narcotics
Eisenach JC, Grice SC, Dewan DM (Wake Forest Univ)
Anesthesiology 68:444–448, March 1988   9–8

Epidural morphine and intravenous patient-controlled analgesia (PCA) are alternatives to the traditional intramuscular administration of analgesics for treating postoperative pain. The few studies that have compared epidural morphine and PCA have usually focused on pain scores. Pain scores, side effects, and patient satisfaction were compared in women receiving epidural morphine, intravenous PCA, or intramuscular narcotics after cesarean section.

Sixty women with American Society of Anesthesiologists physical status I or II, scheduled for elective repeat cesarean section, were studied. All had uncomplicated pregnancies, were taking no medications, and had received intramuscular doses of narcotics after previous cesarean procedures. Immediately after delivery, each woman received 0.5 mg of droperidol intravenously as prophylaxis against nausea and was assigned randomly to receive postoperative analgesia by epidural morphine, intravenous PCA morphine, or intramuscular narcotics.

Hourly morphine consumption remained constant in the PCA and intramuscular groups, but the interpatient variability was large. Total use of narcotics was greater in the PCA group than in the intramuscular group and was greater in the intramuscular group than in the epidural morphine group. Forty percent of those receiving epidural morphine required parenteral narcotics within 12 hours of surgery and 50% required parenteral narcotics within 24 hours. Patients in the intramuscularly treated group were more likely than those in the other 2 groups to report being uncomfortable or in pain. Epidural morphine caused more pruritus than PCA or intramuscular therapy, although the incidence of nausea was comparable in all groups. Patients in both the PCA and epidural morphine groups preferred their therapy over the intramuscular narcotic given after their first cesarean section, but only those receiving epidural morphine perceived better pain relief. Decreased pain scores were correlated with patient satisfaction overall.

Compared with intramuscularly administered narcotics after cesarean section, epidural morphine and PCA provided better analgesia and patient satisfaction. However, epidural morphine caused the most pruritus, and PCA, the most sedation.

▶ It is evident from these studies that epidural morphine provides superior pain relief when compared with patient-controlled analgesia (PCA) or intramuscular administration of narcotics. However, with this success also comes the down side evidenced by side effects. In both studies, the PCA group had approximately double the pruritus of the intramuscular group, whereas the epidural group had more pruritis than the other groups in both studies and more nausea in the Eisenach et al. study (Abstract 9–8) than the PCA group. Whereas the amount of drug administered showed little difference between the PCA and the intramuscular groups, patient satisfaction with PCA was comparable with the pain relief obtained by the epidural morphine group in the Harrison et al. study (Abstract 9–7) and better in the Eisenach et al. study. The authors state that responsible factors may be the increased pain tolerance and satisfaction related to a more uniform level of analgesia, a lack of troublesome side effects, and the ability to provide their own reliable analgesia when required.

Although patients using PCA morphine did not achieve total analgesia, they were able to balance at a level at which the troublesome side effects of increasing sedation, nausea, and pruritus were kept to a minimum. As the authors suggest, the agent for PCA administration may not be morphine but one of the more lipid soluble opioids that are presently being investigated. This is an exciting new area in acute pain management and undoubtedly we will see many studies in the near future with a wide variety of drugs administered by patient-controlled analgesia.— G.W. Ostheimer, M.D.

Development of an Anesthesiology-Based Postoperative Pain Management Service

Ready LB, Oden R, Chadwick HS, Benedetti C, Rooke GA, Caplan RC, Wild LM (Univ of Washington)
Anesthesiology 68:100–106, January 1988   9–9

Effective pain control is a vital aspect of surgical management. Like chronic pain, acute pain deserves a commitment by interested and expert practitioners. An Acute Pain Service (APS) was formed jointly by anesthesiology and nursing services, with the goal of making epidural opiate analgesia constantly available to surgical patients. Patient-controlled analgesia also is part of the program. Standard protocols comprise physician orders, planned nursing care, and communication between anesthesiologists and APS physicians.

The APS cared for 820 patients during the first 18 months. The mean number of days of care provided per patient was 3.8 (range, 1–15). Most patients received epidurally administered narcotics. Teaching ward nurses to inject narcotics has made epidural analgesia much easier. Marked respiratory depression was noted in 4 patients during the first 6 months of APS experience. All these patients were elderly and at high risk, and underwent major, prolonged operations. No serious respiratory depression has occurred since.

The ability to monitor adequacy of ventilation, rather than merely respiratory rate, would improve surgical care. Acute pain management will be part of the year of training recently added to anesthesiology residencies.

▶ This article and the accompanying editorial (1) in the journal *Anesthesiology* should be required reading for anesthesiologists. Clearly the anesthesiologist is the most competent person to deal with pain management. Just as anesthesiologists got out of the operating room and into the intensive care unit in the 1960s, the pain management team is getting out of the operating room and into the management of acute and chronic pain in the 1980s. A perusal of the abstracts at scientific meetings of the major national societies over the last few years will document the inventive approaches by anesthesiologists to the management of pain either by epidural infusions, intrapleural catheter infusions or by patient-controlled analgesic infusions.

The management of chronic pain is often a tedious task and one easily relinquished by the surgeon. The anesthesiologist can make a contribution to chronic pain management; however, the overall management relies on a mul-

238 / Anesthesia

tidisciplinary approach. Conversely, the management of acute pain is and always will be the bailiwick of the practicing anesthesiologist. As Dr. Saidman comments in his editorial, new and inventive ways of providing pain relief coupled with pharmacologic advances in opioid and nonopioid drugs will provide significant advances in pain therapy in the future.—G.W. Ostheimer, M.D.

Reference

1. Saidman LJ: The anesthesiologist outside the operating room: A new and exciting opportunity. *Anesthesiology* 68:1–2, January 1988. Editorial.

Continuous Infection of Bupivacaine via Intrapleural Catheter for Analgesia After Thoracotomy in Children
McIlvaine WB, Knox RF, Fennessey PV, Goldstein M (The Children's Hosp, Denver; Univ of Colorado)
Anesthesiology 69:261–264, August 1988   9–10

Previous studies have demonstrated the efficacy of intrapleural analgesia when used in adults after cholecystectomy, mastectomy, and renal operations, but this form of analgesia has not yet been evaluated in children. The efficacy of continuous intrapleural bupivacaine infusion for analgesia after thoracotomy was assessed in 14 children whose mean age was 129.9 months. All had undergone thoracotomy for coarctation or anterior fusion.

Pain scores were determined before infusion as soon as the patient was alert after the anesthesia and hourly for 32 hours thereafter. Each child was given a 24-hour continuous infusion of 0.25% bupivacaine with 1:200,000 epinephrine via an intrapleural catheter. Rectally administered chloral hydrate and intravenously administered diazepam were given for sedation with acetaminophen given rectally as needed for fever. Narcotic analgesics were given if analgesia at the maximum infusion rate was inadequate. The study was terminated if pain was not controlled within 30 minutes of an infusion rate increase. Intravenously administered morphine was used for analgesia after termination of the infusion.

The pain scores for all 14 children showed a statistically significant difference from baseline scores. There were no statistically significant differences between postoperative and control measurements of vital signs at any time during the study. None of the patients required narcotics during intrapleural infusion.

Infusion of local anesthetics via an intrapleural catheter appears to provide safe and effective postoperative analgesia in children.

▶ This is the first study of the use of the intrapleural catheter to provide analgesia with a continuous infusion of local anesthetic after thoracotomy in children. Although a number of authors have shown efficacy of this technique in certain surgical procedures in adults, the overall assessment of what procedures this technique is best for and whether the procedure is safe enough for current everyday practice is yet to be determined. The reader is referred to the editorial by Dr. Covino in *Anesthesia and Analgesia* (67:427–429, 1988) for a well-presented overview of this technique. Certainly the fact that bupivacaine concentrations exceeded the recommended peak concentrations for adults is of concern. The authors made reasonable recommendations, and I'm sure we will see other recommendations in the near future. The reader is advised to look to further issues of YEAR BOOK OF ANESTHESIA for more articles and commentary on this procedure.—G.W. Ostheimer, M.D.

Intrapleural Administration of 0.25%, 0.375%, and 0.5% Bupivacaine With Epinephrine After Cholecystectomy
Strömskag KE, Reiestad F, Holmqvist ELO, Ogenstad S (Molde County Hosp, Molde, Norway; Pain Control, Clinical Research, and Dept of Biostatistics, Astra, Sweden)
Anesth Analg 67:430–434, 1988   9–11

Pulmonary complications after upper abdominal surgery are minimized by assuring adequate pain relief. Systemic uptake of bupivacaine was estimated after the intrapleural administration of different concentrations in 30 patients undergoing cholecystectomy. The patients received 20-ml volumes of 0.25%, 0.375%, and 0.5% bupivacaine with added epinephrine. Total doses were 50, 75, and 100 mg, respectively. Injections were made into the right pleural space when pain occurred.

Nearly all patients obtained complete pain relief within 15–30 minutes of bupivacaine injection. The duration of analgesia ranged from 4 hours 20 minutes after administration of the lowest dose of bupivacaine to 7 hours 45 minutes after the highest dose. The peak plasma concentration in patients given 100 mg of bupivacaine was 1.20 µg/ml. No side effects occurred.

Intrapleurally administered bupivacaine is an effective method of analgesia after unilateral upper abdominal surgery. Reverse diffusion of local anesthetic from the pleural to the subpleural space and thence to the thin muscles may explain the spread of anesthesia to a large number of intercostal spaces.

Interpleural Catheter Analgesia for Pancreatic Pain
Durrani Z, Winnie AP, Ikuta P (Univ of Illinois, Chicago)
Anesth Analg 67:479–481, 1988   9–12

Interpleural anesthetic instillation is used after cholecystectomy and renal surgery. As both visceral and abdominal wall pain are abolished, this approach might be useful in managing pain caused by abdominal malignancies.

Man, 63, presented a week after exploration for inoperable pancreatic cancer with severe, constant upper abdominal pain radiating to the back. Marked nausea accompanied the pain. Doses of hydromorphine gave relief for 1 hour. Because any position other than sitting made the pain worse, the patient refused procedures involving any but the sitting position. A left interpleural catheter was inserted, and increments of 0.5% bupivacaine were instilled until pain was totally relieved. Oral feedings became possible without undue discomfort. A second injection of 0.5% bupivacaine, 8 ml, was similarly effective. Pain then was controlled adequately by acetaminophen for the next 3 months.

Interpleural injections of local anesthetic provide long-lasting relief of upper abdominal cancer pain. They may be a useful alternative to celiac plexus block in some patients. If pain relief is transient, injections of dilute phenol might be indicated. Many types of pathologic pain in the upper abdomen and thorax may be amenable to this approach.

▶ These 2 articles (Abstracts 9–11 and 9–12) that the pleural administration of local anesthetic produces adequate pain relief in patients undergoing surgical procedures, in this case, cholecystectomy, and in a patient with chronic pain from carcinoma of the pancreas. The reader is referred to the accompanying editorial (1) on interpleural regional anesthesia by Dr. Benjamin Covino. In his editorial, Dr. Covino raises a number of issues that must be addressed concerning this technique. The term intrapleural has been used in some studies, whereas Dr. Covino feels that the correct term should be inter*pleural regional analgesia* because the anesthetic solution is deposited between the parietal and visceral pleura. The reader will note I am using the term *"pleural" analgesia* because the solution is deposited in the pleural space. Both Dr. Covino and I hope that future articles will use a standard terminology so as not to confuse the reader.

The mechanism of analgesia has been suggested to be diffusion of local anesthetic solution from the pleural space through the innermost intercostal muscle to reach the intercostal space where blockade of the intercostal nerve will occur. However, because the blocks reported to date have not been intense enough to provide sensory analgesia, one may question whether this is the mechanism. Dr. Covino raises the issue that the degree of analgesia may be qualitative more than quantitative owing to the concentration of local anesthetic used. Many more studies need to be performed to determine the optimal volume, concentration, and total dosage of local anesthetics required for this technique that are safe for the patient. The most prominent adverse effect is the production of a pneumothorax. However, to date, this has not been a major problem. The question of vascular absorption leading to a toxic reaction is of major concern of all those interested in this technique. High enough levels of bupivacaine have not been recorded to lead one to believe that this is an immediate problem. As with intranasal administration of narcotics, these studies demonstrate that the inventiveness of the anesthesiologist at providing operative conditions and postoperative pain relief will clearly expand in the future.—G.W. Ostheimer, M.D.

Reference

1. Covino BG: Interpleural regional analgesia. *Anesth Analg* 67:427–429, 1988. Editorial.

Transcutaneous Electrical Nerve Stimulation in the Management of Acute Postoperative Pain
McCallum MID, Glynn CJ, Moore RA, Lammer P, Phillips AM (Radcliffe Infirmary, Oxford; Univ of Oxford, England)
Br J Anaesth 61:308–312, 1988   9–13

The effectiveness of transcutaneous electrical nerve stimulation (TENS) in the management of chronic pain has been well established, but its usefulness in the management of acute postoperative pain has been less well documented. Several studies reported that TENS avoided the problems of respiratory depression, sedation, and nausea observed with the use of opioids, and that TENS was associated with a reduced incidence of postoperative ileus and pulmonary complications when compared with extradural analgesia. As TENS has not yet been evaluated in a randomized, double-blind, placebo-controlled study, the efficacy of TENS was assessed prospectively with 2 groups of patients receiving the same anesthetic for identical surgical procedures.

Of 20 patients undergoing decompressive lumbar laminectomy, 10 received active and 10 received inactive TENS for the management of postoperative pain during the first 24 hours after operation. The efficacy of TENS was assessed using morphine demand analgesia by comparing the number of patient demands for analgesia, the total dose of morphine delivered by the demand equipment, and the plasma concentration of morphine attained.

None of the patients experienced complications or difficulties with the use of the TENS system, as all patients had been instructed in its use before operation, and they were sufficiently familiar with the stimulator box and its controls to be able to start using TENS shortly after regaining consciousness. However, there was no statistically significant difference between the 2 groups in the number of patient demands for analgesia, morphine dose, or plasma morphine concentrations.

Transcutaneous electrical nerve stimulation is no better than a placebo in producing relief of acute postoperative pain.

▶ Similar findings have been reported in regard to the use of TENS for the pain of labor. However, the use of TENS in patients with chronic pain conditions may be more promising.—G.W. Ostheimer, M.D.

Meperidine-Induced Delirium
Eisendrath SJ, Goldman B, Douglas J, Dimatteo L, Van Dyke C (Univ of California, San Francisco)
Am J Psychiatry 144:1062–1065, August 1987   9–14

Meperidine was originally developed as an anticholinergic agent, but today it is widely used as an analgesic. Although several other adverse effects have been reported, little has been written about meperidine-induced delirium.

The records of 26 patients with neuropsychiatric disturbances related to meperidine treatment were reviewed. Twenty patients were excluded from the study because of medical causes. Two of 6 patients in the study also suffered seizures. In all but 1 patient, symptoms were induced by less than the maximum recommended dose administered over a period of at least 3 days. Discontinuation of meperidine resulted in disappearance of symptoms within 72 hours.

Delirium must be considered as a possible side effect in patients treated with meperidine, particularly when they are also receiving other drugs with anticholinergic activity. For patients in whom meperidine-induced delirium is suspected, morphine or other analgesics should be substituted. Further study is warranted to investigate the effect of cimetidine on the metabolism of meperidine.

▶ Anesthesiologists are well aware that anticholinergic effects of drugs such as scopolamine and, to a lesser extent, atropine may lead to undesirable central nervous system effects that are often characterized as delirium. Considering these known side effects of anticholinergic drugs, it is surprising that meperidine has escaped notice. The present report calls our attention to the possibility, but the occurrence of these phenomena during the perioperative period seems remote considering the observation in the present report that symptoms did not occur before 3 days of administration.—R.K. Stoelting, M.D.

Dexamethasone Alters Plasma Levels of Beta-endorphin and Postoperative Pain

Hargreaves KM, Schmidt EA, Mueller GP, Dionne RA (Natl Inst of Dental Research; Uniformed Services Univ of the Health Sciences, Bethesda, Md)
Clin Pharmacol Ther 42:601–607, December 1987   9–15

To confirm the hypothesis that secretion of pituitary immunoreactive β-endorphin may modulate the perception of pain, the effects of placebo or dexamethasone in intravenous doses of 0.1 mg, 0.32 mg, or 1.0 mg on suppression of immunoreactive β-endorphin secretion and development of postoperative pain were studied in 48 patients after surgical removal of impacted third molars. Pain was assessed using 3 visual analog scales and a category scale.

Compared with baseline values, circulating levels of immunoreactive β-endorphin nearly doubled in all groups during the stress of oral surgery. All 3 doses of dexamethasone significantly suppressed the postoperative increase in circulating β-endorphin levels compared with placebo (Fig 9–1). Within 60–120 minutes after surgery, patients treated with 0.1 mg of dexamethasone reported more severe pain than those who received placebo. Postoperative pain reported by the groups treated with 0.32 mg and 1.0 mg doses of dexamethasone did not differ from that in the placebo group.

These findings indicate that the increased pain observed after administration of low-dose dexamethasone is probably the result of its inhibition

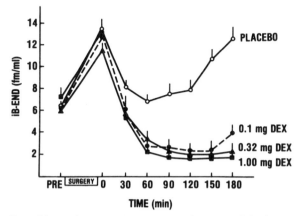

Fig 9–1.—Effects of dexamethasone *(DEX)* (0.1, 0.32, and 1.0 mg) and placebo on circulating levels of immunoreactive β-endorphin. Placebo *(open circles)*, 0.1 mg dexamethasone *(closed circles, hatched lines)*, 0.32 mg dexamethasone *(triangles)*, or 1.0 mg dexamethasone *(squares)* was administered to patients 10 minutes after completion of oral surgery. From 60 through 180 minutes after drug injection, all groups given dexamethasone had significantly lower levels of immunoreactive β-endorphin as compared with the placebo group ($P < .01$; mean ± SE). (Courtesy of Hargreaves KM, Schmidt EA, Mueller GP, et al: *Clin Pharmacol Ther* 42:601–607, December 1987.)

of pituitary β-endorphin secretion. This study supports the hypothesis that pituitary β-endorphin modulates the perception of acute postoperative pain in man.

▶ Many substances, including β-endorphins, are likely to modulate pain. It is surprising in the present study that the lowest dose, but not higher doses, of dexamethasone was associated with more severe pain despite the fact that all doses of the corticosteroid suppressed β-endorphin secretion. This observation makes cause-and-effect conclusions difficult to accept.—R.K. Stoelting, M.D.

Age Predicts Effective Epidural Morphine Dose After Abdominal Hysterectomy
Ready LB, Chadwick HS, Ross B (Univ of Washington)
Anesth Analg 66:1215–1218, December 1987   9–16

Sixty-six patients aged 22–84 years were administered morphine epidurally for pain after abdominal hysterectomy. The initial doses of morphine were 5 mg for patients aged 15–44 years, 4 mg for patients aged 45–65 years, 3 mg for patients aged 66–75 years, and 2 mg for older patients.

The mean requirement for epidurally administered morphine over 24 hours was 11.1 mg. Age was correlated weakly but significantly with the severity of pain; older patients required less morphine. The length of treatment was similar among all age groups, and side effects were no more frequent at any particular age.

Older women require less epidurally administered morphine after abdominal hysterectomy; nevertheless, the dose should be carefully adjusted in each patient for optimal analgesia and maximum safety.

▶ This article confirms an anecdotal impression I have had since I began using epidural morphine: that age is a useful predictor of the dose of epidural morphine. This retrospective study suffers from several deficits. The authors used age to determine their initial dose of epidural morphine and thus prejudiced the results to find what they retrospectively were looking for. In addition, there aren't as many patients as one would like to see in the age groups over 75; exactly 2 of their 66 patients were 75 years of age or older. I believe it is in that group where the age correlation would be strongest. Nevertheless, they did find a correlation with an R value of .4, which means approximately 16% of the difference in effectiveness of the epidural morphine dose was related to age. I would have guessed it would be more, but perhaps the lack of older people and the fact that the majority of their patients were between 40 and 70 account for the lack of a stronger correlation. Nevertheless, the article is important in pointing out that, as with virtually every other drug therapy, the dose of epidural morphine should be modified for the age of the patient.—M.F. Roizen, M.D.

Pulmonary

Subjective Effects of Humidification of Oxygen for Delivery by Nasal Cannula: A Prospective Study

Campbell EJ, Baker MD, Crites-Silver P (Jewish Hosp at Washington Univ, St Louis)
Chest 93:289–293, February 1988   9–17

Humidification of oxygen provided by nasal cannula is an expensive practice that has been justified by the prevention of patient discomfort related to drying of the upper airway mucosa. Routine humidification of low-flow oxygen ($\leq$ 4L/min) through nasal cannula has been challenged recently, based on theoretic and clinical grounds. To evaluate the necessity of oxygen humidification, 185 consecutive patients who received nasal oxygen at relatively high flow rates (5 L/min) were studied during 3 winter months in a hospital heated by hot water/forced air. The subjective complaints of 99 patients who received humidified oxygen and 86 patients who received dry oxygen were recorded. In addition, the policies for humidification of oxygen by respiratory therapy departments were assessed in 55 medium-sized American hospitals

Complaints, especially of dry nose and dry throat, were common in both patient groups. The symptoms were relatively mild and did not increase significantly when dry oxygen was given. The severity of symptoms remained stable or decreased with increasing duration of oxygen therapy. Nearly half of the hospitals surveyed delivered humidified oxygen for all patients, and only 3 did not routinely humidify nasal cannula oxygen.

Routine humidification of oxygen for nasal cannula administration remains a common respiratory care practice in American hospitals. These data indicate that routine humidification of nasal cannula oxygen is not justifiable on grounds of patient comfort, and that cessation of this practice will result in considerable reductions in both time and material costs in respiratory care.

▶ Another cherished tradition in postanesthesia respiratory care appears to have bitten the dust. Of course, a lack of subjective complaints doesn't mean that potential complications won't result if a specific technique is discontinued. However, humidification through nasal prongs, a cannula, or face mask has never been demonstrated to be of benefit. These findings are not applicable to intubated patients in whom natural humidification is bypassed.—R.R. Kirby, M.D.

Postoperative Pulmonary Complications: General Anesthesia With Postoperative Parenteral Morphine Compared With Epidural Analgesia
Jayr C, Mollié A, Bourgain JL, Alarcon J, Masselot J, Lasser P, Denjean A, Truffa-Bachi J, Henry-Amar M (Inst Gustave-Roussy, Villejuif; Hôpital A Béclère, Clamart, France)
Surgery 104:57–63, July 1988   9–18

Pulmonary complications after abdominal surgery are common. Several previous studies suggested that postoperative epidural analgesia may reduce the incidence of pulmonary complications. A comparison was made of the incidence of pulmonary complications in 146 patients who underwent major abdominal cancer surgery with or without postoperative epidural analgesia.

The patients were randomly assigned to either general intravenous fentanyl anesthesia followed by postoperative parenteral morphine on demand or combined general fentanyl and epidural bupivacaine anesthesia followed by postoperative epidural morphine every 12 hours. In the morning of the first 5 postoperative days, each patient was asked to score his or her pain relief on a visual pain scale. Pulmonary status was evaluated on the day before operation and daily during the first 5 postoperative days. Pulmonary evaluation included clinical assessment, chest x-ray studies, and measurement of blood gases and pulmonary volumes.

Epidural doses of morphine produced slightly better pain relief during the first 4 postoperative days than did parenterally administered morphine, but the difference was significant only on the first postoperative day. The incidence of postoperative pulmonary complications was similar in both groups. Clinical pulmonary complications developed in 21% of the patients given parenteral analgesia and in 26% given epidural analgesia. The incidence of radiologic complications was 50% for the parenteral group and 64% for the epidural group. These differences were not statistically significant.

Although postoperative epidural analgesia significantly improved patients' comfort on the first postoperative day after abdominal cancer surgery, it did not decrease the incidence of pulmonary complications.

▶ The results of this study may surprise many anesthesiologists. For years we believed that relief of postoperative pain would improve pulmonary function by, among other things, preventing splinting and atelectasis. Patients would thus be more cooperative, and pulmonary complications would be reduced. A nice scenario! The only problem is that available data don't support the hypothesis. Apparently the factors that predispose to pulmonary difficulties are more complex than was originally thought to be the case, and pain is only one of them. Reflex alterations in diaphragmatic function following abdominal surgery may be important, as are alterations in the distribution of ventilation and perfusion in the supine position. Altered breathing patterns also seem to be important. Thus it is perhaps too much to hope that correction of one problem, pain, will have a major impact. This observation doesn't mean we should not attempt to minimize pain, only that our expectations as to the benefit of those interventions should not be too high.—R.R. Kirby, M.D.

Alterations in the Course of and Histopathologic Response to Influenza Virus Infections Produced by Enflurane, Halothane, and Diethyl Ether Anesthesia in Ferrets

Tait AR, Du Boulay PM, Knight PR (Univ of Michigan)
Anesth Analg 67:671–676, July 1988   9–19

Recent studies indicate that it may not be necessary to postpone surgery because of mild viral infection. Changes in the course of and histopathologic response to influenza viral infections by halothane, enflurane, and diethyl ether anesthesia were investigated in ferrets. Type A influenza virus was used to infect animals aged 8–10 weeks. Animals were exposed to anesthesia 4 days after viral inoculation.

There were no significant clinical differences in fever, rhinorrhea, or sneezing between anesthetized and control animals, and no differences in lung pathology. Changes in the nasal turbinates were, however, significantly more marked in animals given enflurane. Infected animals exposed to enflurane had more epithelial necrosis and sloughing than those given the other anesthetic agents.

General anesthesia carries minimal respiratory morbidity in ferrets infected with influenza A virus. However, the possibility that enflurane may act differently on defensive processes is worth exploring. Further studies on how the volatile anesthetics influence immune responses and clinical manifestations of infection are necessary.

▶ It's unlikely that the response of infected ferrets to anesthetic agents will cause us to completely alter our timing of anesthetic administration for patients with upper respiratory infections. Other factors, such as tracheal intubation, type of operation, etc., must be considered. Nevertheless, this work provides interesting food for thought. The role of enflurane in the possible exacerbation of airway pathology certainly deserves additional investigation.—R.R. Kirby, M.D.

10 Coagulation

Preoperative Evaluation

Evaluation of Risk Factors in Intraoperative Bleeding Tendency

Halonen P, Linko K, Wirtavuori K, Hästbacka J, Ikkala E (Univ Central Hosp, Helsinki; Finnish Red Cross, Helsinki)
Ann Chir Gynaecol 76:298–302, 1987
10–1

Routine preoperative laboratory screening does not always identify risk factors for intraoperative bleeding. Unexpected intraoperative bleeding can often be attributed to either the preoperative administration of certain drugs or to relatively low factor VIII activity. Patients with high rates of factor VIII activity associated with blood group A have a tendency to increased intraoperative thrombosis. Whether patients with low rates of factor VIII activity associated with blood group O have a converse tendency to increased intraoperative bleeding was investigated. The effects of other potential risk factors on intraoperative bleeding, such as the preoperative use of nonsteroidal anti-inflammatory drugs (NSAIDs), the intraoperative use of plasma expanders, and the type of anesthesia, also were analyzed.

In elective abdominal or urologic procedures in 354 patients, the anesthetist measured intraoperative blood loss by weighing the swabs, estimating the amount of blood in the operative field, and measuring the blood in the suction chamber. At the end of the operation the surgeon estimated intraoperative bleeding tendency by grading it on a scale of 1–5, with grades 4 and 5 denoting an increased bleeding tendency.

According to the surgeons' estimates, 42 (12%) of the 354 patients had an increased bleeding tendency. However, the surgeons' estimates of bleeding tendency were correlated only weakly with actual blood loss as measured by the anesthetists. Patients who received dextran infusions during operation tended to have more excessive bleeding than those who received gelatin plasma expanders, but the difference was not statistically significant. Of all of the other potential risk factors assessed, only the preoperative use of NSAIDs was associated with a statistically significant increased bleeding tendency. The type of anesthesia used did not affect bleeding tendency. Patients with low rates of factor VIII activity associated with blood group O did not have a greater tendency toward intraoperative bleeding than did other patients (table).

The disorder of primary hemostasis caused by NSAIDs is common. Therefore, patients with additional risks of hemostasis who are scheduled to undergo surgery should not use NSAIDs before operation, especially if accurate hemostasis is of particular importance in a specific case.

▶ This study looked at the preoperative histories of a series of patients as well

247

The Effect of Analyzed Risk Factors on Estimated
Intraoperative Bleeding Tendency*

Risk factor	Estimated bleeding tendency		Proba-bility
	increased	normal	
NSAID +	24 (17 %)	118	0.016
NSAID −	18 (8 %)	194	
Dextran +	5 (24 %)	16	0.081
Dextran −	36 (11 %)	288	
Gelatin +	5 (15 %)	16	0.587
Gelatin −	36 (12 %)	276	
Halothane +	11 (15 %)	60	0.310
Halothane −	31 (11 %)	248	
Enflurane +	29 (11 %)	290	0.456
Enflurane −	13 (14 %)	79	
Low dose heparin +	2 (8 %)	23	0.535
Low dose heparin −	40 (12 %)	289	
Blood group O+	13 (12 %)	98	0.856
Blood group O−	21 (9 %)	205	
P + P			
< 0.20	0 (−)	2	
0.20−0.50	3 (38 %)	5	
0.50−0.80	4 (18 %)	18	
> 0.80	33 (12 %)	247	0.139

*Pearson chi-square test was used for comparison of number of patients
with given risk factor (+) and that of remaining patients not having this particular risk factor (−) serving as controls. In *parentheses* is the number of
patients having increased bleeding tendency within each group.
(Courtesy of Halonen P, Linko K, Wirtavuori K, et al: *Ann Chir Gynaecol* 76:298–302, 1987.)

as the risk factor based on what type of chronic drug therapy influenced a patient's intraoperative bleeding tendency. They found that the only thing that
correlated well with bleeding tendency was the use of nonsteroidal
anti-inflammatory drugs, including aspirin. Based on this, it seems justifiable to
withdraw nonsteroidal anti-inflammatory drugs before operation. Although they
didn't examine the period of days necessary for withdrawal of drug therapy to
normalize transfusion requirements, it is probable that you need about 3 days
without these drugs in order to have enough platelet aggregation activity to clot
normally.—M.F. Roizen, M.D.

Risk Factors and Transfusion Requirements in Aortic Surgery
Chant ADB, McEleny P, Machin D, Clifford PC (Royal South Hants Hosp,
Southampton; Univ of Southampton, England)
J Cardiovasc Surg 29:208–210, March–April 1988   10–2

To increase efficiency of transfusion practice at 1 institution and to
identify factors that determine individual transfusion requirements, a
study was made of heterologous blood usage by 168 patients, 135 men

Patient Characteristics by Geometric Mean Blood Transfused

		Number of patients	Geometric transfused (units)	z	P
Pre-operative					
Male	—	135	5.2	0.94	0.37
Female	—	33	5.9		
Ischaemic heart disease	No	119	5.1	1.29	0.20
	Yes	49	5.9		
Hypertensive disease	No	120	5.0	1.77	0.08
	Yes	48	6.2		
Diabetes mellitus	No	157	5.2	1.74	0.08
	Yes	11	7.4		
Occlusive disease	—	83	4.9	2.01	0.04
Aneurysm	—	85	5.9		
Anti-platelet drug	No	163	5.3	0.40	0.69
	Yes	4	6.2		
	Unknown	1	—		
Seniority	Consultant	131	5.2	0.97	0.33
	sen. registrar	37	5.9		
Operative					
Graft	Woven	77	4.6	2.77	0.006
	Knitted	80	6.0		
	Unknown	11	—		
Procedure	Bifurcated	148	5.1	1.41	0.16
	tube	20	6.8		
Post-operative					
Operative	No	161	5.2	2.51	0.01
Death	Yes	7	9.3		

(Courtesy of Chant ADB, McEleny P, Machin D, et al: *J Cardiovasc Surg* 29:208–210, March–April 1988.)

and 33 women with a mean age of 65.8 years, who underwent selective aortic reconstruction during a 3-year period. The mean hemoglobin level of these patients was 14.5 g units. Twelve units of blood were routinely ordered for every selective aortic reconstruction.

Patients with hypertensive disease required another 1.2 units of blood, those with diabetes mellitus needed an extra 2.2 units, and patients with an aneurysm required 1.0 extra units (table). The use of knitted rather than woven prostheses increased operative blood requirements by 1.4 units.

Analysis of blood requirements for selective aortic reconstruction resulted in a reduction of the standard blood bank order from 12 units to 9 units. However, it was not possible to predict individual patient requirements on the basis of this analysis.

▶ Whereas this study is interesting in that it correlates the risk factors of transfusion requirements and finds only that repair of aneurysmal disease requires more blood than repair of occlusive disease, that knitted grafts require more blood than woven grafts, and the patients who died required more blood transfusions, the overall use of blood in this series is about 2–3 times that used in America for similar operations now being reported at university centers. I believe our concern with blood, highlighted by the AIDS problem, has caused more conservative surgical practices, and perhaps those could be used by these surgeons as well. For instance, the knitted graft may have been used only for those patients in whom a knitted graft was seen to be better as a long-term vessel substitute, that is, those younger patients who needed more endothelialization, which apparently is granted by knitted graft over woven graft. For some reason, tube grafts required more blood, although not statistically more, than bifurcated grafts, something that shouldn't occur but may be a figment of the surgical technique. I believe surgical technique is probably the most important risk factor for transfusion requirements. However, the multiple regression equation that they used, including hypertensive, diabetes, aneurysm, the type of graft, and the preoperative hemoglobin accounted for only 11% of the total variation in blood given.—M.F. Roizen, M.D.

Cardiopulmonary Bypass

Failure of Prophylaxis With Fresh Frozen Plasma After Cardiopulmonary Bypass

Roy RC, Stafford MA, Hudspeth AS, Meredith JW (Bowman Gray School of Medicine, Winston-Salem, NC; Univ of Newcastle upon Tyne, England)
Anesthesiology 69:254–257, August 1988   10–3

The risks of disease transmission and of noncardiogenic pulmonary edema, associated with the prophylactic use of fresh frozen plasma (FFP) to offset dilution of clotting factors following cardiopulmonary bypass operation, warrant clear documentation of the benefit of FFP to justify its continued routine use. Routine use of FFP was discontinued and was replaced by 5% albumin solution at the authors' institution after noncardiogenic pulmonary edema developed during an infusion of FFP. The records of 100 patients who received either FFP or albumin were reviewed retrospectively.

During a 7-month study period, 52 patients received FFP and 48 patients received 5% albumin postbypass for volume replacement. All patients had normal preoperative prothrombin, activated partial thromboplastin, and bleeding times, normal platelet counts, and hemoglobins greater than 12 gm/100 ml. The prothrombin time and activated partial thromboplastin time were measured immediately upon the patients' arrival in the intensive care unit. Blood loss was defined as the 24-hour mediastinal drainage volume. Both groups of patients were well matched for age, number of grafts, bypass time, heparin and protamine doses, and male:female ratio.

Patients who received FFP had shorter prothrombin times and longer activated partial thromboplastin times than those who received albumin, but the difference was statistically not significant. For both groups, 24-hour blood losses were less than 1,100 ml, except in 1 FFP-treated patient and 2 albumin-treated patients who required reoperation because of bleeding. The difference between the 2 study groups with regard to blood loss and the number of units of whole blood and packed red blood cells transfused was not statistically significant.

The prophylactic use of FFP does not reduce blood loss, and it does not limit the number of patients who need reexploration for bleeding following cardiopulmonary bypass. Therefore, replacing FFP with 5% albumin is recommended because the use of albumin for volume replacement reduces the risk of disease transmission or other untoward reactions.

▶ Despite overwhelming evidence to the contrary, physicians continue to use fresh frozen plasma to treat presumed dilution of clotting factors following cardiopulmonary bypass. A possible solution is the requirement of accrediting agencies and quality assurance committees to document the indications for blood products. It seems unlikely that an expensive blood product with the potential for transmitting disease would be released by blood banks insisting on a recognized and valid indication before dispensing any blood product.—R.K. Stoelting, M.D.

In Vitro Effect of Fresh Frozen Plasma on the Activated Coagulation Time in Patients Undergoing Cardiopulmonary Bypass
Barnette RE, Shupak RC, Pontius J, Rao AK (Temple Univ)
Anesth Analg 67:57–60, January 1988   10–4

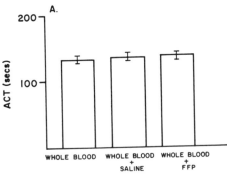

Fig 10–1.—Effect of in vitro addition of fresh-frozen plasma *(FFP)* or saline on whole blood ACT. **A,** before systemic administration of heparin, no prolongation of ACT was observed. **B,** addition of FFP but not saline after systemic administration of heparin resulted in significant prolongation of ACT $(P < .05)$. (Courtesy of Barnette RE, Shupak RC, Pontius J, et al: *Anesth Analg* 67:57–60, January 1988.)

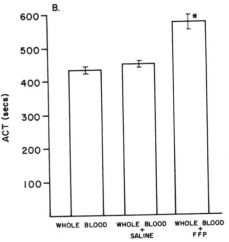

Heparin sometimes fails to prolong the coagulation time in cardiopulmonary bypass patients. Possible explanations include past exposure to heparin and a deficiency in antithrombin-III. Fresh frozen plasma has normalized the response in patients resistant to heparin. The in vitro effects of fresh frozen plasma on the activated coagulation time of whole blood in vitro were investigated in 18 patients undergoing coronary bypass surgery.

The addition of fresh frozen plasma, but not saline, increased the activated coagulation time of postheparin samples (Fig 10–1). Six of the 18 patients were heparin-resistant. Their postheparin activated coagulation time (ACT) was 346 seconds, compared with 470 seconds for the other patients. Three patients failed to obtain an ACT of 400 seconds or longer after the addition of fresh frozen plasma. The mean plasma antithrombin-III activity in all patients was 79%, significantly below normal.

In some heparin-resistant patients, adding fresh frozen plasma to whole blood after heparin administration may fail to adequately prolong the activated coagulation time. The resultant ACT may not be suitable for instituting cardiopulmonary bypass.

▶ Extrapolation of these data to the period following cardiopulmonary bypass might introduce a paradoxical drug interaction. For example, administration of fresh frozen plasma often without clear indications other than continued bleeding could accentuate a problem rather than correct it. Fresh frozen plasma, like other treatments or drugs should only be instituted when specific clinical or laboratory data confirm the need for such an intervention.—R.K. Stoelting, M.D.

Decreased Platelet Number and Function and Increased Fibrinolysis Contribute to Postoperative Bleeding in Cardiopulmonary Bypass Patients

Holloway DS, Summaria L, Sandesara J, Vagher JP, Alexander JC, Caprini JA (Evanston Hosp, Evanston, Ill)
Thromb Haemost 59:62–67, February 1988
10–5

Several changes in hemostatic mechanisms have been reported during and after cardiopulmonary bypass. Platelet and fibrinolytic concentrations were monitored simultaneously in 9 patients undergoing surgery using cardiopulmonary bypass to determine their individual and combined effects on postoperative blood loss. These systems were analyzed during the procedure and until the sixth postoperative day, and findings were correlated with chest tube drainage, the measure of postoperative blood loss.

During bypass, the hematocrit was reduced as were the platelet count and plasminogen α_2-antiplasmin, and antithrombin–III concentrations; the levels of plasminogen and antithrombin–III decreased much more than dilution. During bypass, platelet aggregability to adenosine diphosphate did not change from prebypass levels, but aggregability to arachidonic acid was significantly reduced. After protamine administration, free protease activity increased significantly, the platelet count dropped further, and platelet aggregability was decreased significantly. After protamine administration, infusion of 1 unit of fresh autologous platelets in all patients resulted in an increased circulating platelet count and improved the aggregability of circulating platelets.

The combination of a decreased platelet count and increased free protease activity was correlated significantly with chest tube drainage during the first 4 hours postoperatively. The combination of a decreased platelet count and decreased platelet aggregability was correlated significantly with the total chest tube drainage. None of the measured changes was individually correlated with chest tube drainage.

These data indicate that during the early postoperative period, increased fibrinolytic activity and a decreased platelet count contribute to postoperative blood loss in patients undergoing cardiopulmonary bypass, and that during the entire first 24-hour period postoperatively a decreased platelet count and platelet aggregability are important contributors to blood loss.

▶ This is a well-done study that confirms what many have preached before: that fibrinolytic activity and decreased platelet activity contribute to the coagulopathy associated with cardiopulmonary bypass. Hopefully, this will not encourage clinicians to administer ε-aminocaproic acid.—R.D. Miller, M.D.

Preoperative Aspirin Ingestion Increases Operative Blood Loss After Coronary Artery Bypass Grafting
Ferraris VA, Ferraris SP, Lough FC, Berry WR (Letterman Army Med Ctr, San Francisco; Uniformed Services Univ of Health Sciences, Bethesda, Md)
Ann Thorac Surg 45:71–74, January 1988   10–6

For a variety of reasons, increasing numbers of patients are given aspirin before coronary artery bypass grafting (CABG). Some studies have suggested that preoperative aspirin ingestion is associated with increased perioperative bleeding, but previous authors have not addressed the issue of postoperative blood loss. The factors that affect post-CABG blood loss in patients taking aspirin were investigated.

Thirty-four patients were randomized to receive either 325 mg of aspirin or no aspirin on the day before CABG. Bleeding time was determined in aspirin-treated patients between 2 and 10 hours after ingestion. The level of serum thromboxane B_2 was determined just before surgery.

Preoperative template bleeding time and the serum thromboxane B_2 levels were the only preoperative variables that differed significantly between the 2 groups. Aspirin-treated patients had prolonged bleeding times and decreased serum thromboxane B_2 levels compared with controls. Aspirin-treated patients had significantly increased chest-tube blood loss 12 hours after surgery (table) and required significantly more blood-product transfusions. Six patients treated with aspirin required unusual interventions for postoperative bleeding; 2 of these patients required reoperation.

Parameters of Operative Blood Loss in Aspirin-Treated
and Control Patients*

Variable	Controls	Aspirin-Treated Patients
Recovery room laboratory values		
Change in HCT (%)	−16.2 ± 6.2	−18.6 ± 8.9
Change in PLC (×1,000)	−165 ± 55	−152 ± 40
Change in PTT (sec)	+15.7 ± 11.7	+22.4 ± 21.4
Change in PT (sec)	+2.8 ± 1.1	+3.5 ± 2.2
Chest-tube blood loss in first 12 hr postoperation (ml)	916 ± 482	1,513 ± 977[a]
Transfusion requirements		
PRBC (units)	1.8 ± 1.3	4.4 ± 3.5[a]
FFP (units)	0.7 ± 1.6	3.6 ± 4.9[a]
PLT (× six-donor units)	0.16 ± 0.38	1.3 ± 1.3[a]
Patients requiring reoperation for bleeding	0	2
Patients requiring EACA or desmopressin acetate for excessive blood loss	0	4

[a]$P \leq .05$, compared with control values, by Student's t test.
*Most values are means ± SD. HCT, hematocrit; PLC, platelet count; PTT, partial thromboplastin time; PT, prothrombin time; PRBC, packed red blood cell transfusions; FFP, fresh-frozen plasma transfusions; PLT, platelet six-pack transfusions; EACA, e-aminocaproic acid.
(Courtesy of Ferraris VA, Ferraris SP, Lough FC, et al: Ann Thorac Surg 45:71–74, January 1988.)

Aspirin ingestion increases postoperative bleeding and transfusion requirements. A subset of patients is particularly sensitive to aspirin and has significantly longer bleeding times. Aspirin therapy should be discontinued before CABG.

▶ The authors of this study have examined an old question and concluded that aspirin ingestion increases postoperative blood loss and transfusion requirements. How did they test this possibility? They gave approximately half of the patients 1 aspirin (325 mg) 1 day before the operation. Although statistical significance was achieved, the data are inadequately reported, in this reviewer's opinion. For example, the aspirin-treated patients had a mean blood loss of 1513 ± 977 ml versus 916 ± 482 ml in the patients who did not receive 1 aspirin tablet. Obviously, the variability was tremendous. The authors should have provided the data for each individual patient, which would be easy to plot. Also, they recommend that preoperative measurement of template bleeding times be performed although they were unable to demonstrate a linear relationship between bleeding time and blood loss. This reviewer suggests that the entire article is read thoroughly before the authors' recommendation is followed.—R.D. Miller, M.D.

Heparin and Protamine

Heparin-Induced Thrombocytopenia and Thromboembolism in the Postoperative Period

Rizzoni WE, Miller K, Rick M, Lotze MT (Natl Cancer Inst, Bethesda, Md)
Surgery 103:470–476, April 1988   10–7

Heparin-induced thrombocytopenia and thrombosis syndrome is associated with hemorrhage as well as development of systemic thrombosis. A posthepatectomy patient was seen with probable heparin-induced thrombocytopenia complicated by venous thrombosis and pulmonary emboli after receiving low doses of heparin as line flushes.

Woman, 59, underwent extensive right-hepatic lobectomy for metastatic colon cancer. Internal jugular and radial artery catheters were placed and low doses of heparin were used as line flushes (total dose, approximately 6,000 units). Six days later, profound thrombocytopenia developed complicated by iliofemoral thrombosis, renal vein thrombosis, and pulmonary emboli. An extensive evaluation implicated heparin as the probable causative agent. This was evidenced by immediate platelet aggregation on mixing citrated plasma and heparin from the patient with platelet-rich plasma from a normal donor. Additional platelet-aggregation studies with the use of HLA-matched platelets and the patient's plasma were performed and showed aggregation only if heparin was added, probably secondary to the presence of strong HLA antibodies in addition to heparin-dependent antiplatelet antibodies. The patient's platelet count reached a nadir 12 days after initiation of heparin flushes and returned to normal 1 week after discontinuation of heparin, a clinical course that was consistent with heparin-induced thrombocytopenia. The patient was observed closely for hemorrhage and recurrent pulmonary emboli. The patient received HLA-matched platelets and the platelet count rose; warfarin therapy was then initiated. The patient's coagulation data, such as decreased fibrinogen and elevated cross-linked derivatives, indicated a consumptive coagulopathy, which cleared without treatment.

Because of the frequent use of heparin, heparin-induced thrombocytopenia is not rare and thrombosis can occur. Platelet counts should be closely observed in patients who receive heparin for any reason. If thrombocytopenia with or without thrombosis develops, heparin should be discontinued and bed rest, close observation, and subsequent anticoagulation with warfarin when platelet count rises above 50,000/mm^3 should be given. If anticoagulation is contraindicated and lower-extremity thrombosis exists, an inferior vena cava filter should be placed. If heparin is used therapeutically, it is recommended that anticoagulation with warfarin should be initiated simultaneously to minimize exposure time to heparin.

▶ Paradoxical responses to heparin are always intriguing although they seem unlikely to be manifest during the immediate postoperative period. The uniqueness of the present observation is the role of heparin flushes, presumably a small total dose, in evoking thrombocytopenia and thromboembolism. If this is even a rare occurrence, it should be recognized as a possible complication during the intraoperative or early postoperative period.—R.K. Stoelting, M.D.

Heparin-Induced Hyperkalemia

Busch EH, Ventura HO, Lavie CJ (Ochsner Clinic and Alton Ochsner Med Found, New Orleans)
South Med J 80:1450–1451, November 1987   10–8

Hyperkalemia developing during heparin therapy may be more common than previously appreciated. Three patients were seen in whom severe hyperkalemia developed during heparin therapy. All 3 had diabetes and renal insufficiency. Two patients received low doses of heparin subcutaneously for prevention of deep venous thrombosis, and 1 received intravenous doses of heparin in treatment of deep venous thrombosis. Hyperkalemia developed in all 3 patients, and atrioventricular block, in 1. Serum potassium levels returned to normal on cessation of heparin therapy.

Twelve patients with heparin-induced hyperkalemia, including the 3 already described, have now been reported in literature. Serum potassium concentrations ranged from 6.1 mEq/L to 8.3 mEq/L. Seven patients had diabetes mellitus, 8 had renal insufficiency, and 5 had both diabetes and renal insufficiency. Nine were given heparin subcutaneously, with low doses in 8. Aldosterone levels were decreased in 6 of 7 patients tested. Renin levels were increased in 4 of 6 patients tested, possibly representing a compensatory, but inadequate, increase in renin production.

Heparin-induced hyperkalemia is a potentially life-threatening problem that is more common than previously reported. Although heparin therapy is associated with decreased aldosterone production in all patients, stimulation of the renin-angiotensin-aldosterone axis occurs in most patients, thus causing kaliuresis, and preventing hyperkalemia. However, patients with diabetes or renal insufficiency who are incapable of a compensatory increase in renin production may be particularly susceptible to heparin-induced hypoaldosteronism and thus heparin-induced hyperkalemia. The serum potassium level should be monitored frequently during heparin therapy in these high-risk patients.

▶ This is an important potential drug interaction that is not commonly appreciated. It seems unlikely, however, that the acute administration of heparin, as occasionally utilized in the operating room, would produce hyporeninemia sufficient to cause hyperkalemia. Indeed, in the 3 patients described in detail by the authors, the onset of hyperkalemia occurred after 5, 10, and 14 days of heparin therapy.—R.K. Stoelting, M.D.

Hemodynamics of Protamine Administration: Comparison of Right Atrial, Left Atrial, and Aortic Injections

Katz NM, Kim YD, Siegelman R, Ved SA, Ahmed SW, Wallace RB (Georgetown Univ)
J Thorac Cardiovasc Surg 94:881–886, December 1987   10–9

Protamine injection for heparin reversal after cardiopulmonary bypass is occasionally associated with mild to severe hemodynamic deterioration, ranging from mild hypotension to cardiovascular collapse. Several studies have suggested that changing the protamine injection site to the left side of the circulation might avoid hypotensive reactions. This suggestion was based on the hypothesis that passage of concentrated protamine through the pulmonary bed would be avoided. To determine whether the injection site influences hemodynamic deterioration, the hemodynamic effects of protamine injection into the right atrium, left atrium, and aorta were compared.

The study group consisted of 68 patients who underwent isolated coronary artery bypass grafting. After the venous drainage cannula had been removed, protamine was injected in the right atria of 23 patients, the left atria of 22 patients, and the aortas of 23 patients. The 3 groups were matched as to age, sex, and clinical characteristics. Hemodynamic measurements were recorded before cannulation, after removal of the venous drainage catheter, and 1 minute, 5 minutes, and 10 minutes after protamine administration.

Eleven patients experienced a 20% decrease in systolic blood pressure, 2 in the right atrium group, 4 in the left atrium group, and 5 in the aorta group. Hypotension occurred during protamine administration in patients who received protamine via the aortic route. However, none of the differences between the 3 groups was statistically significant. A further analysis for type II error indicated that it was unlikely that an important difference had been missed.

The route of administration does not affect the hemodynamic changes associated with protamine administration.

▶ Rate of administration and the patient's intravascular fluid volume are probably more important than the actual site of injection of protamine. Nevertheless, if protamine-induced histamine release occurs in the lungs, a peripheral venous injection site or, alternatively, a site distal to the pulmonary circulation would be logical. There are data supporting a peripheral venous injection site (*Anesth Analg* 65:78–80, 1986) although this benefit is not supported by left atrial or aortic injection sites, which initially exclude the lungs from the highest blood concentrations of the drug.—R.K. Stoelting, M.D.

Desmopressin

1-Desamino-8-D-Arginine Vasopressin (Desmopressin) Decreases Operative Blood Loss in Patients Having Harrington Rod Spinal Fusion Surgery: A Randomized, Double-Blinded, Controlled Trial
Kobrinsky NL, Letts RM, Patel LR, Israels ED, Monson RC, Schwetz N, Cheang MS (Univ of Manitoba; Children's Hosp of Winnipeg, Man; Manitoba Cancer Treatment and Research Found, Winnipeg)
Ann Intern Med 107:446–450, October 1987   10–10

Desmopressin improves the bleeding time in hemostatically impaired patients undergoing surgery. This might also be true in hemostatically

Preoperative Desmopressin-Related Changes in Hemostatic Values

	Mean Values		Mean Change	95% Confidence Interval	p Value
	Before Desmopressin Therapy	After Desmopressin Therapy			
Plasma factors *†, %					
Prothrombin time	99	99	0	−0.02 to 0.02	0.770
Partial thromboplastin time	98	85	−13	−16.0 to −10.5	0.0001
Factor VIII coagulant activity	116	267	151	127 to 174	0.0001
von Willebrand antigen	106	183	78	65 to 90	0.0001
Platelet factors					
Platelets ‡, × 10^9/L	314	303	−11	−19 to −2	0.018
Platelet volume ‡, fL	9.3	8.9	−0.37	−0.52 to −0.22	0.002
Glass-bead platelet retention §, %	43	79	36	30.7 to 41.6	0.0001
Other factors					
Bleeding time *, min	5.8	4.5	−1.3	−1.8 to −0.8	0.0003
Prothrombin consumption ‖, %	82	91	9	5.8 to 12.2	0.0001
Hematocrit ‡, L/L	0.401	0.380	−0.022	−0.027 to −0.017	0.0001

*Number of patients tested was 33.
†Data are expressed as percentage of control values.
‡Number of patients tested was 29.
§Determinations were done in 30 patients.
‖ Measurements were taken in 22 patients.
(Courtesy of Kobrinsky NL, Letts RM, Patel LR, et al: Am Intern Med 107:446–450, October 1987.)

normal patients. Operative blood loss was evaluated in a trial of desmopressin in patients with scoliosis undergoing spinal fusion surgery.

Seventeen of 35 patients scheduled for spinal fusion with Harrington rod instrumentation were randomized to receive desmopressin. The remaining patients received placebo.

Preoperatively, desmopressin increased factor VIII coagulant activity, von Willebrand antigen concentrations, prothrombin consumption, and glass-bead platelet retention; and it decreased the partial thromboplastin and bleeding times (table). Intraoperative blood loss was reduced by 32% in patients receiving desmopressin. The need for concentrated erythrocyte transfusions was reduced by 25%, and the need for postsurgical analgesia was reduced by 13% in these patients. The best predictors of intraoperative blood loss and transfusion requirements were bleeding time, glass-bead platelet retention, and the use of desmopressin.

The use of desmopressin in surgical procedures associated with significant blood loss is recommended. Blood loss and requirements for transfusion may be reduced as may the need for postoperative analgesia.

▶ This is a well-conducted study, although this reviewer has some concern that we are on a desmopressin bandwagon. Can administration of desmopressin be that good in reducing operative blood loss? Increased experience and multiple studies will ascertain whether these initial reports are valid. Nevertheless, the results of this study are encouraging.—R.D. Miller, M.D.

Treatment of Refractory Thrombocytopenic Bleeding With 1-Desamino-8-D-Arginine Vasopressin (Desmopressin)
Kobrinsky NL, Tulloch H (Univ of Manitoba; Manitoba Cancer Treatment and Research Found, Winnipeg, Man)
J Pediatr 112:993–996, June 1988 10–11

To provide surgical hemostasis, desmopressin is commonly used in patients with von Willebrand's disease, uremia, liver cirrhosis, and primary or acquired platelet function defects. An attempt was made to determine whether desmopressin would also be useful in providing hemostasis for patients with acute thrombocytopenic bleeding.

During a 2-year study period, 6 thrombocytopenic patients aged 7–16 years, including 5 with epistaxis, 2 with menorrhagia, and 1 with gingival bleeding secondary to leukemia, aplastic anemia, and other hematologic disorders, were treated with desmopressin. The drug was diluted in 0.9% saline solution and administered in a dose of 10 $\mu g/m^2$ by intravenous infusion for 20 minutes. ϵ-Aminocaproic acid was administered in a dose of 1,500 mg/m^2 by intravenous infusion for 30 minutes to 1 patient and orally in a dose of 1.5 gm in 3 divided doses to another.

During desmopressin infusion, epistaxis stopped in all 5 patients. After desmopressin infusion, menorrhagia decreased in both patients, as did gingival bleeding. None of the 5 patients had a recurrence of epistaxis. However, 1 boy who was in terminal care for acute lymphocytic leukemia died 12 hours later. Menorrhagia also remained controlled without further therapy.

Desmopressin for the control of acute thrombocytopenic bleeding can be used immediately in an emergency setting, carries no risk of virus transmission, and appears to be immediately effective. Desmopressin therapy should be considered in the management of acute thrombocy-topenic bleeding when standard therapeutic therapy has failed.

▶ This represents another application for the use of desmopressin. It can't be that good!—R.D. Miller, M.D.

General

Clotting Factor Levels and the Risk of Diffuse Microvascular Bleeding in the Massively Transfused Patient

Ciavarella D, Reed RL, Counts RB, Baron L, Pavlin E, Heimbach DM, Carrico CJ
(Harborview Med Ctr, Seattle)
Br J Haematol 67:365–368, November 1987   10–12

Previous studies have shown that patients who require massive blood transfusions may suffer diffuse microvascular bleeding (MVB), which is not surgically correctable. This type of generalized bleeding is the result of a primary failure of hemostasis, for which the cause has not yet been established. A study was conducted to determine to what extent abnormalities in clotting factor levels and coagulation mechanisms are involved in the development of microvascular bleeding and to assess the effects of infusion of prophylactic platelet concentrate and fresh frozen plasma in the prevention of microvascular bleeding associated with massive transfusion in trauma patients. The diagnostic value of coagulation screening tests are also assessed.

The study population consisted of 36 trauma patients who were resuscitated with lactated Ringer's solution and modified whole-blood formulas. Clotting factor activities and coagulation profiles were measured af-

Predictive Indices of Diffuse Microvascular Bleeding*

	Sensitivity (%)	Specificity (%)	Predictive value Positive (%)	Negative (%)
PT ratio				
$\geqslant 1\cdot3$	89	50	33	94
$\geqslant 1\cdot8$	44	96	80	84
PTT ratio				
$\geqslant 1\cdot3$	56	56	26	82
$\geqslant 1\cdot8$	56	96	83	87
$\geqslant 1$ Factor $\leqslant 30\%$	67	48	30	82
$\geqslant 1$ Factor $\leqslant 20\%$	44	96	67	84
Platelet count $\leqslant 50 \times 10^9/l$ or fibrinogen $\leqslant 50$ mg/dl	89	93	73	96

*PT, prothrombin; PTT, partial thromboplastin.
(Courtesy of Ciavarella D, Reed RL, Counts RB, et al: *Br J Haematol* 67:365–368, November 1987.)

ter administration of every 12 units of blood and whenever diffuse microvascular bleeding developed.

Microvascular bleeding developed in 9 of the 36 patients. Its cause in 3 patients appeared to be thrombocytopenia. Severe hypofibrinogenemia was the most significant finding in 2 patients. Four patients had multiple and severe hemostatic abnormalities, including thrombocytopenia, hypofibrinogenemia, and a decrease in the level of at least 1 clotting factor to less than 15% of normal. The platelet count and fibrinogen level were the most sensitive diagnostic tests for predicting microvascular bleeding (table).

The results of this study suggest that commonly used replacement formulas of modified blood, which contain different ratios of whole blood to fresh frozen plasma or packed red cells, do not prevent the development of MVB. Although most patients did well with modified whole blood, patients whose platelet counts fall below 50×10^9 per liter should be given platelet transfusions, and patients whose fibrinogen levels fall below 0.8 gm/L should be given fresh frozen plasma or cryoprecipitate. Whole blood, rather than modified blood-replacement formulas, should be used in patients who require massive transfusions.

▶ This study provides additional information regarding the hemostatic defects associated with massive transfusions. In general, the conclusions of previous studies have been substantiated and extended in a more sophisticated manner. Also the reader should recognize that the authors were using modified whole blood rather than pure whole blood or packed red cells.—R.D. Miller, M.D.

Hemostatic Evaluation of Patients Undergoing Liver Transplantation
Owen CA Jr, Rettke SR, Bowie EJW, Cole TL, Jensen CC, Wiesner RH, Krom RAF (Mayo Clinic and Found, Rochester, Minn)
Mayo Clin Proc 62:761–772, September 1987   10–13

The Mayo Clinic began its liver transplantation program in March 1985, and detailed coagulation and thromboelastographic (TEG) studies were performed on the first 50 such procedures in 44 patients. Most of the patients had primary sclerosing cholangitis, primary biliary cirrhosis, or chronic active hepatitis. Seven required a second liver transplant, and 6 patients died, none intraoperatively.

Pronounced hemostatic abnormalities developed during all of the liver transplantation procedures; this was expected, because the liver generates most of the clotting factors. The outstanding exception was factor VIII, which was usually in the high-normal or an even higher range. During reperfusion of the donor liver, substantial deterioration in coagulation factors was noted; this trend was corrected within 1 hour in some instances, but platelet counts continued to decrease and some coagulation factors rebounded only partially. Serial factor VII determinations appeared to have prognostic value; successive reductions in factor VII levels were noted beginning from the anhepatic phase in 1 patient who died, whereas increasing values were noted in 1 patient who survived.

Close inspection of the TEG data showed a rough approximation of 4 conventional clotting tests. Fibrinogen levels and platelet counts were correlated fairly well with TEG:reaction time (TEG:r), which reflects whole blood clotting times, and better with TEG:angle, a function of the rate of clotting. Modest negative correlations were observed between both the activated partial thromboplastin time and the prothrombin time on one hand and TEG:angle and TEG:maximum amplitude (TEG:MA), which evaluates the amount of clot, on the other.

Because TEG tracings are quickly available to the liver transplant team and because they tend to forewarn of impending hemostatic problems, TEG is a reasonably effective procedure for monitoring coagulation during liver transplantation. With continuous monitoring, any prolongation of TEG:r and TEG:r + k (the whole blood clotting times), or reduction of TEG:angle, or decrease of TEG:MA can be detected early and treated appropriately before overwhelming bleeding occurs. However, TEG studies cannot reveal specifically whether platelets, fresh frozen plasma, or cryoprecipitate is most needed.

▶ This is one of several articles that have followed the coagulation variables associated with liver transplantation. Obviously, the coagulopathy depends on multiple factors, including the preexisting condition of the patient, number of units of blood given, and so on. Also it is of interest that many liver transplant teams are attempting to provide a rebirth to the thromboelastograph.—R.D. Miller, M.D.

Surgery in Patients With Congenital Antithrombin III Deficiency
Tengborn L, Bergqvist D (Univ of Lund, Malmö, Sweden)
Acta Chir Scand 154:179–183, March 1988   10–14

It is well known that decreased antithrombin (AT)-III activity predisposes to venous thrombosis. However, no data have as yet been collected on the outcome in AT-III-deficient patients who undergo surgery. This retrospective study was done to assess postoperative clinical signs and symptoms of thromboembolic complications in AT-III-deficient patients who underwent a variety of surgical procedures, with or without thromboprophylaxis.

The study population consisted of 23 patients with confirmed congenital AT-III deficiency who underwent a total of 57 procedures, including 11 who had 21 gynecologic procedures, 8 patients who underwent 19 procedures for varicose or incompetent perforating veins, and 12 who underwent 17 various other operations. Thromboprophylaxis consisting of dextran alone was given before 18 of the 57 operations, whereas dextran with AT-III concentrate was given before 10 operations.

Thromboembolic complications developed after 5 of the 29 operations for which no thromboprophylaxis was provided. In 2 patients deep vein thrombosis developed after 3 procedures, 1 patient had postoperative thrombophlebitis, and in 1 patient pulmonary embolism was suspected. Four of the 18 operations for which dextran thromboprophylaxis, but no AT-III concentrate, was given were followed by thromboembolic complications. However, none of the 10 more recent operations for which prophylactic AT-III concentrate was available was followed by thromboembolic complications.

The data from this retrospective review show that the incidence of postoperative thromboembolic complications in patients with congenital AT-III deficiency is not affected by dextran thromboprophylaxis. However, none of the patients given prophylactic AT-III concentrate had clinical signs of thrombosis postoperatively.

▶ This is a useful article for those anesthesiologists who might have to take care of patients with this rare deficiency.—R.D. Miller, M.D.

Tissue Plasminogen Activator Antigen and Activity in Disseminated Intravascular Coagulation: Clinicopathologic Correlations

Francis RB Jr, Seyfert U (Los Angeles County–Univ of Southern California Med Ctr, Los Angeles)

J Lab Clin Med 110:541–547, November 1987   10–15

The fibrinolytic response to disseminated intravascular coagulation (DIC) has been considered important in preventing thrombosis and in contributing to hemorrhage. To define clearly the mechanisms of the fibrinolytic response in DIC, tissue plasminogen activator (t-PA) antigen and activity levels were measured with the use of sensitive, specific assays in 74 patients with DIC, 53 hospitalized patients with similar illnesses without DIC, and 36 healthy subjects.

In most disease categories studied, mean t-PA antigen levels were significantly higher in patients with DIC than in either hospitalized controls or healthy persons (table). Markedly elevated t-PA antigen levels were

Tissue Plasminogen Activator Antigen Levels in Hospitalized Patients With and Without Disseminated Intravascular Coagulation*

	DIC		No DIC		
Diagnosis	ng/ml	n	ng/ml	n	P
Liver disease	51.6 ± 36.5	8	23.1 ± 20.6	11	<0.05
Sepsis	34.6 ± 22.3	11	10.3 ± 6.9	8	<0.01
Solid tumors	18.4 ± 10.4	7	10.2 ± 5.2	11	<0.05
Leukemia-lymphoma	21.2 ± 16.2	7	8.6 ± 5.1	16	<0.01
Liver disease with sepsis	48.5 ± 40.4	24	43.9 ± 37.6	2	NS
Leukemia-lymphoma with sepsis	12.3 ± 5.9	7	7.0 ± 0.6	2	NS
Leukemia-lymphoma with liver disease	41.9 ± 38.9	3	16.5 ± 10.6	3	NS
Solid tumors with liver disease	20.3 ± 7.1	7		0	
All subjects	35.0 ± 32.5	74	13.9 ± 15.4	53	<0.001

*DIC, disseminated intravascular coagulation; NS, not significant. Values are expressed as mean ± SD.
(Courtesy of Francis RB Jr, Seyfert U: *J Lab Clin Med* 110:541–547, November 1987.)

seen in patients with liver disease both with and without DIC, with the highest levels seen in patients with DIC and associated liver disease. Detectable free t-PA activity was infrequently seen in patients with DIC. There was no significant correlation between the levels of t-PA antigen or activity and the presence of thrombotic or hemorrhagic complications. However, 2 patients with intracranial hemorrhage complicating DIC had detectable free t-PA activity. Bleeding complications were caused primarily by underlying anatomical lesions, and thrombotic complications occurred almost exclusively in patients with other known predisposing factors, such as metastatic carcinoma and atherosclerosis.

Increased circulating t-PA antigen levels are typically present in DIC, but free t-PA activity is infrequently seen, most likely because of increased levels of t-PA inhibitor. The presence or absence of free t-PA activity does not appear to be useful in predicting which patients with DIC will suffer hemorrhage or thrombosis.

▶ Are the authors guilty of setting up a straw man and then proceeding to knock him down?—R.D. Miller, M.D.

11 Ventilation

Methods of Ventilatory Support

Acute Left Ventricular Dysfunction During Unsuccessful Weaning From Mechanical Ventilation

Lemaire F, Teboul J-L, Cinotti L, Giotto G, Abrouk F, Steg G, Macquin-Mavier I, Zapol WM (Hôpital Henri Mondor, Paris; Massachusetts Gen Hosp, Boston)
Anesthesiology 69:171–179, August 1988   11–1

Some patients with chronic obstructive pulmonary disease (COPD) become totally dependent on mechanical ventilation. Attempts to wean such patients from ventilatory support can result in hypercapnea and hypoxia. Some begin wheezing, which is a sign of cardiac asthma or bronchospasm. This suggests that acute left ventricular dysfunction may prevent successful weaning. To test this hypothesis, 15 patients with cardiovascular disease and COPD were examined who could not be weaned from mechanical ventilation despite the apparent ability for spontaneous respiration.

Pulmonary and systemic hemodynamic measurements and blood gas

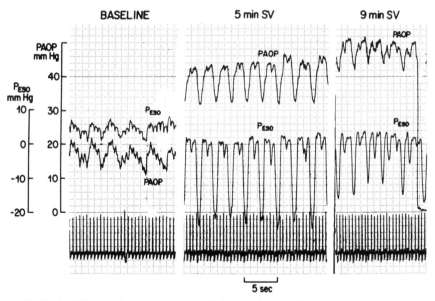

Fig 11–1.—Weaning of patient from mechanical ventilation *(baseline)* to spontaneous ventilation *(SV₁)*. There is progressive increase of pulmonary artery occlusion pressure *(PAOP)* from 14 mm Hg *(baseline)* to 50 mm Hg *(9 min SV)*. Esophageal pressure is reduced during SV with marked negative inspiratory excursions. (Courtesy of Lemaire F, Teboul J-L, Cinotti L, et al: *Anesthesiology* 69:171–179, August 1988.)

tensions were recorded before and after 10 minutes of spontaneous ventilation without positive end-expiratory pressure. All patients showed a progressive increase of pulmonary artery occlusion pressure (Fig 11–1). The mean increase was from 7.5 mm Hg to 24.5 mm Hg. Spontaneous ventilation increased the left ventricular end-diastolic volume index with left ventricular ejection fraction remaining the same.

After a 10-day course of diuretics, blood volume and body weight were reduced. Nine of the patients were then able to breathe alone with unchanged pulmonary artery occlusion pressure. An increase in left ventricular filling pressure may narrow small airways and bring about rapid respiratory muscle fatigue. A decrease in circulating blood volume can prevent respiratory failure when transferring patients with impaired left ventricular function and COPD from mechanical ventilation to spontaneous ventilation.

▶ One of the more interesting aspects of this study was that during the 10-minute period of spontaneous breathing the hemodynamic measurements appeared to have improved (cardiac index and blood pressure increased). However, the large increase of pulmonary artery occlusion pressure showed that acute left ventricular dysfunction was clearly present. The study shows once again the complex cardiovascular and pulmonary interactions that are so important in the successful resolution of acute exacerbations of COPD.—R.R. Kirby, M.D.

Do Periodic Hyperinflations Improve Gas Exchange in Patients With Hypoxemic Respiratory Failure?
Novak RA, Shumaker L, Snyder JV, Pinsky MR (Univ of Pittsburgh)
Crit Care Med 15:1081–1085, December 1987   11–2

Prolonged artificial ventilation may lead to worsening gas exchange and pulmonary compliance in patients with otherwise healthy lungs. Prolonged hyperinflation to 40 cm H_2O can completely reverse gas exchange deterioration. Similar efforts have effectively recruited atelectatic lung areas in patients who are critically ill. Sustained exaggerated hyperinflation may succesfully open collapsed lung units when standard recruitment techniques fail. The effects of the directed recruitment technique were compared with standard bag-sigh-suctioning (BSS) in 16 stable patients aged 36–85 years with hypoxemic respiratory failure treated by mechanical ventilation for more than 24 hours.

Periodic hyperinflation of 40 cm H_2O lasting for 15–30 seconds associated with body positioning (the directed recruitment technique) were compared with BSS, and their effects on gas exchange and pulmonary compliance were noted. Patients were sequentially alternated between directed recruitment and BSS.

Neither technique, alone or in sequence, produced sustained improvement or deterioration in either gas exchange or pulmonary compliance. Although recruitment procedures may mitigate subsequent deterioration of gas exchange, the routine application of standard BSS to these patients periodically in an attempt to improve gas exchange is of unproven value.

▶ Not surprising! As soon as either directed recruitment or BSS is released, whatever factors led to the problem in the first place are once again unopposed, and alveolar collapse, fluid-filling, etc. recur almost immediately. The same findings were demonstrated in "sigh" therapy so popular in mechanical ventilation during the 1960s and 1970s. There also the benefit of sighing and/or the provision of extra large, mechanical tidal volumes (15–25 ml/kg) were found to have no significant effect on gas exchange, correction of atelectasis, and reduction of intrapulmonary shunt.—R.R. Kirby, M.D.

Improving Arterial Oxygenation During One-Lung Ventilation
Slinger P, Triolet W, Wilson J (Montreal Gen Hosp, McGill Univ)
Anesthesiology 68:291–295, February 1988   11–3

It is often difficult to maintain adequate oxygenation during 1-lung ventilation for thoracic surgery. A study was conducted to determine

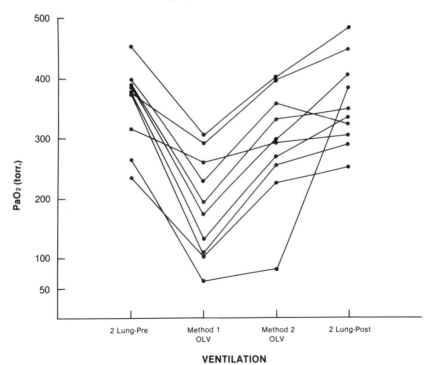

VENTILATION

Fig 11–2.—Intraoperative arterial oxygen pressure (tension) (Pa_{O_2}) changes in group A patients. Individual patient's values are connected by *lines. 2 Lung-Pre* indicates initial Pa_{O_2}; *OLV*, 1-lung ventilation; and *2 Lung-Post*, Pa_{O_2} 15 minutes after resuming 2-lung ventilation (15 minutes after ligation of pulmonary artery in pneumonectomies). (Courtesy of Slinger P, Triolet W, Wilson J: *Anesthesiology* 68:291–295, February 1988.)

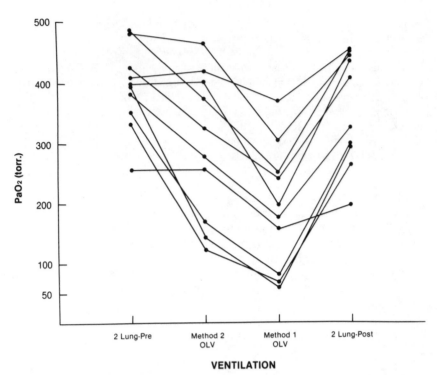

VENTILATION

Fig 11–3.—Intraoperative Pa_{O_2} changes for group B patients. (Courtesy of Slinger P, Triolet W, Wilson J: *Anesthesiology* 68:291–295, February 1988.)

whether the method in which continuous positive airway pressure (CPAP) is applied affects PaO_2 during OLV and whether altering the method of CPAP application can improve subsequent arterial oxygenation.

Twenty patients were randomized to 2 equal groups. Group A patients underwent treatment with method 1, in which after a tidal volume inflation to an airway pressure of 20 cm of water, the nondependent lung was allowed to deflate to 0 cm of water CPAP for 5 minutes; CPAP was then increased to 5 cm of water for 20 minutes. After this period, surgery was halted, and the nondependent lung was reinflated to an airway pressure of 30 cm of water until all visible atelectatic areas were reexpanded. The lung was then inflated to an airway pressure of 20 cm and allowed to deflate to a CPAP of 2 cm of water for 5 minutes; CPAP was increased to 5 cm of water for 20 minutes (method 2). The same procedure was used in group B except that methods 1 and 2 were reversed.

One patient in group A and 2 patients in group B experienced hypoxemic episodes during 1-lung ventilation with method 1 CPAP (Figs 11–2 and 11–3). The mean PaO_2 values for groups A and B combined during 1-lung ventilation with CPAP 5 cm of water using method 1 were 202 mm Hg at 5 minutes and 187 mm Hg at 20 minutes. For method 2, the

PaO$_2$ results were 329 mm Hg for 5 minutes and 294 mm Hg for 20 minutes.

The method by which CPAP is applied to the nondependent lung affects the subsequent arterial oxygenation during 1-lung ventilation. Continuous positive airway pressure can be applied in a controlled way that will reduce the risk of intraoperative hypoxemia without harm to surgical conditions.

▶ There can be no doubt that statistically significant differences in PaO$_2$ occurred between methods 1 and 2. However, the clinical significance is difficult to ascertain. Even the "low" values obtained with method 1 were certainly acceptable for the groups as a whole. Whether enough information is available to decide that the 3 patients who became hypoxemic with method 1 are representative of patients in general is not answered by this small study. However, further work is indicated. John Benumof's book, *Anesthesia for Thoracic Surgery* (New York, Churchill Livingstone, 1986) addresses this question in considerable detail.— R.R. Kirby, M.D.

Effect of Positive End-Expiratory Pressure on Right Ventricular Performance: Importance of Baseline Right Ventricular Function
Schulman DS, Biondi JW, Matthay RA, Barash PG, Zaret BL, Soufer R (Yale Univ; West Haven VA Med Ctr, West Haven, Conn)
Am J Med 84:57–67, January 1988   11–4

Application of positive end-expiratory pressure (PEEP) has a variable effect on right ventricular function, as PEEP increases both pulmonary vascular resistance and intrathoracic pressure. The hemodynamic responses to mechanical ventilation with PEEP have been well studied in experimental animals. In an effort to understand the hemodynamic responses to PEEP in human beings more clearly, 36 patients with diverse baseline right ventricular functions were studied prospectively during incremental PEEP application.

The study population consisted of 22 men and 14 women aged 18–80 years (mean age, 52 years) who required PEEP and mechanical ventilation. Eight patients had cardiogenic pulmonary edema; 11 had adult respiratory distress syndrome secondary to aspiration pneumonia, sepsis, bacterial and nonbacterial pneumonia; 9 had received low-level PEEP as a prophylactic measure following abdominal surgery; and 8 had multilobar pneumonia and severe hypoxemia. Systemic hemodynamics were monitored with indwelling radial arterial catheters, and pulmonary hemodynamics were monitored with indwelling pulmonary arterial catheters. Right heart pressures, cardiac output, right ventricular ejection fractions, and ventricular volumes were obtained at each PEEP level. Right ventricular peak systolic pressure-end-systolic volume ratios were analyzed as an index of contractile function.

Patients with severely depressed baseline right ventricular ejection fractions of 30% or less had increased end-diastolic and end-systolic volumes. These patients also had a decline in estimated right ventricular contractile function at 20 cm water PEEP. Patients with normal baseline right ventricular ejection fractions of 40% or more, or with moderately depressed baseline right ventricular ejection fractions of 31% to 40% showed no change in right ventricular volumes or estimated contractile function.

These results indicate that the effect of PEEP on right ventricular function differs in relation to the baseline right ventricular ejection fraction.

▶ A decade ago, Dr. Myron Laver pointed out that right ventricular function was a critical determinant of outcome in patients treated with mechanical ventilation and PEEP. This paper confirms and expands his observations. Of interest, however, is the now well-established fact that what may be deleterious to right ventricular performance can benefit that of the left ventricle. Thus, an increase of pleural pressure, which reduces venous return to the right ventricle and increases its afterload, simultaneously decreases left ventricular afterload and improves left ventricular performance. In critically ill patients with respiratory failure, one must walk a fine line to find a suitable ventilator strategy that preserves optimal cardiac function.—R.R. Kirby, M.D.

Effect of Positive End-Expiratory Pressure on Alveolar Capillary Perfusion
Nieman GF, Paskanik AM, Bredenberg CE (State Univ of New York, Syracuse)
J Thorac Cardiovasc Surg 95:712–716, April 1988   11–5

The dead space-tidal volume ratio could increase with positive end-expiratory pressure (PEEP) because of a net reduction in pulmonary perfusion caused by a lowered cardiac output. Alternately, the increased alveolar pressure might compress capillaries in the interalveolar septa, creating regions of reduced capillary flow and a high alveolar ventilation-perfusion ratio. The impact of each of these mechanisms was assessed in anesthetized dogs by restoring the cardiac output to baseline values with dextran 70 after the application of 15 cm water of PEEP. Alveolar capillary perfusion was studied by in vivo photomicroscopy through the visceral pleura.

Positive end-expiratory pressure led to a fall in cardiac output and alveolar capillary perfusion, with a rise in the alveolar dead space-tidal volume ratio and the arterial carbon dioxide tension. Dextran infusion only slightly increased alveolar capillary perfusion; the dead space-tidal volume ratio and Pa_{CO_2} remained significantly elevated. The alveolar capillaries were compressed and flattened by PEEP, whereas extraalveolar vessels continued to be perfused.

Most of the effects of PEEP on the dead space-tidal volume ratio and Pa_{CO_2} persisted despite normalization of the cardiac output. Compression of alveolar capillaries by high intraalveolar pressure appears to be chiefly responsible for the PEEP-induced decrease in capillary perfusion in the normal canine lung.

▶ It's the presence of parallel alveolar and extra-alveolar vessels that prevent us from manipulating the pulmonary circulation the way we would like during mechanical ventilation and PEEP. As lung volume is increased with positive pressure, the cross-sectional diameter of the extra-alveolar vessels increase, whereas that of the septal capillaries is reduced. Blood flow will thus pass through the extra-alveolar vessels whose resistance is less, even in the presence of an augmented intravascular volume. Nieman et al. have demonstrated this basic concept very nicely.—R.R. Kirby, M.D.

Effects of Expiratory Flow Resistance on Inspiratory Work of Breathing
Banner MJ, Downs JB, Kirby RR, Smith RA, Boysen PG, Lampotang S (Univ of Florida; Ohio State Univ; Mem Med Ctr, Jacksonville, Fla)
Chest 93:795–799, April 1988   11–6

Work of breathing is affected by fluctuations in both inspiratory and expiratory pressures during spontaneous breathing with continuous positive airway pressure. Flow resistance in the inspiratory limb of the breathing circuit and an inadequate continuous gas flow rate result in airway pressure fluctuation and increased work of breathing. However, the effects of resistance offered by the expiratory pressure value on inspiratory airway pressure and work of breathing are still speculative. To evaluate these effects, 3 types of expiratory pressure valves were compared: a threshold resistor with low resistance to flow, an inflatable balloon (mushroom) valve with moderate resistance to flow, and a variable-orifice flow resistor with a high resistance to flow (Fig 11–4).

With a continuous flow of 40 L/min, inspiratory airway pressure decreased less with the threshold resistor, more with the balloon valve, and most with the variable-orifice flow resistor (Fig 11–5). Compared with

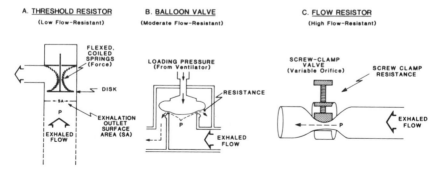

Fig 11–4.—**A,** threshold resistor expiratory pressure valve. Expiratory positive pressure *(P)* is generated through constant force exerted by flexion of multiple coiled springs against plastic disk with constant surface area *(SA)*. **B,** inflatable balloon valve. Inflatable balloon is pressurized by loading pressure from ventilator, set by operator. Exhaled flow is opposed by balloon loading pressure and is directed through narrow openings between bottom of balloon and valve seat; i.e., resistance to flow. *P* is proportional to loading pressure plus resistance times flow. **C,** flow resistor valve (variable orifice) determines *P* by resistance times flow. The smaller the orifice size, the greater the resistance; hence, the greater the *P* (assuming flow is constant). (Courtesy of Banner MJ, Downs JB, Kirby RR, et al: *Chest* 93:795–799, April 1988.)

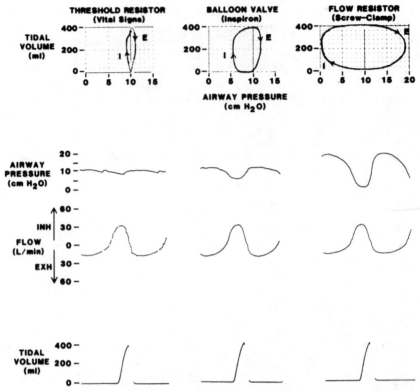

Fig 11–5.—Airway pressure, flow rate, and tidal volume recordings for 3 types of expiratory pressure valves with end-expiratory pressure of 10 cm H_2O. During all conditions, peak inspiratory and expiratory flow rates, inhalation-to-exhalation time ratio, breathing frequency, spontaneous tidal volume, and flow rate (40 L/min) directed through continuous positive airway pressure breathing circuit were constant. Variations in airway pressure during inhalation *(I)* and exhalation *(E)* were directly proportional to flow resistance of valves. Circumscribed area within pressure-volume loops represents work *(W)*. Because tidal volume was constant, the greater the change in airway pressure, the greater the W. (Courtesy of Banner MJ, Downs JB, Kirby RR, et al: *Chest* 93:795–799, April 1988.)

the threshold resistor, work of breathing was significantly increased up to threefold with the balloon valve and more than tenfold with the flow resistor.

To apply continuous positive airway pressure, expiratory pressure valves with low-flow resistance should be used to minimize fluctuations in airway pressure and thus in the work of spontaneous breathing. It appears that the greater the resistance of the valve, the greater the decrease in airway pressure and work of breathing.

▶ The effect of flow resistor PEEP values on expiratory work of breathing has been recognized for several years. This is the first report concerning an increase of inspiratory work when such valves are used. A knowledge of the operational characteristics of such valves is important when they are used in the management of spontaneously breathing patients with respiratory insufficiency. The increased work of breathing caused by expiratory/PEEP valves, when combined with that generated by many high resistance ventilator circuits, may preclude successful weaning with intermittent mandatory ventilation (IMV)/synchronized IMV in some patients.— R.R. Kirby, M.D.

Effect of Positive End-Expiratory Pressure on Extravascular Lung Water in Porcine Acute Respiratory Failure

Myers JC, Reilley TE, Cloutier CT (Ohio State Univ)
Crit Care Med 16:52–54, January 1988   11–7

Recent studies in acute respiratory failure suggest that positive end-expiratory pressure (PEEP) promotes the accumulation of extravascular lung water. Increments of PEEP were provided to pigs after acute respiratory failure was produced by infusion of live *Pseudomonas aeruginosa*. The ventilated animals received Ringer's lactate in varying amounts, and PEEP was added in increments of 5 cm of H_2O every 30 minutes, beginning an hour after infusion of the microorganism.

The PaO_2 increased significantly at higher levels of PEEP (Fig 11–6). The shunt fraction decreased with the level of PEEP (Fig 11–7). Cardiac output declined in all animals except for those given the largest amount of Ringer's lactate. Extravascular lung water was lower when PEEP was delivered, and it did not increase despite administration of large amounts of fluid.

The addition of PEEP protected against an increase in extravascular lung water in this porcine model of acute respiratory failure. Its use may therefore allow the infusion of more crystalloid when acute lung injury is present.

▶ For years, we've been told that extravascular lung water is increased by PEEP. Now we are told that PEEP may protect against an increase of extravas-

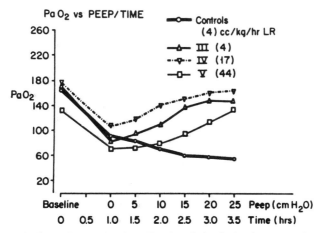

Fig 11–6.—As shown, PaO_2 increased significantly at higher levels of PEEP. *LR,* lactated Ringer's solution. (Courtesy of Myers JC, Reilley TE, Cloutier CT: *Crit Care Med* 16:52–54, January 1988.)

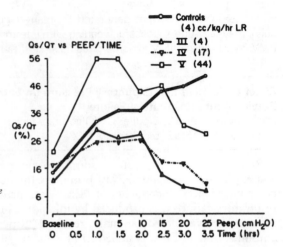

Qs/QT vs PEEP/TIME

Controls
(4) cc/kg/hr LR
III (4)
IV (17)
V (44)

Fig 11–7.—Shunt fraction (Q̇s/Q̇t) decreased with level of PEEP. *LR*, lactated Ringer's solution. (Courtesy of Myers JC, Reilley TE, Cloutier CT: *Crit Care Med* 16:52–54, January 1988.)

cular lung water. I've always doubted the former postulate because our work in the 1970s showed improved lung function, even with large volume infusions, so long as PEEP was high enough. Of course one always likes to see his or her personal biases confirmed, because they so often are formed with a substantial lack of facts! Nevertheless, this study is persuasive and deserves further attention.—R.R. Kirby, M.D.

A Hazard of Pressure Support Ventilation

Black JW, Grover BS (Madigan Army Med Ctr, Tacoma, Wash)
Chest 93:333–335, February 1988   11–8

Many newer models of mechanical ventilators feature pressure support as an option for ventilation or weaning or both. The mechanism for termination of a pressure support breath varies considerably among the various ventilators, but most use a decreased inspiratory flow rate to terminate each pressure support breath. The potential for the sudden inadvertent application of a high, unremitting pressure support breath or continuous positive airway pressure (CPAP) exists with some ventilators. In 2 patients, air leak around the endotracheal tube cuff resulted in sudden sustained application of CPAP associated with adverse consequences.

Both patients were successfully weaned and extubated after thoracostomy tube insertion for pneumothorax in the first patient and thoracotomy for a lung cancer in the second. Reintubation was necessary for recurrent pneumothorax in 1 patient and atelectasis in the other, but attempts at weaning were unsuccessful. While receiving pressure support of 20 cm of water, the ventilator alarms indicated a high respiratory rate and low exhaled tidal volume. In both patients tachypnea, tachycardia, and a decrease in blood pressure developed. Continuous escape of air around the endotracheal tube cuff was noted. Cuff pressure was increased with resolution of the leak, decrease in the CPAP reading to 5 cm of water, and rapid clinical improvement.

Sudden inadvertent application of CPAP is a potential hazard of pressure support ventilation, which may produce significant adverse hemodynamic effects. Standard ventilator monitoring systems that do not include mean airway pressure monitoring may not detect this problem before significant adverse consequences have occurred. Physicians using this mode of ventilation must be familiar with the terminating mechanism of their particular ventilator and choose an appropriate monitoring or alarm system.

▶ Pressure support ventilation is an increasingly popular and useful technique for stand-alone ventilatory support or as an adjunct to synchronized intermittent mandatory ventilation. These case reports emphasize the importance of knowing the mechanisms by which increasingly sophisticated modes of mechanical ventilation operate. High rate and low exhaled volume alarms alerted intensive care unit personnel to the fact that a problem had occurred. However, the nature of the difficulty was not immediately apparent. Such problems may be expected to increase as more ventilators incorporate pressure support and the technique becomes more widespread. At least 1 ventilator capable of pressure support (Hamilton Veolar) "releases" its pressure if the spontaneous inspiration lasts more than 3 seconds. This complication could not occur with the Hamilton. All pressure support ventilators should incorporate a similar design.—R.R. Kirby, M.D.

High-Frequency Ventilation

Tracheal and Bronchial Injury in High-Frequency Oscillatory Ventilation and High-Frequency Flow Interruption Compared With Conventional Positive-Pressure Ventilation

Wiswell TE, Clark RH, Null DM, Kuehl TJ, deLemos RA, Coalson JJ (Brooke Army Med Ctr, Wilford Hall Air Force Med Ctr, Univ of Texas Health Science Ctr, Southwest Found for Biomedical Research, San Antonio, Tex)
J Pediatr 112:249–256, February 1988   11–9

Necrotizing tracheobronchitis, a severe and often fatal airway injury, has been associated with the use of high-frequency jet ventilation. Its association with other types of mechanical ventilation, including oscillatory ventilation, has been controversial. The histopathologic changes in the airways of premature baboons treated with conventional positive-pressure ventilation (PPV) were compared with those seen after high-frequency oscillatory ventilation (HFOV) and high-frequency flow interruption (HFFI). Ventilation in the HFOV and HFFI groups was at a frequenc of 10 Hz. Twenty-six animals were treated with ventilation for 24 hours (5 PPV, 10 HFOV, 11 HFFI), and 18 were treated with ventilation for 96 hours (6 PPV, 6 HFOV, 6 HFFI). Tissue changes in the trachea, carina, and both mainstem bronchi were graded using a semiquantitative scoring system.

All 3 forms of mechanical ventilation produced airway injury. The degree of injury was similar and relatively mild for the PPV- and HFOV-treated animals at 24 and 96 hours. There was significantly more severe damage, characterized by diffuse submucosal necrosis, extensive hemorrhage, dense polymorphonuclear leukocyte infiltration, sloughed epithelium, focal basophilia, and intraluminal debris, in 11 of 17 baboons treated with HFFI at 24 and 96 hours, compared with PPV- and HFOV-treated animals. There was no significant difference in airway injury scores between PPV and HFOV-treated animals.

In conclusion, HFOV results in no greater tracheobronchial injury than conventional PPV, whereas HFFI is associated with a far greater degree of damage than either PPV or HFOV.

▶ The authors previously have shown that their premature baboon model is almost identical to hyaline membrane disease in human babies. Thus their studies, unlike many which use animal models, are clinically relevant. In this case, the problem with HFFI may relate to the larger tidal volumes and pressures that can be generated compared with HFOV. In addition, the lack of an active expiratory phase with HFFI appears to predispose to air trapping and occult PEEP. The conclusion that a ventilator strategy which is useful for one mode of support or a particular disease process may be dangerous for another is applicable to all devices and disorders.—R.R. Kirby, M.D.

Ultra-High-Frequency Jet Ventilation in a Bronchopleural Fistula Model
Orlando R III, Gluck EH, Cohen M, Mesologites CG (Hartford Hosp, Hartford, Conn; Univ of Connecticut, Farmington)
Arch Surg 123:591–593, May 1988   11–10

Conventional high-frequency jet ventilation (CHFJV) has been shown to decrease air leakage from bronchopleural and tracheoesophageal fistulas in experimental animals and in a clinical setting. However, CHFJV does not always achieve adequate oxygenation and ventilation. Current regulations of the Food and Drug Administration limit high-frequency ventilation to maximum ventilatory rates of 150 breaths per minute. A newly developed ventilator design for ultra-high-frequency jet ventilation (UHFJV) that is capable of rates as high as 900 breaths per minute is presently in the investigative stage. The effect of jet ventilator frequency on hemodynamics, gas exchange, and bronchial-stump gas flow was investigated in an animal model of bronchopleural fistula.

Ten pigs underwent right-sided thoracotomy and right-sided upper pulmonary lobectomy with cannulation of the upper lobe bronchus to enable measurement of bronchial fistula flow rates. Each animal underwent ventilation with a random sequence of conventional positive-pressure ventilation at 12–20 breaths per minute, CHFJV at 12–20 breaths per minute, and UHFJV at 450 breaths per minute. Arterial blood gas levels, hemodynamic data, and bronchial fistula flow rates were recorded as the animal was given ventilation in the different modes.

Hemodynamic measurements, including mean arterial pressure, mean pulmonary artery occlusion pressure, and mean cardiac output were similar with all 3 ventilatory modes. However, oxygenation was best with UHFJV, as the highest oxygen tensions were observed with UHFJV, and the lowest were seen with conventional positive-pressure ventilation. Bronchial fistula flow was greatest with conventional ventilation, intermediate with CHFJV, and lowest with UHFJV.

The UHFJV resulted in superior oxygen loading, adequate carbon dioxide elimination, and the lowest flow through the bronchial fistula. These findings suggest that both the design of the new ventilator and its ventilatory rate are important therapeutic variables in the treatment of major bronchial disruption.

▶ The main problem with this study is that the pigs' lungs were normal. In the clinical setting, however, bronchopleural fistula is frequently associated with severe respiratory insufficiency and decreased lung compliance. Under those circumstances, control of fistula flow by any means is difficult and often unsuccessful. Any method that resolves this problem and maintains satisfactory oxygenation and ventilation in such patients will represent a major forward step in respiratory care. Ultra-high-frequency jet ventilation has not yet been shown to do so.—R.R. Kirby, M.D.

12 Aspiration of Gastric Contents

Haemodynamic Effects of the I.V. Administration of Cimetidine or Raniti-dine in the Critically Ill Patient: A Double-Blind Prospective Study
Smith CL, Bardgett DM, Hunter JM (Royal Liverpool Hosp, England)
Br J Anaesth 59:1397–1402, November 1987   12–1

In an attempt to decrease the incidence of acute upper gastrointestinal tract hemorrhage, histamine H_2-receptor antagonists are used to reduce the acidity of gastric contents in critically ill patients not receiving enteral nutrition. Deleterious changes in heart rate and arterial pressure have occurred in such patients after cimetidine is given intravenously. A double-blind, crossover study was done to compare the hemodynamic effects of intravenous doses of cimetidine and ranitidine in 20 critically ill patients.

Cimetidine, 200 mg, or ranitidine, 50 mg, was administered intravenously. Both agents produced transient decreases in mean arterial pressure and systemic vascular resistance, although no significant change was noted in either group with regard to heart rate, cardiac output, central venous pressure, pulmonary artery wedge pressure, or pulmonary vascular resistance. Hypotensive systemic vasodilatory effects occurred more commonly after cimetidine than after ranitidine administration. Also, these effects were significantly greater after cimetidine treatment.

In this series, both cimetidine and ranitidine caused transient decreases in the mean arterial pressure and systemic vascular resistance. Both histamine H_2-receptor antagonists may produce hypotension in critically ill patients.

▶ The H_2-receptors are widespread in the body, including the heart. The need for rapid intravenous administration of an H_2-receptor antagonist would seem to be infrequent and should be tempered by concern for significant, and not so infrequent, adverse hemodynamic effects.—R.K. Stoelting

13 Critical Care

Respiratory Distress Syndrome and Respiratory Care

Pulmonary Toxicity After Treatment With Bleomycin Alone or in Combination With Hyperoxia: Studies in the Rat

Blom-Muilwijk MC, Vriesendorp R, Veninga TS, Hofstra W, Sleyfer DT, Wieringa RA, Konings AWT (Academic Med Ctr, Amsterdam; Univ Hosp Groningen, the Netherlands)
Br J Anaesth 60:91–97, 1988
13–1

Bleomycin treatment followed by a high concentration of oxygen may contribute to pulmonary toxicity in patients postoperatively. Bleomycin seems to act by generating oxygen radicals that destroy cellular DNA. Pulmonary changes were studied in rats given doses of bleomycin comparable to those used clinically, in the presence or absence of hyperoxia. Hyperoxia was produced by exposure for 4 hours to 50% oxygen-enriched air.

A mild reaction was seen in the lungs of rats in all groups. Intra-alveolar macrophages were increased in rats treated with bleomycin, whether or not hyperoxia was produced, but the effect was most marked in hyperoxic animals. The numbers of type II pneumocytes did not differ significantly, nor were there differences in levels of superoxide dismutase or glutathione peroxidase activity.

Bleomycin in clinical doses did not produce significant pulmonary damage in rats in this study, even when combined with hyperoxia.

▶ It's interesting to find out how the problem with bleomycin and the concern of using increased oxygen in patients who had been treated with bleomycin began. This obviously began with a concerned anesthesiologist who noted a problem after surgery. This problem has largely been put to rest by 2 excellent studies: (1) a retrospective study by Douglas et al. (*Can Anaesth Soc J* 27:449–452, 1980) and (2) a study by Ken LaMantia (*Anesthesiology* 60:65–67, 1984). In those studies, they found no significant increase in morbidity related to giving oxygen to patients previously treated with bleomycin. This study in the rat confirms that lack of increase in morbidity caused by oxygen. Although I am still not totally comfortable giving increased oxygen levels to patients who have received bleomycin, these data are more reassuring than previously and allow one to breathe easier when one gives supplemental oxygen to a patient who has received bleomycin. Nevertheless, there is still an uneasiness with the data, as the absence of morbidity hasn't been demonstrated; consequently, until I feel more comfortable, I'll continue to monitor such patients with both a pulse oximeter and transcutaneous oxygen meter and continue to try to keep the PaO_2 in the 80 to 100 range for patients who have previously received bleomycin. While such may be just giving weight to my biases, the technologies available allow us to do that and, until the question is more completely resolved, I will continue to do so.—M.F. Roizen, M.D.

▶ Obviously rats are not people, but an increasing body of evidence now suggests that the adverse effects previously ascribed to oxygen and bleomycin were overrated. How many bleomycin-treated patients were subjected to the potential or actual risks of hypoxia because of clinicians' fears that irreversible pulmonary damage would result if they were given even low levels of oxygen support? Who knows? *If*, indeed, there is no adverse synergistic effect, then how in the world were we persuaded that there was? For that matter, how will we resolve the discrepancies in apparently well-conducted research coming to such different conclusions? This problem of course, is at the core of all medical therapeutic controversies.—R.R. Kirby, M.D.

Upper Airway Obstruction Following Adult Respiratory Distress Syndrome: An Analysis of 30 Survivors
Elliott CG, Rasmusson BY, Crapo RO (LDS Hosp, Salt Lake City; Univ of Utah)
Chest 94:526–530, September 1988   13–2

Patients who have been treated for adult respiratory distress syndrome (ARDS) are at risk for injury to the upper airway. Thirty survivors of ARDS were studied to determine the frequency of upper airway obstruction and the factors that might lead to this complication.

The patients completed a respiratory disease questionnaire, underwent a physical examination, and performed inspiratory and expiratory maximal flow-volume curves. The mean follow-up examination took place at 4 years. At the time of treatment for ARDS, the patients' mean age was 28 years. Tracheal intubation was administered for 3–35 days.

Four patients experienced exertional dyspnea more than 6 months af-

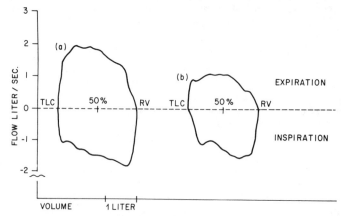

Fig 13–1.—Flow-volume curves of patient demonstrate progressive upper airway obstruction caused by laryngotracheal stenosis at 5(a) and 6 months (b) after extubation. (Courtesy of Elliott CG, Rasmusson BY, Crapo RO: *Chest* 94:526–530, September 1988.)

ter the onset of ARDS, but no evidence of central airway obstruction could be found. Three patients, however, did have symptomatic upper airway obstruction, and all 3 required more than 1 operation for laryngotracheal reconstruction. In 1 of these patients fibrous adhesions of the subglottic larynx and superior trachea were seen. Two flow volume curves showed progressive upper airway obstruction (Fig 13–1).

These 3 patients did not differ from the 27 others in age or length of intubation. But 1 patient had a prolonged and difficult intubation, and another required tracheal tube cuff pressures in excess of 35 cm of H_2O. When progressive dyspnea occurs in the first year after ARDS, laryngotracheal obstruction should be suspected.

▶ We have tended to assume that the use of high-volume, low-pressure cuffs and nontoxic materials in endotracheal and tracheotomy tubes has significantly reduced airway injury. In patients who require high ventilator pressure, I don't believe this is true. This article seems to substantiate this view. Much work involving improved cuff design is necessary.—R.R. Kirby, M.D.

Variables Affecting Outcome in Blunt Chest Trauma: Flail Chest vs. Pulmonary Contusion
Clark GC, Schecter WP, Trunkey DD (Univ of California, San Francisco; San Francisco Gen Hosp)
J Trauma 28:298–303, March 1988   13–3

Flail chest and pulmonary contusion are 2 potentially life-threatening chest injuries. The optimal methods of treatment for these conditions are controversial. The variables affecting outcomes of patients with pulmonary contusion or flail chest or both are identified.

The factors adversely affecting morbidity and mortality were analyzed in 144 consecutive patients with pulmonary contusion or flail chest injuries, most of which were sustained in motor vehicle or motorcycle accidents. Ninety-two percent of the patients with combined pulmonary contusion and flail chest and 67% with either injury alone had associated intrathoracic injuries.

Overall mortality was 25%. More than half of all deaths were caused by central nervous system injuries; another third were caused by massive hemorrhage. For either flail chest or pulmonary contusion alone, mortality was 16%, but when both injuries were suffered, the rate jumped to 42%. The Injury Severity Score was 32 for survivors and 60 for those who died. One quarter of the patients requiring mechanical ventilation died.

Higher morbidity and mortality were associated with a high Injury Severity Score, severe associated thoracic injuries, the presence of shock, falls from heights, and the combination of pulmonary contusion and flail chest.

▶ The message in this paper is a bit confusing. I think it is *not* so much a comparison of flail chest and pulmonary contusion mortality as is suggested by the title. Instead, the data presented show that injuries which produce both abnormalities tend to be more severe and are associated with other major problems, such as intrathoracic vascular injuries and CNS dysfunction. Ultimately, the latter probably are more important determinants of outcome than are the chest wall and pulmonary injuries. Thus, one may view flail chest and pulmonary contusion as sentinel events, indicative of other potentially more serious and immediately life-threatening conditions.

Of interest was the discussion following the paper in which the participants seemed to agree that the mortality from the lung-thorax injuries, per se, was reduced compared with that reported in earlier studies (*J Trauma* 28:303–304, March 1988). The conclusion seemed to be that respiratory failure was handled more effectively than a decade earlier, i.e., that patients die with these injuries rather than because of them.—R.R. Kirby, M.D.

Use of the Oxygen Cost of Breathing as an Index of Weaning Ability From Mechanical Ventilation
McDonald NJ, Lavelle P, Gallacher WN, Harpin RP (Toronto Western Hosp)
Intensive Care Med 14:50–54, January 1988   13–4

The appropriate time to initiate the weaning of critically ill patients from mechanical ventilatory support is based on subjective as well as objective factors. The time course and eventual outcome of weaning are hard to predict. One research team found that the oxygen cost of breathing (OCB) was significantly greater in postoperative patients in whom extubation failed than in those who were successfully extubated. The relationship between OCB and the derived variable—the OCB as a percentage of total oxygen consumption during spontaneous ventilation ($OCB/\dot{V}_{O_2}$-SV%)—and weaning ability was investigated in 16 females and 14 males aged 17–96 years.

All 30 patients were recovering from a critical illness that necessitated mechanical ventilation for at least 24 hours. The OCB was measured at commencement of weaning from the mechanical ventilation. Weaning was done conventionally in 13 patients and with intermittent mandatory ventilation in 17.

The $\dot{V}_{O_2}$-SV% was greater than the $\dot{V}_{O_2}$ during controlled ventilation. The mean difference between the 2 measurements of $OCB/\dot{V}_{O_2}$-SV% done in each patient was 3.69%. A significant exponential correlation was found between the OCB in milliliters per square meter per minute and the duration of weaning in days. Again, a significant exponential relationship was noted between the $OCB/\dot{V}_{O_2}$-SV% and the duration of weaning.

▶ Here is one of those studies in which the statistical significance must be weighed against the clinical significance. The difference in OCB between spontaneous and controlled ventilation was only 3.69 ± 3.06%. The exponential correlation between OCB and the duration of weaning was questionable at best (based upon 2 patients out of 30 who required more than 20 days of weaning). I don't believe an analysis of OCB adds a great deal of information to what we already know about the problems of weaning. In this regard, see Kemper M et al. (Metabolic and respiratory changes during weaning from mechanical ventilation. *Chest* 92:979–983, 1987).—R.R. Kirby, M.D.

Bedside Assessment of the Work of Breathing
Lewis WD, Chwals W, Benotti PN, Lakshman K, O'Donnell C, Blackburn GL, Bistrian BR (New England Deaconess Hosp, Boston; Harvard Univ)
Crit Care Med 16:117–122, February 1988   13–5

Because clinical signs of an increase in the work of breathing develop long before exhaustion and worsening arterial blood gases, many clinicians believe that clinically apparent increased respiratory work may be an indication for the institution or continuation of mechanical ventilation. The oxygen consumption ($\dot{V}_{O_2}$) of 8 healthy volunteers and 30 patients recovering from respiratory failure in the intensive care unit was measured by indirect calorimetry with the use of the Sensormedics Horizon system and the Utah MGM/TWO system during complete mechanical and spontaneous ventilation. The work of breathing was calculated as the difference in $\dot{V}_{O_2}$ between spontaneous and mechanical ventilation and was expressed as a percentage of mechanical ventilation (%$\Delta\dot{V}_{O_2}$).

The average %$\Delta\dot{V}_{O_2}$ for the normal healthy volunteers was 3.7%. Among patients who were recovering from respiratory failure average %$\Delta\dot{V}_{O_2}$ was 7.7% for patients who were weaned successfully from respiratory support that was based on clinical criteria within 24 hours of metabolic study and was 24.7% for patients who were not weaned successfully. An increase in %$\dot{V}_{O_2}$ of less than 15% was evident in 14 of 16 (88%) patients who were weaned, compared with only 1 of 14 (7%) of those who were not weaned. Those patients with increases in $\dot{V}_{O_2}$ of greater than 15% during spontaneous ventilation were unable to be weaned. The average $\dot{V}_{O_2}$ did not differ significantly between patients who were measured with the different systems.

The oxygen cost of breathing is a reliable predictor of weaning and extubation in patients who are recovering from respiratory failure. Bedside measurement of the oxygen cost of breathing by indirect calorimetry may be clinically useful in identifying patients who cannot sustain spontaneous ventilation because of excessive respiratory work.

▶ These investigators also report that increased $\dot{V}_{O_2}$ is associated with difficult weaning. However, compare and contrast their findings and those of McDonald et al. (Abstract 13–4) with the article by Kemper et al. (Abstract 13–6), which minimizes the value of this measurement. Pay your money and take your choice.—R.R. Kirby, M.D.

Metabolic and Respiratory Changes During Weaning From Mechanical Ventilation
Kemper M, Weissman C, Askanazi J, Hyman AI, Kinney JM (Columbia Univ)
Chest 92:979–983, December 1987   13–6

Weaning from mechanical ventilation is performed daily in intensive care units. A study was done to determine whether among postoperative patients there were any differences in the changes in oxygen consumption and carbon dioxide production between successfully extubated patients and those in whom ventilation was continued or reinstituted.

Of 35 patients given mechanical ventilation after surgery, 18 were successfully weaned and 17 were not. The weaning method used was a stepwise reduction in mandatory breaths—from 10–12 to 4–6—followed by a period of continuous positive airway pressure (CPAP). In patients successfully weaned, oxygen consumption and carbon dioxide production increased by a mean of 10%. Minute ventilation decreased by a mean of 9% and the $PaCO_2$ was unchanged when values at an intermittent mandatory ventilation rate of 10–12 were compared with those on CPAP. In patients who were not weaned successfully, the mean oxygen consumption and carbon dioxide production increased by 8% and 6%, respectively, and the mean $PaCO_2$ rose significantly from 38 to 42.5. A significantly greater decrease in minute ventilation was observed in this group than in the other group.

In this study, no difference between the change in oxygen consumption and carbon dioxide production was found in patients who were or were not successfully weaned from mechanical ventilation. Further studies are needed to determine whether results would be similar in other patient populations.

▶ This study arrives at conclusions different from those of McDonald et al. (Abstract 13–4), who found that an increased oxygen cost of breathing occurred in patients who were difficult to wean. Kemper et al., however, noted that changes in neither V_{O_2} nor V_{CO_2} correlated with predictability of the success of weaning. I think we must conclude that at best these measurements provide interesting but not particularly relevant information for the average patient who is mechanically ventilated.—R.R. Kirby, M.D.

Capnography in Mechanically Ventilated Patients
Carlon GC, Ray C Jr, Miodownik S, Kopec I, Groeger JS (Mem Sloan-Kettering Cancer Ctr, New York)
Crit Care Med 16:550–556, May 1988   13–7

Capnography is the technique of displaying changes in carbon dioxide levels during respiratory cycles. Infrared capnographers and mass spectrometers are the instruments generally used for this purpose. Some clinical and technical problems that may be easily resolved with mass spectrometry and capnography were reviewed.

The shape of the capnogram after a mechanical breath in an individual with healthy lungs is similar to that of a spontaneous breath. The pattern is different in a patient undergoing mandatory ventilation. Mechanical failures during ventilation can be detected by capnography. The effectiveness of respiratory support can be evaluated immediately using capnogra-

0cm H₂O PRESSURE SUPPORT

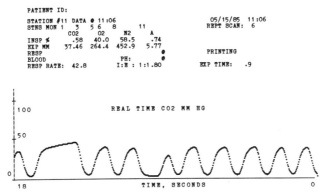

Fig 13–2.—Intermittent mandatory ventilation without pressure support. Note irregular respiratory pattern, tachypnea, absence of alveolar plateau, low end-tidal carbon dioxide (Pet$_{CO_2}$), and high baseline CO$_2$. (Courtesy of Carlon GC, Ray C Jr, Miodownik S, et al: *Crit Care Med* 16:550–556, May 1988.)

phy. For example, after initiation of pressure support ventilation, normalization of respiratory patterns are illustrated in Figures 13–2 through 13–4. When a lower level of support is provided 24 hours later, the mass spectrometry tracings of Figure 13–5 are obtained. This tracing verifies clinical improvement over time. Capnographs can also be used to follow up lung function in patients with neuromuscular dysfunction.

Capnography can provide useful guidelines for the management of mechanically ventilated patients. It can be used to identify mechanical failures noninvasively and to monitor patient progress. An expanded role for capnography in the monitoring of mechanically ventilated pa-

PRESSURE SUPPORT 20cm H₂O
5 min Later

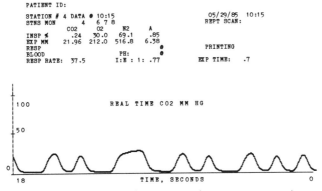

Fig 13–3.—Five minutes after addition of 20 cm water of pressure, support respiratory rate has decreased and baseline CO$_2$ has returned to normal, although alveolar plateaus are still absent and Pet$_{CO_2}$ is low. (Courtesy of Carlon GC, Ray C Jr, Miodownik S, et al: *Crit Care Med* 16:550–556, May 1988.)

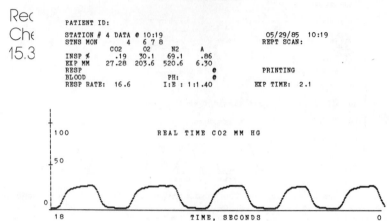

PRESSURE SUPPORT 20cm H₂O
15 min Later

Rec
Che
15.3

PATIENT ID:

STATION # 4 DATA @ 10:19   05/29/85 10:19
STNS MON   4   6 7 8   REPT SCAN:
             CO2   02   N2   A
INSP %   .19   30.1 69.1   .86
EXP MM   27.28 203.6 520.6 6.30
RESP   θ
BLOOD   PH: θ   PRINTING
RESP RATE: 16.6   I:E : 1:1.40   EXP TIME: 2.1

100   REAL TIME CO2 MM HG

50

0
18   TIME, SECONDS   0

Fig 13–4.—Fifteen minutes after addition of 20 cm water of pressure support, normal capnogram and respiratory rate can be observed. (Courtesy of Carlon GC, Ray C Jr, Miodownik S, et al: *Crit Care Med* 16:550–556, May 1988.)

tients would increase the role of mass spectrometers in the intensive care unit.

▶ I'm a firm believer in the use of capnography to ensure correct endotracheal tube placement and that ventilation is occurring. I'm less certain that one needs it to regulate the way the ventilator is used. Nevertheless, this article and the study by Yamanaka and Sue (Abstract 13–8) demonstrate the potential

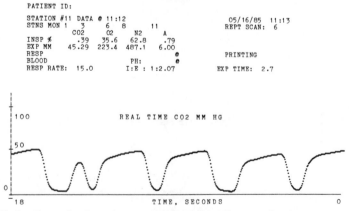

24 HOURS LATER
4cm H₂O PRESSURE SUPPORT

PATIENT ID:

STATION #11 DATA @ 11:12   05/16/85 11:13
STNS MON 1   3   6   8   11   REPT SCAN: 6
             CO2   02   N2   A
INSP %   .39   35.6 62.8   .79
EXP MM   45.29 223.4 487.1 6.00
RESP   θ
BLOOD   PH: θ   PRINTING
RESP RATE: 15.0   I:E : 1:2.07   EXP TIME: 2.7

100   REAL TIME CO2 MM HG

50

0
18   TIME, SECONDS   0

Fig 13–5.—Twenty-four hours later, respiratory conditions have significantly improved. Adequate gas exchange can now be maintained at lower pressure support. (Courtesy of Carlon GC, Ray C Jr, Miodownik S, et al: *Crit Care Med* 16:550–556, May 1988.)

usefulness of capnography in this regard. It's probably only a matter of time until every intensive care unit bed is equipped with an infrared capnometer. A few representative capnographic tracings and the way they may be used to gauge the efficacy of ventilatory support are shown in the 4 selected figures.— R.R. Kirby, M.D.

Comparison of Arterial-End-Tidal P_{CO_2} Differences and Dead Space-Tidal Volume Ratio in Respiratory Failure
Yamanaka MK, Sue DY (Harbor-UCLA Med Ctr, Torrance; Univ of California, Los Angeles)
Chest 92:832–835, November 1987   13–8

Measuring the end-tidal carbon dioxide pressure ($PetCO_2$) is often used as a noninvasive substitute for arterial CO_2 pressure (Pa_{CO_2}) in evaluating patients with respiratory failure. However, in patients with lung disease, the $PetCO_2$ can differ from Pa_{CO_2} because of ventilation-perfusion ($\dot{V}A/Q$) mismatching, and changes in $PetCO_2$ may be seen with corresponding increase, decrease, or no change in Pa_{CO_2} depending on what happens to $V\dot{A}/Q$ mismatching. To determine the role of $PetCO_2$ in assessing the effectiveness of ventilation, comparisons of individual and mean Pa_{CO_2}, $PetCO_2$, arterial end-tidal-Pa_{CO_2} difference ($P[a-et]CO_2$), and dead space/tidal volume (VD/VT) were undertaken in 17 patients undergoing mechanical ventilation.

There was considerable variation in $PetCO_2$ for values of Pa_{CO_2} in individual patients. The $P(a-et)CO_2$ varied from 0 to 39 mm Hg and correlated closely with VD/VT. The VD/VT was calculated from the mixed-expired Pa_{CO_2} ($P\bar{e}CO_2$) from an inline mixing box without actually "collecting" expired gas. The mean $P\bar{e}CO_2$ values obtained were comparable to the measured $P\bar{e}CO_2$ from bag collection and the values of VD/VT were nearly identical.

These findings indicate that $PetCO_2$ is a poor estimate of Pa_{CO_2} in patients with respiratory failure. However, the difference between them, the $P(a-et)CO_2$ which is closely correlated with VD/VT, can be used to assess the efficiency of ventilation. In addition, VD/VT can be calculated from $P\bar{e}CO_2$ by the use of a simple mixing box system.

▶ In view of the current popularity of $PetCO_2$ monitoring, this study is pertinent. Whether the $P(a-et)CO_2$ gradient can be used to optimize ventilator settings remains to be seen. It is useful in demonstrating the alterations that can result from inappropriate mechanical ventilation, however.—R.R. Kirby, M.D.

Attenuation of the Hemodynamic Responses to Chest Physical Therapy
Klein P, Kemper M, Weissman C, Rosenbaum SH, Askanazi J, Hyman AI (Columbia Univ, New York Univ)
Chest 93:38–42, January 1988   13–9

Chest physiotherapy (CPT), a commonly used technique in mechanically ventilated critically ill patients, has been shown to be a stressful procedure that may have significant metabolic and hemodynamic effects. Twenty-three postoperative mechanically ventilated patients were studied on 26 occasions to determine the hemodynamic and metabolic changes that occur with CPT and to determine whether narcotic analgesics can attenuate these responses. Three groups of patients were examined: 10 patients in group 1 received fentanyl, 1.5 μg/kg, or placebo intravenously in random order before each of 2 CPT sessions; 10 patients in group 2 received fentanyl, 3 μg/kg, or placebo before CPT; and 6 patients in group 3 received only placebo before CPT.

During CPT, heart rate, systolic and mean blood pressures, cardiac output, oxygen consumption, and carbon dioxide production were all increased compared with placebo. In some groups, arterial pH decreased significantly and carbon dioxide pressure (tension) increased, wehreas minute ventilation decreased or did not change. There was a significant reduction in the increase in blood pressure and heart rate with the higher, but not the lower, fentanyl dose. With the higher dose, no substantial hemodynamic changes occurred once CPT was stopped. The higher fentanyl dose did not alter the metabolic response during CPT.

These data show that CPT produces significant major hemodynamic and metabolic changes. The hemodynamic response to CPT can be attenuated, but not abolished, by prior intravenous administration of a moderate dose of fentanyl. Further studies are needed to assess whether higher doses of fentanyl or other narcotic agents can further suppress or possibly abolish this response without causing major hemodynamic disruption once the procedure has been completed.

▶ The problem with the fentanyl technique described is that it practically guarantees a longer period of mechanical ventilation and weaning because of the associated respiratory depression. Thus, one must weigh the risks of the hemodynamic stress response to CPT against that of a longer period of tracheal intubation and ventilatory support. Patient selection would appear to be a major determinant of which route one pursues.—R.R. Kirby, M.D.

Variability of the Breathing Pattern Before and After Extubation

Krieger BP, Chediak A, Gazeroglu HB, Bizousky FP, Feinerman D (Univ of Miami at Mt Sinai Med Ctr, Miami Beach)
Chest 93:767–771, April 1988   13–10

The decision to extubate is primarily influenced by a stable breathing pattern and gas exchange during unassisted ventilation through an endotracheal tube before extubation. To assess the variability of breathing patterns and to establish guidelines for the interpretation of changes in the breathing pattern, 50 spontaneously breathing patients who were being weaned from mechanical ventilation were monitored with respiratory inductive plethysmography for 1 hour before and after successful extubation.

Immediately after extubation, mean respiratory rates, tidal volumes, minute ventilation, and mean inspiratory flow increased slightly. These parameters returned to preextubation values by 30 minutes postextubation. There was no significant change in variability of respiratory rate or tidal volume.

These results highlight the relative stability of the breathing pattern in critically ill patients. The spontaneous breathing pattern of a stable patient before extubation is almost identical to the postextubation pattern. Prospective studies are warranted to establish whether changes in the spontaneous breathing will be clinically helpful in predicting respiratory failure or weaning success.

▶ I'm not sure of the clinical usefulness of this paper. The problems with weaning and tracheal extubation occur not in stable patients but in those who are not stable, yet for whom extubation may still be desirable. In such individuals, there are marked differences in preextubation and postextubation patterns, and it is for them that predictions of respiratory failure or weaning success are needed most.—R.R. Kirby, M.D.

Incidence and Morbidity of Extubation Failure in Surgical Intensive Care Patients

Demling RH, Read T, Lind LJ, Flanagan HL (Brigham and Women's Hosp, Boston; Harvard Univ)
Crit Care Med 16:573–577, June 1988   13–11

Reintubation is required when patients fail to tolerate the removal of ventilator support. The rate of extubation failure in the general surgical critical care population has never been determined, and the reason for extubation failure or extubation-associated complications have not been identified.

The rate of extubation failure was determined for 700 consecutive intubated patients, 400 of whom were admitted to a general surgical intensive care unit (ICU) and 300 who were admitted to a burn/trauma ICU. Patients were weaned from mechanical ventilation using an intermittent mandatory ventilation mode with subsequent placement on either a T piece or continuous positive airway pressure before extubation. Extubation failure was defined as a patient requiring reintubation within a 7-day period.

Thirty-two extubation failures occurred in 30 patients, for an overall reintubation incidence of 4%. Of 400 extubations in the general surgical ICU, there were 22 reintubations in 20 patients. Most of these patientswere elderly, with an average age of 65 years. The need for positive-pressure ventilation was the major reason for reintubation. Eight (40%) of the 20 patients requiring reintubation died in the hospital. The major cause of death was progressive cardiopulmonary failure. The morbidity rate from failed extubation was close to 50%.

Of 300 extubations in the burn/trauma unit, there were 10 extubation failures in 9 patients whose mean age was 44 years. Five failures occurred in patients with smoke inhalation and burns. Air maintenance and pulmonary toilet were the main reason for reintubation. There was only 1 death in this group.

The incidence, reasons for, and outcome of reintubations in surgical ICU patients vary greatly and are dependent on the underlying disease process. Predictors of extubation failure could not be identified.

▶ The results of this study suggest that the authors were very good at selecting the appropriate time to extubate, notwithstanding their disclaimer that predictors of extubation failure could not be identified. It appears that they were even better than they assumed. That extubation failure was defined by a need to reintubate within 7 days of extubation seems too stringent. Many things can occur in burn and surgical ICUs that are completely unrelated to the original problem that necessitated intubation. In most cases, I would consider extubation that "lasts" for 7 days to be successful as contrasted with extubation of 24 hours or less, followed by reintubation.—R.R. Kirby, M.D.

Neonatal and Pediatric

Necrotizing Tracheobronchitis in Intubated Newborns: A Complication of Assisted Ventilation

Metlay LA, Macpherson TA, Doshi N, Milley JR (Univ of Rochester, NY; Univ of Pittsburgh)
Pediatr Pathol 7:575–584, 1987

13–12

It is well known that direct contact of an endotracheal tube with the trachea can cause acute and chronic airway damage. A newly recognized type of iatrogenic tracheal lesion was recently described. Although this lesion is also associated with conventional mechanical ventilation in intubated neonates, it differs from previously described tracheal lesions in that it is most severe distal to the tip of the endotracheal tube. This lesion, necrotizing tracheobronchitis (NTB), is manifested as a basophilic necrosis of the tracheal mucosa. Sloughing of the tracheal mucosa occurring in the later stages can cause respiratory obstruction. In an effort to identify additional patients with NTB, the autopsy records from the 2 previous years were retrospectively reviewed and 45 perinatal autopsies were prospectively studied.

Necrotizing tracheobronchitis was found in 20 of the 45 prospective autopsies and 18 retrospective autopsies. Patients with NTB had birth weights ranging from 700 to 4,000 gm, and gestational ages ranging from 25 to 43 weeks. Survival ranged from 40 minutes to 13 days, with a mean survival of 5 days. All but 1 of the newborns with NTB had received conventional mechanical ventilation for periods ranging from 3 hours to 13 days. One infant with NTB had lived for 40 minutes during which he had been intubated because of meconium aspiration.

Necrotizing tracheobronchitis was graded on a scale of 1 to 4 according to severity. A relationship was found between the length of survival and the grade of endotracheal damage. Diagnosis of NTB requires examination of the trachea distal to the endotracheal tube, as the macroscopic lesion is not striking, and might not be seen when only the routine proximal laryngeal sample is taken.

The etiology of NTB has not yet been established, but mechanical ventilation appears to be implicated in the pathogenesis of the lesion. Its morphological appearance suggests a drying effect, possibly caused by inadequate humidification and heat.

▶ The authors suggest that necrotizing tracheal bronchitis (NTB) may be a common lesion and perhaps would be better diagnosed if there were more extensive sampling of the distal tracheobronchial tree at autopsy or perhaps tracheobronchial cytology examination during life. Inadequate humidification of respiratory gases may produce a drying effect and thus be considered as a possible etiology of NTB. Further investigation could focus on accurate means of assessing humidification, and commercially produced humidifiers may have to be redesigned to provide adequate distal humidification.— G.W. Ostheimer, M.D.

End-Tidal, Transcutaneous, and Arterial P_{CO_2} Measurements in Critically Ill Neonates: A Comparative Study

McEvedy BAB, McLeod ME, Mulera M, Kirpalani H, Lerman J (The Hosp for Sick Children, Toronto; Univ of Toronto)
Anesthesiology 69:112–116, July 1988   13–13

Noninvasive estimates of arterial carbon dioxide (Pa_{CO_2}) based on end-tidal ($PetCO_2$) and transcutaneous ($PtcCO_2$) carbon dioxide measurements are used routinely in the monitoring of critically ill neonates. However, several investigators who questioned the accuracy of $PetCO_2$ measurements in neonates have shown that $PetCO_2$ measurements taken from the distal end of the endotracheal tube are significantly more accurate than those taken from the proximal end. The accuracy of $PetCO_2$ and $PtcCO_2$ measurements as estimates of Pa_{CO_2} in preterm and full-term mechanically ventilated neonates was assessed.

Twenty-seven neonates with a mean gestational age of 34.0 weeks, a mean postnatal age of 3.9 days, and a mean postnatal weight of 0.9 kg were studied. None of the neonates was in shock at the time of the study. All neonates were either mechanically ventilated with a pressure-limited ventilator or breathing spontaneously with continuous positive airway pressure. In all, 46 sets of distal $PetCO_2$, $PtcCO_2$, and Pa_{CO_2} measurements, and 36 sets of proximal and distal $PetCO_2$ measurements were recorded.

Distal $PetCO_2$ measurements were significantly greater than all corresponding proximal $PetCO_2$ measurements, and more closely approximated Pa_{CO_2} values than did the corresponding proximal measurements. The $PtcCO_2/Pa_{CO_2}$ ratio was the most accurate ratio determined, with the $PetCO_2$ distal/Pa_{CO_2} ratio being significantly less accurate than the $PtcCO_2/Pa_{CO_2}$ ratio. No complications from the presence of the sampling catheter within the endotracheal tube occurred.

These results confirm that in critically ill neonates, distal $PetCO_2$ measurements more accurately approximate Pa_{CO_2} than do proximal $PetCO_2$ measurements.

▶ It would appear that we are approaching a time when only a selected few critically ill neonates will require umbilical arterial or intra-arterial monitoring with its attendant morbidity.—G.W. Ostheimer, M.D.

Neurologic Status in Infants Treated With Extracorporeal Membrane Oxygenation: Correlation of Imaging Findings With Developmental Outcome
Taylor GA, Glass P, Fitz CR, Miller MK (Children's Hosp Natl Med Ctr, Washington, DC; George Washington Univ)
Radiology 165:679–682, December 1987   13–14

Extracorporeal membrane oxygenation (ECMO) is a very recent, increasingly important technology in the treatment of severely ill neonates. Newborn infants currently considered candidates for ECMO are usually near-term infants with severe respiratory failure who have not responded to maximal medical therapy. Because perinatal asphyxia, hypoxia, and hypotension are commonly associated with the conditions that lead to respiratory insufficiency, these infants are already at high risk for abnormal developmental outcome even before EMCO bypass therapy is initiated. Factors associated with the use of ECMO per se pose an additional risk for neurologic impairment.

In this study, the intracranial images obtained within the newborn period in 46 infants who had been treated with ECMO were retrospectively reviewed. In all patients, cranial ultrasonography had been performed before and daily during ECMO bypass treatment. Computed tomography was performed within 3 weeks after completion of ECMO. A neuroimaging score was determined for each infant based on the extent and severity of findings on both ultrasonographic and computed tomographic scans. The infants were reevaluated at a mean age of 11.8 months at which time the neuroimaging scores were correlated with findings of neurodevelopmental evaluation.

Of the 46 infants who were reevaluated, 27 (59%) were normal, 8 (17%) were suspect for neurodevelopmental delay, and 11 (24%) had neurodevelopmental delay. However, none of the infants had severe developmental delay. Of 28 infants (61%) with normal neuroimaging findings, 20 (71%) were developmentally normal, 5 (18%) were suspect for delay, and 3 (11%) were developmentally delayed. Of 18 infants with abnormal neuroimaging findings, 7 (39%) were normal, 3 (17%) were suspect, and 8 (44%) were delayed. Thus, there was a significant inverse correlation between neuroimaging scores at the time of ECMO and neurodevelopmental delay.

Individual neurodevelopmental outcomes after ECMO cannot be predicted on the basis of neuroimaging. However, neuroimaging scores are useful for assigning surviving patients to risk categories for developmental outcome.

▶ Long-term prospective studies of neurodevelopment must be performed on newborns who receive major interventions such as ECMO at the time of birth. Only by these types of studies will we be able to demonstrate whether these interventions are appropriate for the newborn. Centers that are unable to do long-term follow-up should consider whether they should pursue these programs of aggressive intervention.—G.W. Ostheimer, M.D.

Airway Management of Acute Supraglottitis at The Children's Hospital, Boston: 1980–1985
Crockett DM, Healy GB, McGill TJ, Friedman EM (Harvard Univ; The Children's Hosp, Boston)
Ann Otol Rhinol Laryngol 97:114–119, March–April 1988   13–15

Since 1970, nasotracheal intubation has been the sole method of airway management of acute supraglottitis at The Children's Hospital in Boston. Experience there during the past 5 years was compared with results obtained elsewhere. Hospital charts were reviewed for 80 patients managed for acute supraglottitis. Parents of 30 children provided additional follow-up information on stridor, recurrent croup, upper respiratory infection, exercise intolerance, or other symptoms of upper-airway disease. Follow-up ranged from 2 months to 5 years.

The management protocol begins with auscultation of the heart and lungs and visual examination. Manipulation is kept to a minimum. After nasotracheal intubation, the patient is sedated with chloral hydrate and placed in a humidified tent. Hand restraints are applied, and intubation is maintained for 36–60 hours. When a sufficient air leak can be found, the patient is extubated. Laryngoscopy is not performed.

Intubation averaged 2.2 days, and hospitalization, 7.5 days. Six children extubated themselves and were successfully reintubated. Tubes were changed without difficulty in 10 patients. No patient required reintubation after planned extubation. The only death resulted from complicating meningitis. Immediate complications included atelectasis, pneumonia, pulmonary edema, and pleural effusion. All problems eventually resolved without sequelae. Estimated complications from otitis media, exudative pharyngitis or tonsillitis, and cervical lymphadenopathy were less than 20%. There were no recorded delayed complications; by parents' reports, all 30 children remained healthy.

This method of airway management of acute supraglottitis has been successful and will be continued.

▶ One cannot argue with success. It would behoove every hospital dealing with acute pediatric airway management problems to develop protocols such as this to effectively deal with these emergencies in its pediatric population.— G.W. Ostheimer, M.D.

Shock and Trauma

Wasted Blood in Trauma Resuscitation
Troop B, Myers RAM, Dawson RB, Britten JS (Univ of Tennessee; Maryland Inst for Emergency Med Services Systems, Baltimore)
Infect Surg 7:242–248, April 1988   13–16

Trauma centers that treat patients with multiple injuries require ready access to blood for rapid transfusion in the treatment of patients admitted in hemorrhagic shock. Because of the emergency situation, there is always a potential for blood wasting. Earlier data suggested that 15% of all cross-matched blood units were being wasted through delay in use, spillage, or error. This study was done to investigate the problem of blood wasting in a major trauma center.

Blood utilization was evaluated in the cases of 150 consecutive patients admitted for resuscitation after hemorrhagic injury. A total of 1,033 units of packed cells were cross-matched. Of the 150 patients, 67 (45%) did not receive transfusions and 83 (55%) did receive transfusions. For the 67 patients who did not receive transfusions, 281 units of packed cells were cross-matched, of which 4 (1.4%) were discarded (table). For the 83 patients who did receive transfusions, 752 units of packed cells were cross-matched, of which 478 units were actually delivered and 15 (2.0%) were discarded. For these 150 patients, an average of 6.9 units of blood was cross-matched per admission, and the total waste was 19 (1.8%) of the 1,033 units cross-matched. Of 308 units of fresh frozen plasma ordered for the 83 patients who received transfusions, 291 (94.5%) were used, and 9 (2.9%) were discarded. Of 55 units of platelets requested, 52 (94.5%) were used, and 3 (5.5%) were discarded. All 3 types of blood components were equally likely to be wasted. Reasons for wasting of blood components included technical administration errors, time delays, and loss by spillage. Units were sometimes rendered useless

Data on Discarded Packed Cells

Patient Type	Number of Patients	Number	Average Per Patient	Crossed-matched Units Units Transfused	Units Discarded	Total Units Used	Discarded per Cross-matched (%)
Transfused	83	752	9.1	478	15	493	2.0
Not transfused	67	281	4.2	0	4	4	1.4
Totals	150	1033	6.7	478	19	497	1.8

(Courtesy of Troop B, Myers RAM, Dawson RB, et al: *Infect Surg* 7:242–248, April 1988.)

after proper preparation, mostly when patients died before the blood could be administered.

The amount of blood wasted because of reasons such as delays in administration and loss of bags within the patient's linens could be reduced by providing patients with a small ice chest in which dispensed units could be kept until infusion. Increased training of personnel involved in blood handling should further reduce the number of technical errors, such as accidental puncture of infusion bags.

▶ This type of cost analysis is obviously important. There are several suggestions that should be taken seriously by those emergency room personnel who deal extensively with trauma.—R.D. Miller, M.D.

Is Advanced Life Support Appropriate for Victims of Motor Vehicle Accidents: The South Carolina Highway Trauma Project
Reines HD, Bartlett RL, Chudy NE, Kiragu KR, McKnew MA (Med Univ of South Carolina; Univ of South Carolina; South Carolina Dept of Health and Environmental Control; Clemson Univ)
J Trauma 28:563–570, May 1988   13–17

Advanced Life Support (ALS) is controversial in the treatment of multisystem injury. To define the proper role of ALS in motor vehicle accidents, 538 ambulance run reports and their corresponding hospital reports were examined in South Carolina in 1983. A trauma review committee examined 248 of these records in depth.

Paramedics were present in the ambulance in 81% of cases. Basic Life Support crews arrived in an average of 18.1 minutes, whereas ALS crews arrived in an average of 24.8 minutes. Total response time was 46 ± 20 minutes. Extrication and rural location increased response time. Endotracheal intubations were successful in only 67% of patients and intravenous lines were successfully placed in 88% of patients. Blood pressure increased in 32% of patients with ALS and in 12% of patients with basic life support en route to the hospital. The trauma review committee determined that the care was beneficial to 85% of patients and inadequate to 11.7% of patients.

Advanced Life Support appears to be beneficial to victims of motor vehicle accidents with multisystem trauma even in a rural state such as South Carolina. Further research is necessary to optimize the care dispensed by ALS teams.

▶ The basic controversy centers on the question whether time taken to resuscitate trauma victims is better spent in transporting them. The answer seems to involve the location of the trauma. In rural areas, where transport times may be prolonged, many studies such as this one support the view that ALS is beneficial. In urban settings with very short transit times, ALS is felt by many to be counterproductive in that it delays the provision of definitive care.—R.R. Kirby, M.D.

Increased Survival After Major Thermal Injury: A Nine Year Review

Merrell SW, Saffle JR, Sullivan JJ, Larsen CM, Warden GD (Univ of Utah)
Am J Surg 154:623–627, December 1987   13–18

The survival of patients with major thermal injury has improved considerably as a result of better understanding and treatment of burn shock, burn wounds, respiratory failure, prevention of sepsis, and advances in intensive care and metabolic support. To assess the impact of these factors on burn mortality, data on 1,458 acutely injured patients admitted to the burn center from 1978 through 1986 were reviewed. Specifically, patient mortality and hospital length of stay were assessed among patients with burns over at least 30% of the total body surface area. Two study periods were evaluated: 1978 through 1981, and 1982 through 1986. Management consisted of isotonic fluid resuscitation, immediate mechanical débridement of burn wounds with topical application of antimicrobials, and enteral alimentation through nasoduodenal feeding.

In the total population, the burn covered a mean of 51% of the total body surface area; the patient age was a mean of 24.4 years. The overall survival rate was 92%. Among patients with burns of at least 30% of the total body surface area, patient survival increased from 59% before 1982 to 77% afterward, mostly as a result of a significantly reduced late mortality rate. Causes of late mortality were sepsis, respiratory failure or acute respiratory distress syndrome, and sudden cardiopulmonary arrest, among others. In contrast, mortality related to burn shock changed little during the 2 study periods. Mortality in patients with inhalation injury decreased less than that in patients without inhalation injury. Death caused by burn injuries of less than 30% of the total body surface area

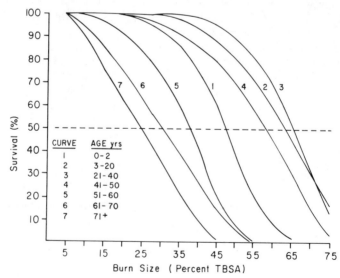

Fig 13–6.—Patient survival and burn size according to patient age. *TBSA*, total body surface area. (Courtesy of Merrell SW, Saffle JR, Sullivan JJ, et al: *Am J Surg* 154:623–627, December 1987.)

was unusual in patients aged 3–40 years, whereas survival was uncommon for patients aged 60 or more years with burns in excess of 45% of the total body surface area (Fig 13–6). The mean length of hospital stay increased from 28.1 days before 1982 to 35.2 days afterward.

These data demonstrate increased survival rates after major thermal injury as a result of improvements in prevention and treatment of sepsis and other late complications of thermal injury.

▶ I believe this experience mirrors that of most major burn centers. The authors of this study used isotonic fluid resuscitation. Could the outcome related to burn shock have been altered by the use of hypertonic saline as has been suggested by other investigators.—R.R. Kirby, M.D.

Comparison of Peripheral and Central Infusions of 7.5% NaCl/6% Dextran 70
Hands R, Holcroft JW, Perron PR, Kramer GC (Univ of California, Davis, Sacramento)
Surgery 103:684–690, June 1988   13–19

Experimental studies have shown that central venous injections of small volumes of a hypertonic solution containing 7.5% sodium chloride and 6% dextran 70 quickly restores blood pressure, cardiac output, oxygen consumption, and urine output in animals in moderately severe hemorrhagic shock. When given to animals in severe shock, this form of resuscitation improved survival rates. To find widespread application in a prehospital setting, hypertonic solutions would have to be given through a peripheral vein, but to date, only central infusions have been used in the animal studies.

In this study, 7.5% NaCl/6% dextran 70 was administered as a 2-minute infusion into the cephalic vein, femoral artery, or superior vena cava of 9 chronically instrumented, conscious sheep in moderately severe hemorrhagic shock. The salt solution was given in a volume of 5 ml/kg of body weight.

All 3 routes of injection gave equivalently good results. Peripheral injection of the resuscitation fluid promptly reestablished arterial blood pressure and cardiac output within 3 minutes of initiation of resuscitation, restored plasma volume by 10 minutes, and fully reestablished urine output by 30 minutes. No vein damage occurred, and all sheep responded well to the infusions, as evidenced by the fact that they were back on their feet shortly after injection.

Peripheral injection of 7.5% NaCl/6% dextran 70 is safe and effective in the resuscitation of sheep in moderately severe hemorrhagic shock. The favorable findings of this study suggest that peripheral injection with hypertonic salt solution will find a place in the prehospital resuscitation of selected trauma patients.

▶ Hypertonic saline is receiving increasing attention as a means to resuscitate victims from shock. If this regimen proves to be as valuable an adjunct as most studies suggest, the ability to administer the fluid through peripheral vascular cannulas is of great importance. We have seen no evidence of phlebitis in patients to whom we have administered 3% to 7.5% saline peripherally for up to 12 hours.—R.R. Kirby, M.D.

Tandem 8.5-French Subclavian Catheters: A Technique for Rapid Volume Replacement

Jones TK, Barnhart GR, Gervin AS (Univ of Iowa, Virginia Commonwealth Univ)
Ann Emerg Med 16:1369–1372, December 1987   13–20

Patients with hemorrhagic shock are treated with rapid restoration of intravascular volume. The celerity with which volume is restored can influence survival and is dependent on the time needed to obtain venous access and on the conduit resistance. Multiple peripheral intravenous lines may be difficult to start in profoundly hypovolemic patients with collapsed peripheral circulation. A technique was developed for the ipsilateral insertion of tandem 8.5-French catheters for subclavian catheters.

Technique.—The patient is put in the Trendelenburg position and a rolled towel is placed vertically behind the upper thoracic spine. After the infraclavicular region is prepared and draped in the usual manner, an insertion site is selected at the junction of the medial and middle third of the clavicle. The 18-gauge insertion needle is inserted infraclavicularly and directed at the apex of the sternal notch. The metal stylet is withdrawn, and a guide wire is advanced into the superior vena cava after venous blood return is obtained. The plastic cannula is removed, and the site of the second catheter is chosen about 1 cm lateral to the first insertion site. After both guide wires are inserted, the skin opening around each wire is enlarged by making small stab incisions. The first 8.5-French catheter with its dilator is then inserted over the guide wire. Dilator and guide wire are withdrawn, and intravenous tubing is connected to the catheter. This maneuver is repeated with the second 8.5-French catheter, and both are quickly secured with 1 suture. To avoid catheter kinking at the junction of the subclavian and internal jugular veins, about 2 cm of each catheter may be left outside the skin and secured. When tandem catheters are inserted in the left subclavian positions, they can usually be secured fully advanced without risk of kinking.

The method allows rapid volume administration while minimizing the risk associated with bilateral subclavian insertions.

▶ The increasing incidence of civilian trauma demands that vigorous resuscitation be carried out early. There seems to be no doubt that hemorrhagic shock at the time of admission to the hospital has a high association with later multiorgan failure and death. Furthermore, up to 20% of "DOAs" may be saved if they manifest any signs of life, either at the trauma site or en route to the hospital. Vascular access is always a problem. Although I have no personal experi-

ence with the technique described herein, it appears to merit further investigation.—R.R. Kirby, M.D.

Head Injury and Hemorrhagic Shock: Studies of the Blood Brain Barrier and Intracranial Pressure After Resuscitation With Normal Saline Solution, 3% Saline Solution, and Dextran-40
Gunnar W, Jonasson O, Merlotti G, Stone J, Barrett J (Univ of Illinois; Hektoen Inst for Med Research, Chicago)
Surgery 103:398–407, April 1988   13–21

Many neurologic deaths of head-injured patients result from intracranial hypertension. Increased intracranial pressure is closely related to a poor neurologic outcome and long-term disability in surviving patients. Beagle dogs had a subarachnoid bolt in place to measure intracranial pressure as an epidural balloon was inflated to mimic closed head injury. After removing 40% of the blood volume for 1 hour, animals received the shed blood along with normal saline, 3% saline solution, or 10% dextran 40 in a volume equal to the amount of shed blood.

Arterial pressure was best restored by dextran 40. The cardiac index increased most with hypertonic saline. Fluid resuscitation markedly increased the intracranial pressure in the normal saline and dextran 40 groups (Fig 13–7). When the dogs were killed after 2 hours of resuscitation, wet brain weight was least in the hypertonic saline group.

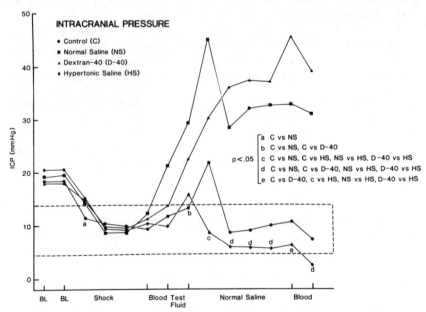

Fig 13–7.—Intracranial pressure measurements with intracranial epidural balloon inflated. Resuscitation was initiated with one-half shed blood volume followed 15 minutes later by volume of test fluid, either NS, D-40, or HS equal to amount of shed blood. (Courtesy of Gunnar W, Jonasson O, Merlotti G, et al: *Surgery* 103:398–407, April 1988.)

An intracranial mass enhances brain ischemia through direct pressure and impaired cerebral autoregulation. Increased cerebral edema is the result. Conventional resuscitation with normal saline or colloid solution does not repair these functions. However, hypertonic saline, given early in the course of resuscitation, promotes the return of cerebral perfusion and cell membrane function.

▶ In view of the lethal nature of brain dysfunction following shock and trauma, any modality that maintains cerebral perfusion pressure *and* reduces cerebral edema merits enthusiastic evaluation. Hemorrhagic shock and fluid resuscitation in beagles is obviously different from closed head trauma in patients. However, the problems faced by the clinician are similar. Thus, attempts to restore intravascular volume with large amounts of blood, colloid, and crystalloid in a massively traumatized patient may be associated with worsening of cerebral edema and intracranial pressure. Because of the other beneficial effects of hypertonic saline, including positive inotropy, decreased systemic vascular resistance, and improved renal function, the salutary CNS effects make it an attractive alternative to more conventional regimens.—R.R. Kirby, M.D.

Effect of Moderate Hypothermia in the Treatment of Canine Hemorrhagic Shock
Meyer DM, Horton JW (Univ of Texas, Dallas)
Ann Surg 207:462–469, April 1988   13–22

Hypothermia reduces oxygen consumption and has been used protectively in neurologic and cardiovascular surgery. After 15 minutes of hemorrhagic shock in dogs hypothermia was initiated, and it was maintained for 1 hour after fluid resuscitation. Iced normal saline was instilled into the peritoneal cavity. Some animals received sodium bicarbonate to correct acidosis.

Heart rate and respiratory rate remained lower in hypothermic animals throughout shock. Myocardial oxygen consumption tended to be lower in hypothermic animals. Normothermic animals had negative myocardial lactate balance. Subendocardial perfusion was better maintained in the hypothermic dogs. However, acidosis persisted in hypothermic dogs when bicarbonate was withheld.

Modern hypothermia lowers the metabolic needs of the heart in dogs subjected to severe hemorrhagic shock. Cardiovascular function and myocardial perfusion are maintained. Hypothermia may have a role in the treatment of severe hemorrhagic shock as long as correction of acid-base disturbances is carried out.

▶ Induced hypothermia, except in cardiac surgical procedures, generally has been relegated to the category of historical interest. Nevertheless, under conditions in which energy depletion is a major concern (i.e., shock), its use has theoretical merit. Twenty years ago we lacked the ability to monitor bodily

function to the extent we can today. Hence, complications might go undetected and organ perfusion might be severely impaired before we are aware anything is wrong. Today, our capabilities are much improved as are our life support techniques. The likelihood of such problems probably is less. Thus the intrinsic limitations of hypothermia are reduced. This paper suffers from 1 major flaw, namely, that *moderate hypothermia* was never defined. Nevertheless, further study seems to be indicated.— R.R. Kirby, M.D.

Prognostic Factors in Severe Accidental Hypothermia: Experience From the Mt. Hood Tragedy
Hauty MG, Esrig BC, Hill JG, Long WB (Oregon Health Sciences Univ)
J Trauma 27:1107–1112, October 1987   13–23

A climbing tragedy on Mt. Hood in May 1986 presented an opportunity to evaluate rapid extracorporeal rewarming by cardiopulmonary bypass in 10 severely hypothermic patients, only 2 of whom survived. The weather conditions were those of a severe late winter storm, with temperatures of 15 to 25 F, winds of up to 60 mph, and more than 4 ft of snowfall in 2 days. The victims spent nearly 72 hours in a snow cave after a 16-hour attempt at ascent.

The 2 survivors had been near the top of the snow cave and were the only ones with obvious signs of life at the time of rescue. No survivor had a core temperature lower than 20 C. In 3 patients, including the survivors, cardiac electric activity was noted before resuscitation. The survivors had initial serum levels of potassium lower than 7 mEq/L, whereas nonsurvivors had marked hyperkalemia. Four nonsurvivors had laboratory findings of disseminated intravascular coagulopathy. Both survivors incurred cold injury to soft tissues of the extremities; 1 required bilateral amputation of the lower extremities.

Severe accidental hypothermia is best managed by rapid core rewarming on cardiopulmonary bypass. Significant prognostic indicators include serious underlying medical illness, duration of exposure to cold, and presence of vital functions. Intravascular thrombosis and signs of irreversible cell lysis are poor prognostic signs.

▶ No editorial comment is necessary here. The article speaks for itself. Most of us will never be called upon to deal with such large numbers of severely hypothermic patients, but perhaps the information presented here can be successfully applied to individual cases.— R.R. Kirby, M.D.

Beneficial Effects of a Hypertonic Solution for Resuscitation in the Presence of Acute Hemorrhage
Cone JB, Wallace BH, Caldwell FT Jr, Smith SD, Searcey R (Univ of Arkansas at Little Rock)
Am J Surg 154:585–588, December 1987   13–24

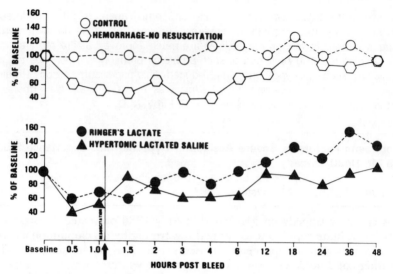

Fig 13–8.—Pulmonary shunt fraction demonstrates that hemorrhage alone produced no pulmonary injury; however, between 18 and 48 hours after hemorrhage, those animals resuscitated with Ringer's lactate solution had small but significant elevation of shunt fraction. (Courtesy of Cone JB, Wallace BH, Caldwell FT Jr, et al: *Am J Surg* 154:585–588, December 1987.)

Hypertonic solutions are useful in resuscitating burn injury victims by expanding the extracellular space at the expense of the intracellular space. In addition, myocardial contractility improves and peripheral vasodilation takes place. Splenectomized dogs were bled to a fixed volume for 1 hour and then given either Ringer's lactate or a hypertonic lactated saline solution containing sodium, 250 mEq/L.

The cardiac index fell to 48% of baseline after bleeding. Significantly less hypertonic solution than Ringer's lactate was needed to maintain the cardiac index, and urine output was better in these animals. Dogs given Ringer's lactate had a significantly elevated intrapulmonary shunt fraction (Fig 13–8). Serum potassium levels were comparable in the 2 groups of dogs, and the solutions were similarly effective in restoring blood volume.

Hypertonic lactated saline solution was effective in this awake canine model, which is analogous to the clinical situation. Pulmonary dysfunction occurred in dogs treated with Ringer's lactate but not in those given hypertonic solution.

▶ Hypertonic saline resuscitation makes sense! Study after study confirms its efficacy in trauma and shock when comparison is made with standard crystalloid resuscitation regimens. Yet clinicians still seem reluctant to employ such therapy. Why this should be so escapes me. Sure, you have to be careful not to "overdo" it and be willing to monitor closely and conscientiously, but any more so than with other protocols? I think not! In this study, the fluid was very conservative, hardly hypertonic compared with some methods, yet the results were still impressive.—R.R. Kirby, M.D.

Heat Related Illnesses During the Hajj (Pilgrimage): Emerging Role of the Anesthesiologist

Seraj MA, Channa AB, Sharif AYM, Kadiwal GH, Jamjoom A (King Saud Univ, Riyadh, Saudi Arabia)
Middle East J Anesth 9:255–276, 1987   13–25

The Hajj is a sacred act of worship in Islam, which takes place in a sandy valley where temperatures range from 38 to 50 C, with a relative humidity of 25%–50%. When the Hajj falls in the hot summer season, pilgrims are exposed to extremely high ambient temperatures, which often cause heat-related illnesses.

Minor heat-related illnesses seen during the Hajj are sunburn, prickly heat, heat intertrigo, heat fatigue, heat edema, and unspecified heat exhaustion. Major illnesses include heat cramps, heat syncope, heat exhaustion, and heatstroke. Most patients suffer from heat exhaustion. This condition may proceed to potentially lethal heatstroke, which is characterized by disturbances of all organ systems, particularly the central nervous system (Table 1). Factors predisposing the heatstroke include high ambient temperature plus humidity; excessive physical exercise; lack of acclimatization; salt and water depletion; fever and acute infections, such as respiratory infections; gastrointestinal disorders, such as vomiting and diarrhea; cardiovascular disease, such as congestive heart failure; and endocrine disorders, such as obesity, diabetes, and thyrotoxicosis. Heatstroke is common in the elderly and is more common in men than in women.

Management of minor heat-related illnesses consists of balanced intra-

TABLE 1.—Systemic Consequences of Heatstroke

Central Nervous System	stupor, delirium, coma and convulsions from thermic stress and cerebrovascular accident
Respiratory System	hyperventilation, cyanosis (hypoxic)
Cardiovascular System	tachycardia, hypotension, cardiogenic shock may follow myocardial infarction or peripheral circulatory collapse
Gastrointestinal System	vomiting and diarrhoea
Renal System	oliguria, glycosuria, haematuria and proteinuria, acute renal failure due to rhabdomyolysis
Electrolytes, Acid Base	hyponatraeemia, hypernatraemia hypokalaemia, hyperkalaemia and metabolic acidosis
Haematological	petechial haemorrhage, disseminated intravascular coagulation

(Courtesy of Seraj MA, Channa AB, Sharif AYM, et al: *Middle East J Anesth* 9:255–276, 1987.)

TABLE 2.—Principles Governing the Treatment
of Heatstroke

Maintenance of airway and ventilation

Control of body temperature

**Management of electrolyte, acid–base
disturbances and fluid therapy**

**Management of cardiovascular complications
such as hypotension, myocardial infarction**

**Management of gastrointestinal disturbances such as
vomiting, diarrhoea, gastrointestinal bleeding**

**Management of central nervous system disturbances -
such as convulsions, coma**

**Management of bleeding diatheses - disseminated
intravascular coagulation**

(Courtesy of Seraj MA, Channa AB, Sharif AYM, et al: *Middle East J
Anesth* 9:255–276, 1987.)

venous salt solutions or dextrose drip or both; rest in a quiet, cool atmosphere; and use of conventional methods of cooling, such as wetting and
fanning. Table 2 summarizes the principles governing the treatment of
heatstroke. While transporting the patient, a clear airway should be
maintained, and oxygen, 4–6 L/minute, can be administered by mask or
endotracheal tube. Core body cooling, which is more effective than vigorous surface cooling, can be achieved with intravenous infusion of
ice-cold saline; bladder, stomach or rectal irrigation with ice-cold saline;
peritoneal dialysis; or extracorporeal circulation. Because these methods
are too complex to implement during the Hajj, surface cooling by means
of the Makkah Al-Mukarramah Body Cooling Unit or conventional cooling methods are currently used. Cooling is stopped when the body temperature has dropped to 38.5–39 C. Central venous pressure serves as an
index of individual fluid requirements; administration of 1–1.5 L of fluid
during an average cooling time of 45 minutes is optimal. Intravenous diazepam, 10–20 mg, can be given initially to control restlessness, shivering, delirium, agitation, and convulsions. Intravenous heparin or platelet
concentrates or both, fresh frozen plasma, or fresh blood is given to correct bleeding diathesis.

There is an increased need for anesthesiologists trained in intensive
care management to cover the multitude of emergency heat-related illnesses during the Hajj pilgrimage.

▶ For those individual involved with critical care medicine, this is an interesting
article if you might treat patients who have been subjected to severe heat.—
R.D. Miller, M.D.

Continuous Epidural Fentanyl Analgesia: Ventilatory Function Improvement With Routine Use in Treatment of Blunt Chest Injury
Mackersie RC, Shackford SR, Hoyt DB, Karagianes TG (Univ of California, San Diego)
J Trauma 27:1207–1212, November 1987   13–26

Studies have demonstrated that the epidural administration of narcotics can provide sustained relief of pain. Continuous epidural fentanyl analgesia (CEFA) is particularly useful because of its rapid onset, short serum half-life, and low incidence of complications. The safety and utility of CEFA were evaluated with regard to providing pain relief and improving postinjury ventilatory function in 40 patients with flail chest or multiple rib fractures.

All patients had serious impairment of ventilatory capacity or poor pain control with systemic narcotics. Ventilatory function tests before and after administration of CEFA were performed.

Eighty-five percent of patients had pain relief ranging from good to excellent with CEFA. Four patients had poor pain relief and required supplemental narcotics; 2 of these later had good relief with epidural catheter replacement. Ventilatory function also improved with the administration of CEFA. Pruritus was the most common complication; 3 patients had transient hypotension. One patient had a suspected episode of systemic narcosis, and 10 contracted pneumonia.

The CEFA is a safe, effective means of pain control that also improves ventilatory function in patients with blunt chest injury. There is a low incidence of complications and no significant associated respiratory depression.

▶ That CEFA provides relief of pain in patients with blunt chest trauma is not surprising in view of its efficacy for postoperative pain relief. Because blunt chest trauma may be associated with other significant injuries and blood loss, a technique to provide pain relief without significant cardiorespiratory compromise (sympathetic blockade, respiratory depression) is potentially of great value. The authors make a persuasive case for the use of CEFA, and I expect that we will see increasing applications of this technique.—R.R. Kirby, M.D.

Cardiopulmonary Resuscitation

Myocardial Oxygen Delivery/Consumption During Cardiopulmonary Resuscitation: A Comparison of Epinephrine and Phenylephrine
Brown CG, Taylor RB, Werman HA, Luu T, Ashton J, Hamlin RL (Ohio State Univ)
Ann Emerg Med 17:302–308, April 1988   13–27

Epinephrine is the vasopressor agent of choice for cardiopulmonary resuscitation (CPR). The α-adrenergic properties of the drug are responsible for its beneficial effects; its β-adrenergic properties, on the other hand, may be harmful in cardiac arrest. Thus a pure α-agonist may be better than epinephrine during CPR. The effect of high-dose epinephrine was compared with the effect of the pure α-agonist phenylephrine on regional myocardial blood flow (MBF), myocardial oxygen delivery (MDO_2), myocardial oxygen consumption (MVO_2), and defibrillation rates during CPR.

Fifteen swine that weighed more than 15 kg were instrumented for measuring regional MBF by using radiolabeled tracer microspheres. Regional MBF, MDO_2, and MVO_2 were measured during normal sinus rhythm. Ventricular fibrillation was induced and continued for 10 minutes.

Then CPR was started by using a pneumatic compression device, and regional MBF, MDO_2, and MVO_2 were measured again.

After 3 minutes of CPR 5 animals were given epinephrine, 0.2 mg/kg; 5 were given phenylephrine, 0.1 mg/kg; and 5 were given phenylephrine, 1 mg/kg. Regional MBF, MDO_2, and MVO_2 were measured again after the drug was given, and extraction ratios were calculated for normal sinus rhythm, CPR, and after drug administration. Defibrillation was attempted 3.5 minutes after the drug was given. No significant differences in MBF, MDO_2, MVO_2, and extraction ratio during normal sinus rhythm and CPR were noted among the groups.

Total mean MBF after administration of drug for the first, second, and third groups was 67.2 ml/minute/100 gm, 7 ml/minute/100 gm, and 36.7 ml/minute/100 gm, respectively. Mean extraction ratios were 76.6%, 94.6%, and 90.7%, respectively. The extraction ratio for the animals who received epinephrine was significantly better than that of the 2 phenyl-ephrine groups. Defibrillation rates for each group were 80%, 0%, and 0%, respectively.

These findings demonstrate that epinephrine in doses that are higher than currently recommended improved MBF and oxygen extraction ratios during CPR when compared with the effect of the pure α-agonist phenylephrine.

▶ Although the anesthesia literature of the early to mid-1960s was replete with articles that suggested that the α-adrenergic effects of pressor agents were all important in CPR, this view has been challenged repeatedly in the 1980s. Epinephrine clearly is the drug of choice. The dosage employed in this study, if it proves applicable to human resuscitation, is remarkable. How many clinicians would employ 14 mg of epinephrine in a 70-kg patient (or 70 mg of phenylephrine)? Similar results were published in the 1988 YEAR BOOK OF ANESTHESIA.—R.R. Kirby, M.D.

A Physiologic Comparison of External Cardiac Massage Techniques
Newton JR Jr, Glower DD, Wolfe JA, Tyson GS Jr, Spratt JA, Fenely MP, Rankin JS, Olsen CO (Duke Univ)
J Thorac Cardiovasc Surg 95:892–901, May 1988   13–28

Some authors suggest that, during cardiopulmonary resuscitation (CPR), blood flow occurs by a thoracic pump mechanism rather than by direct cardiac compression. Both mechanisms may contribute to total cardiac output during CPR, but the relative contribution of each may be related to technique. Five approaches to CPR were compared using both mechanisms to see which technique optimizes hemodynamics.

Dogs were used for the study; the methods studied were high-impulse manual chest compression at 150 per minute; mechanical compression at 60 per minute with concurrent ventilation; mechanical compression at 60 per minute with simultaneous ventilation and either systolic or diastolic abdominal compression, and pneumatic vest compression at 60 per minute.

With high-impulse manual compression, the average cardiac output was 662 ml per minute; with mechanical compression and simultaneous ventilation, it was 340 ml per minute; it was 336 ml per minute with mechanical compression and concurrent ventilation accompanied by systolic abdominal compression; with mechanical compression and simultaneous ventilation along with diastolic abdominal pressure, it was 366 ml per minute; and with vest resuscitation, it was 196 ml per minute. High-impulse manual compression also provided the greatest brachiocephalic blood flow and the highest coronary perfusion pressure.

High-impulse manual compression was superior to other methods of CPR statistically and physiologically. This method generated superior hemodynamics when compared with other techniques.

▶ If there is a more confusing subject in cardiopulmonary resuscitation than how to provide chest compression, I don't know what it is. For the past several years, every combination of chest and abdominal compression at high and low rates, with variable durations, and with or without synchronous mechanical lung inflations have been extolled, condemned, or found to be of no consequence. One problem is that dogs are not very representative of human beings. Thus one must be very careful about data extrapolation. Also, increased brachiocephalic blood flow does not equate with increased cerebral perfusion. Thus, measurement of the former as an indication of the adequacy of resuscitation can be misleading. Finally, the augmentation of cardiac performance by drugs such as epinephrine must be considered. This paper provides additional information for consideration. However, I don't believe we should assume that the case for high-impulse manual compression has been established.—R.R. Kirby, M.D.

Carbicarb: An Effective Substitute for NaHCO₃ for the Treatment of Acidosis
Sun JH, Filley GF, Hord K, Kindig NB, Bartle EJ (Univ of Colorado, Denver)
Surgery 102:835–839, November 1987   13–29

Although sodium bicarbonate (NaHCO₃) has many undesirable side effects, it has traditionally been the treatment of choice for acidosis in conjunction with cardiopulmonary arrest, hemorrhagic shock, and other life-threatening conditions. A new buffer, Carbicarb (CBC), which does not generate carbon dioxide as $NaHCO_3$ does, was compared with $NaHCO_3$, 1 mole/L, and sodium chloride, 1 mole/L, in the treatment of mixed respiratory and metabolic acidosis.

Mixed respiratory and metabolic acidosis was produced by asphyxia in 40 rats, which were divided into 3 groups to receive either CBC, $NaCHO_3$, or hypertonic saline solution in clinically appropriate doses.

Intravenously administered $NaCHO_3$ increased arterial pH only 0.03, elevated carbon dioxide pressure, and increased lactate concentration twofold. With CBC, the pH elevation was 3 times as great, and the blood lactate level remained stable.

Because CBC does not generate carbon dioxide, it should eliminate the increase in the work of respiratory muscles and the potential for intracellular acidosis that is associated with $NaCHO_3$ therapy in cardiopulmonary failure. Another benefit is that lower sodium doses are possible with CBC than with $NaCHO_3$; in addition, CBC does not change the blood lactate level.

▶ Who would have anticipated a few years ago that sodium bicarbonate would have fallen into such disfavor for the treatment of metabolic (nonrespiratory) acidosis. Carbicarb (equimolar solution of sodium bicarbonate and sodium carbonate) appears experimentally to resolve some of the problems of standard bicarbonate administration: evolution of CO_2 and intracellular acidosis. Sodium dichloroacetate is another substance reputed to be more effective than in bicarbonate, and of course, TRIS buffer (THAM) has been touted similarly for many years. What must not be lost sight of is that, regardless of which buffer is used, attention still must be directed toward the basic problem producing the acidosis. Nevertheless, any complications related to therapy should be avoided, and one must suppose that sodium bicarbonate will be used far less frequently as knowledge concerning the complications of such therapy is increasingly disseminated.—R.R. Kirby, M.D.

Improved Hemodynamic Function During Hypoxia With Carbicarb, a New Agent for the Management of Acidosis
Bersin RM, Arieff AI (VA Med Ctr, San Francisco; Univ of California, San Francisco)
Circulation 77:227–233, January 1988   13–30

Bicarbonate is used conventionally to correct lactic acidosis in hypoxic states, but depressed cardiac function and accelerated lactate production may result and the blood pH may even decline. Probably, CO_2 generated by bicarbonate administration is responsible for these effects. Carbicarb, an equimolar solution of sodium carbonate and sodium bicarbonate, buffers excess hydrogen ion in the blood without altering the PCO_2 level. Dogs were ventilated with a hypoxic mixture to induce hypoxic lactic ac-

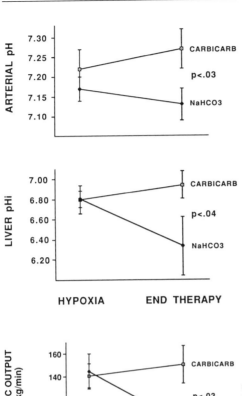

Fig 13–9.—Effects of carbicarb and sodium bicarbonate on arterial pH and liver intracellular pH during hypoxia. The mean values ±SEM are shown. (Courtesy of Bersin RM, Arieff AI: *Circulation* 77:227–233, January 1988.)

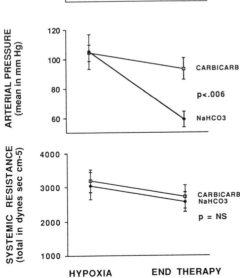

Fig 13–10.—Effects of carbicarb and sodium bicarbonate on cardiac output, arterial blood pressure, and systemic vascular resistance during hypoxia. Mean values ±SEM are shown. (Courtesy of Bersin RM, Arieff AI: *Circulation* 77:227–233, January 1988.)

idosis. After 1 hour they received either sodium bicarbonate or carbicarb, 2.5 mEq/kg.

The arterial pH declined with bicarbonate but improved significantly with carbicarb (Fig 13–9). Treatment did not alter the arterial PO_2 in either group. Cardiac output did not change when carbicarb was given, but it decreased substantially after bicarbonate administration (Fig 13–10). Carbicarb increased whole-body oxygen delivery and oxygen consumption. Net lactate production improved with carbicarb, but worsened with sodium bicarbonate.

In experimental hypoxic lactic acidosis, carbicarb improves the blood pH without adversely affecting myocardial function or the circulation. Trials are warranted in the treatment of clinical acidotic states, especially cardiopulmonary arrest.

▶ Sodium bicarbonate has taken a number of "hits" in recent years, probably justifiably. Carbicarb and other "lactate busters" may be useful and appear to avoid the problems of bicarbonate therapy. However, the correction of a metabolic abnormality (acidosis) does not equate with improved outcome. Fifteen or 20 years ago, people raved about TRIS buffer (THAM) in similar fashion. Where is it today? Clinical trials certainly are indicated.—R.R. Kirby, M.D.

Reservations and Recommendations Regarding Sodium Bicarbonate Administration in Cardiac Arrest
Young GP (Highland Gen Hosp, Oakland, Calif)
J Emerg Med 6:321–323, July–August 1988   13–31

Sodium bicarbonate has been a standard part of the resuscitation of cardiac arrest victims. But the American Heart Association's (AHA) revised Standards and Guidelines for Cardiopulmonary Resuscitation and Emergency Cardiac Care recommends hyperventilation, not sodium bicarbonate, for treating acidosis in cardiac arrest patients. The literature on metabolic acidosis and bicarbonate therapy was examined.

A buildup of carbon dioxide and lactic acid brings about the combined respiratory and metabolic acidosis seen in cardiac arrest. But bicarbonate results in an elevated PCO_2 and a worsening of central venous acidosis. Sodium bicarbonate may also induce hyperosmolarity and hypernatremia. There is little evidence that bicarbonate aids in the ability to defibrillate. Furthermore, 1 animal study showed that successful resuscitation was associated with a greater degree of acidosis than was found in animals with unsuccessful resuscitation.

The new AHA guidelines suggest that bicarbonate be considered only after other proven methods have been tried. Those patients with preexisting acidosis or hyperkalemia may be helped by sodium bicarbonate, but arterial blood gases may not give an accurate assessment of the severity of tissue acidosis during cardiac arrest. The AHA's change in its recommendation is correct, although this is a significant modification in the management of acidosis in cardiac arrest. It may be difficult, however, to convince physicians to abandon the use of sodium bicarbonate.

▶ Here is additional information, if more is necessary, that sodium bicarbonate is ineffective (and perhaps detrimental) in CPR.—R.R. Kirby, M.D.

Using the Heimlich Maneuver to Save Near-Drowning Victims
Heimlich HJ, Patrick EA (Heimlich Inst, Cincinnati; Univ of Cincinnati)
Postgrad Med 84:62–73, August 1988   13–32

Most drowning victims aspirate significant amounts of water as well as foreign materials such as mud, sand, or algae. When water and other substances obstruct the airway, mouth-to-mouth resuscitation may be unsuccessful. The Heimlich maneuver, which expels water from the tracheobronchial tree, should be the first emergency treatment for a near-drowning victim.

Hypoxemia, caused by water in the lungs, is the primary reason for death in drowning. In mouth-to-mouth resuscitation, the rescuer's exhaled air cannot reach the alveoli when obstruction exists, just as a straw filled with water will not empty as long as one end is covered.

Some older techniques of treating near-drowning victims used the principle of intermittent subdiaphragmatic pressure. The Schafer method, introduced in 1903, was the standard procedure from 1929 until 1959. The Heimlich maneuver, a refinement of the prone pressure method, is recommended in the American Heart Association's 1986 Standards and Guidelines for Cardiopulmonary Resuscitation and Emergency Cardiac Care.

The victim should be placed on his or her back with the face to one side. The rescuer, facing the victim, kneels astride the victim's hips and places the heel of 1 hand on the victim's abdomen, slightly above the navel and below the rib cage. With the second hand on top of the first, the rescuer presses into the victim's abdomen with a quick upward thrust, repeating as long as water flows from the mouth. In a number of victims reported here, the Heimlich maneuver was the only form of treatment needed. If the victim does not regain consciousness, cardiopulmonary resuscitation and ventilation techniques should be initiated.

▶ I selected this article for abstracting and editorial comment because it is misleading in several areas that need clarification and correction. I was particularly concerned because Dr. Jerome H. Modell, Chairman of the Department of Anesthesiology at the University of Florida, was alleged to support the findings reported by Dr. Heimlich. In fact, for the most part, this was not true. In addition, several statements made by Dr. Heimlich concerning the pathophysiologic changes in near-drowning are erroneous. These include the following:
  1. "Aspirated water obstructing the airway to 1 or more lobes or to multiple small areas of the lungs leads to hypoxemia." This statement is false. Foreign matter (solids) obstruct, not water.

2. According to Heimlich, flooding of the lungs is a routine occurrence. Again, this statement is erroneous. In fresh water near-drowning, aspirated water is rapidly absorbed into the pulmonary circulation. In sea water near-drowning, lung water increases at the expense of the blood volume.

3. Studies other than those of Heimlich have *not* shown any advantage of the Heimlich maneuver after sea water aspiration in dogs.

4. The delay in initiating standard resuscitative maneuvers, including CPR, can result in irreversible cerebral hypoxia.

5. Performance of the Heimlich maneuver increases the risk of pulmonary aspiration of gastric contents.

According to Modell, the Heimlich maneuver should be reserved for cases in which airway obstruction by foreign material, not water, precludes successful use of conventional methods. I was particularly concerned by the use of a figure showing water in a straw obstructed on 1 end by a finger in an effort to portray what happens in the near-drowning victim. A finger obstructing the distal end of the straw absolutely prevents the fluid from moving. This situation is not analogous to a small airway, which is distensible with positive airway pressure and is connected to alveoli that are expandable. This is just 1 example of shoddy "science" that is used to justify an unproven means of resuscitation for near-drowning. I am afraid that blind following of the recommendations in this article will result in unnecessary loss of life.—R.R. Kirby, M.D.

Crystalloids, Colloids, and Electrolytes

Elevated Urinary Specific Gravity in Acute Oliguric Renal Failure Due to Hetastarch Administration
Haskell LP, Tannenberg AM (Metropolitan Hosp Ctr, New York)
NY State J Med 88:387–388, July 1988   13–33

The specific gravity of urine is commonly measured in the diagnostic evaluation of acute oliguric states. However, the true measure of concentration is the number of particles in solution, which is determined by measuring osmolality. If high-molecular-weight compounds are present in the urine, the specific gravity can be elevated out of proportion to the actual concentration of the urine, resulting in a discrepancy between specific gravity and osmolality values. A number of endogenously produced and exogenously administered substances are known to significantly raise the specific gravity while affecting urinary osmolality to a much lesser degree. One of those substances is hetastarch, which is commonly administered for volume expansion in hemorrhage-induced hypotension.

Man, 54, an alcoholic, was found to have aspiration pneumonia that necessitated mechanical ventilation. Upper gastrointestinal tract bleeding with hypotension developed, and hetastarch was given for volume expansion. Oliguria and progressive azotemia then developed. The specific gravity of the urine was 1.035 4 hours after hetastarch administration and stayed approximately the same in urine samples collected 8, 23, and 24 hours after hetastarch administration

Specific Gravity and Urinary Osmolality Determinations After Hetastarch Administration in 1 Case

Time Interval	Specific Gravity*	Urinary Osmolality	Dipstick Proteinuria
4 hrs after hetastarch	1.035	350	2+
8 hrs	1.035	325	3+
12 hrs	1.030	313	not determined
24 hrs	1.035	320	not determined

*Determined by urinometer and refractometer
(Courtesy of Haskell LP, Tannenberg AM: *NY State J Med* 88:387–388, July 1988.)

(table). On the basis of these findings, a diagnosis of prerenal azotemia due to volume loss was made. However, the urinary osmolality determined in the same urine samples by the freezing point depression technique ranged from 313 to 350 milliosmols (mOsm)/kg of water. These values are more consistent with a diagnosis of acute tubular necrosis than with one of prerenal azotemia. The patient died the day after hetastarch administration.

In patients with intrinsic renal damage, hetastarch can elevate the urinary specific gravity with little effect on urinary osmolality or true urinary concentration ability. Reliance on misleading specific gravity values may well lead to administration of inappropriate fluid therapy. Measurement of urinary osmolality, rather than specific gravity, should be the standard procedure for determining urinary concentration, especially when high-molecular-weight colloid solution has been administered.

▶ This study further substantiated that hetastarch is not as innocuous a plasma expander as once thought.—R.D. Miller, M.D.

The Effects of Hespan on Serum and Lymphatic Albumin, Globulin, and Coagulant Protein
Lucas CE, Denis R, Ledgerwood AM, Grabow D (Wayne State Univ)
Ann Surg 207:416–420, April 1988   13–34

Previous studies found that the addition of human serum albumin to the resuscitation regimen for hemorrhagic shock in man decreases serum concentrations of albumin and nonalbumin proteins, e.g., globulins, immunoglobulins, and coagulant proteins. The effects of hydroxyethyl starch (Hespan) resuscitation on serum and lymphatic proteins after hemorrhagic shock were studied in 34 splenectomized dogs. After the shock insult, the animals were randomly assigned to receive the shed blood plus salt solution, 50 ml/kg, or salt solution with varying concentrations of Hespan (0.22, 0.45, 0.9, and 1.5 gm/kg). Each animal received the test solution, 50 ml/kg/day, for 3 days after the shock.

The levels of all serum proteins, including albumin, globulin, and coagulant proteins, were significantly decreased in all 4 Hespan-supplemented groups. The lymphatic concentrations of proteins increased after Hespan supplementation.

Hespan induces an oncotically controlled extravascular protein relocation. The clinical significance of reduced intravascular protein after Hespan resuscitation needs to be assessed further. Pending such studies, Hespan-supplemented resuscitation should be suspected as a cause of multiple alterations in circulatory protein concentrations and functions.

▶ Obviously Hespan has multiple activities and is not quite as inert as initial studies indicated.—R.D. Miller, M.D.

Hydroxyethyl Starch: An Alternative to Plasma for Postoperative Volume Expansion After Cardiac Surgery
Munsch CM, MacIntyre E, Machin SJ, Mackie IJ, Treasure T (Middlesex Hosp, London)
Br J Surg 75:675–678, July 1988   13–35

Plasma protein fraction (PPF) is generally used for postoperative volume expansion in patients undergoing open heart surgery, but its relative expense and short supply limit its use. Hydroxyethyl starch (HES), a synthetic colloid derived from amylopectin, is available as a 6% solution with an average molecular weight of 450,000. Because of concerns that HES may have an adverse effect on the coagulation mechanism, a study was undertaken to compare its efficacy with PPF after coronary artery surgery, as well as to investigate its effects on coagulation.

Forty patients undergoing elective coronary artery bypass graft surgery were randomly assigned to receive either HES (n = 20) or PPF (n = 20) as non-blood volume replacement according to standard hemodynamic criteria. The 2 groups were comparable in clinical characteristics.

Median volumes of colloid used during the first 24 hours were comparable in the 2 groups: HES, 950 ml (range, 500–1,500), and PPF, 975 ml (range, 350–2,000). Blood use, urine output, and blood loss did not differ between groups. Although there was a more marked shortening of thrombin time in patients who received HES than in those who received PPF, the difference between the 2 groups was not significantly different. All other changes in hemostatic parameters, such as prothrombin time, activated partial thromboplastin time, fibrinogen concentration, platelet function, and factor VIII and von Willebrand factor activity, were similar in both groups and represented the postoperative changes expected in cardiac surgical patients. There was no clinical evidence of excessive bleeding in patients who received HES. There were no hypersensitivity reactions or other deleterious side effects attributable to HES.

Hydroxyethyl starch is a safe and effective volume expander for postoperative cardiac surgical patients. Its relative lack of expense and ease of availability make it an attractive alternative to PPF after cardiac surgery.

▶ These are reassuring data in view of the low cost of the synthetic volume expander. Absence of changes in coagulation despite infusion of up to 2,000 ml of hydroxyethyl starch negates one of the problems alleged to occur with this material.—R.K. Stoelting, M.D.

Costs of Alternative Colloid Solutions
Muñoz E (Long Island Jewish Med Ctr, New Hyde Park, NY)
Infections in Surgery 6:634–638, November 1987   13–36

The ability to predict costs allows medical administrators to identify the types of care that put the greatest strain on the institution's resources and to develop treatment models for achieving maximal cost-benefit ratios. An analysis was undertaken to quantify the cost versus benefit of dextran and starch as substitutes for albumin in colloid therapy.

The unit cost of each 500-cc dose was $10 for dextran, $30 for starch, and $75 for albumin. Rates of anaphylactoid reactions were determined for each of the colloids, as well as hospital and physician costs for each morbidity. Starch was associated with the highest incidence of anaphylactoid reactions, followed by albumin. The average cost of an anaphylac-

TABLE 1.—Cost-Effectiveness Analysis of Alternative Colloids

Comparison*	Value		
Dextran vs starch			
Scenario 1 (1:50,000)	$\frac{\$82.5 - \$23.0}{20}$	=	$2,975,000/life
Scenario 2 (1:5000)	$\frac{\$82.5 - \$23.0}{200}$	=	297,500/life
Scenario 3 (1:500)	$\frac{\$82.5 - \$23.0}{2000}$	=	29,750/life
Dextran vs albumin			
Scenario 1 (1:50,000)	$\frac{\$81.5 - \$23.0}{20}$	=	$2,925,000/life
Scenario 2 (1:5000)	$\frac{\$81.5 - \$23.0}{200}$	=	292,500/life
Scenario 3 (1:500)	$\frac{\$81.5 - \$23.0}{2000}$	=	29,250/life
Starch vs albumin			
Scenario 1 (1:50,000)	$\frac{\$81.5 - \$82.5}{20}$	=	$405,000/life
Scenario 2 (1:5000)	$\frac{\$81.5 - \$82.5}{200}$	=	40,500/life
Scenario 3 (1:500)	$\frac{\$81.5 - \$82.5}{2000}$	=	4,050/life

*One million doses of colloid.
(Courtesy of Muñoz E: *Infections in Surgery* 6:634–638, November 1987.)

TABLE 2.—Cost Analysis Under No Incremental Mortality
Assumption

Comparison	Value* ($ millions)
Dextran vs starch	$82.5–23.0 = $59.5
Dextran vs albumin	$81.5–23.0 = $58.5
Starch vs albumin	$81.5–82.5 = $–1.0

*One million doses of colloid.
(Courtesy of Muñoz E: *Infections in Surgery* 6:635–638, November 1987.)

toid reaction was calculated to be $500. A cost-effective analysis was developed to determine the dollar value saved for each life lost from use of alternative colloids (Table 1), and a comparison made of the agents assuming no incremental mortality (Table 2).

Some incremental mortality was predicted if dextran and starch were substituted for the higher-cost albumin; however, the risks of complication or death associated with the use of these alternative colloids are relatively low, but the savings are substantial—an aggregate of $300 million would be saved annually if dextran were used for volume expansion.

If costs of medical care have to be limited, significant savings could be achieved through the use of alternative colloids in patients receiving colloid resuscitation. Each physician should evaluate the potential savings against the potential risk in patients requiring colloid therapy.

▶ This epidemiologic study is important but leaves many gaps. First is whether we even need to use colloids in resuscitative therapy. Perhaps this can be entirely accomplished with crystalloids. Second, the dextrans are well known to produce more reactions than the starches, which was not reflected in this study. Overall, the main value of this study is to indicate that, in an atmosphere of cost containment, such approaches will be increasingly used. It will be important for physicians to use them in the proper direction.—R.D. Miller, M.D.

Evaluation of Dressing Regimens for Prevention of Infection With Peripheral Intravenous Catheters: Gauze, a Transparent Polyurethane Dressing, and an Iodophor-Transparent Dressing

Maki DG, Ringer M (Univ of Wisconsin, Madison)
JAMA 258:2396–2403, Nov 6, 1987   13–37

Catheter-related septicemia is the most common life-threatening complication of infusion therapy. A prospective randomized study was done of 2,088 peripheral venous catheters to determine tolerance and efficacy for prevention of phlebitis and infection of 4 dressing regimens.

The regimens investigated were sterile gauze and tape replaced every 48 hours; gauze left on for the lifetime of the catheter; a polyurethane transparent dressing left on until the catheter was removed; and a novel transparent dressing with an iodophor antiseptic incorporated in the adhesive, also left on indefinitely.

The 4 dressing regimens provided comparable coverage, except that moisture accumulated more frequently under the transparent dressing. Cutaneous colonization under the dressing was low level and similar with all 4 types, ranging from $10^{0.58}$ to $10^{0.70}$ colony-forming units. The rate of local catheter-related infection also was low and did not differ significantly among dressing types, with a range of 4.6% to 5.9%. No catheter caused bacteremia. Stepwise logistic multivariate analysis demonstrated cutaneous colonization of the insertion site, contamination of the catheter hub, moisture under the dressing, and prolonged catheterization to be significant risk factors for catheter-related infection.

It is not cost effective to redress peripheral venous catheters periodically. For most patients, sterile gauze or a transparent dressing can be used and left in place until the catheter is removed.

▶ This is an excellent study, which showed that whether you put on a transparent polyurethane dressing on an iodophor-containing transparent dressing, just carried it with gauze, or had gauze replaced every other day did not affect the wound infection rate. One of the things that was exceptionally interesting was the confirmation that phlebitis develops in approximately 75% of patients no matter what technique is used after a catheter is in place for 4 days as opposed to about 30% after 2 days. Second, the infection rate is much smaller with these Teflon catheters than in the old days when catheters were made of polyvinylchloride or polyethylene. This difference may be related to the difference in adherence of bacteria to the catheter, and Teflon is more resistant to adherence, or it may just be a result of historical change with time.

Several other things should be noted in this study. First is that an iodine-containing mix was used for placement of all catheters, and I believe it's been shown that that is significantly better than just alcohol swabbing. That change alone may contribute to the very low rate of infection of 5% or less after 72 hours in place (note: phlebitis is not infection). Second is that this test, although it started out with approximately 500 catheters in each group, really was testing only 125 catheters in each group because only that number were in place for more than 48 to 72 hours, the time at which the normal gauze would be changed. The power of this test is much smaller than the power of a 500-catheter test, and my crude statistics show that a 50% difference between groups in the rate of local infection would only have a power of about 20% with this size of 125 catheters in each group as a sample. Third, although 50% of the IVs are placed in the operating room, no mention or credit is given to the anesthesia coordinator or whoever in the department of anesthesia coordinated this process. Whereas such cooperation is to be admired, one cannot help but wonder whether better data would have been obtained were there a responsible anesthesiologist involved in helping design, carry out, and be given credit for those roles in the study.—M.F. Roizen, M.D.

Blood Transfusions

Red Blood Cell Survival Following Admixture With Heated Saline: Evaluation of a New Blood Warming Method for Rapid Transfusion

Wilson EB, Knauf MA, Donohoe K, Iserson KV (Univ of Arizona)
J Trauma 28:1274–1277, August 1988   13–38

Rapid replacement of red blood cells (RBCs) during hemorrhagic shock is limited by the amount of time needed to warm the RBCs from their storage temperature of 4 C. A technique of adding RBCs to saline heated to 70 C was tested in 5 volunteers.

The 5 healthy men each gave 1 unit of blood that was then prepared by standard methods and stored for 14 days. The RBCs were added to saline bags heated by water bath to 70 C. Saline transfer and hand-rocking agitation of the blood bags were completed in 45 seconds. Investigators labeled aliquots of the warmed RBCs with chromium 51 before injection into the autologous donor. Samples of the volunteers' blood were taken at 1 hour and 24 hours, and about 3 times a week for a 3-week period.

Survival of RBCs after transfusion was in the normal range for 2-week storage: The mean survival at 24 hours was 90.2%, and the mean radiolabeled RBC half-life, 25.3 days. Thus saline heated to substantially higher temperatures than previously tried does not impair RBC survival.

Rapid infusion devices require that packed cells be diluted with saline. The technique described here yields mixture temperatures of 35–39 C. No change in plasma hemoglobin or osmotic fragility occurs because the exposure time to elevated temperatures is brief. The blood-warming process seems promising for use in transfusion therapy.

▶ This will certainly be an attractive technique if the logistics of it can be worked out.—R.D. Miller, M.D.

Warming of Resuspended Packed Red Cells With a New Microwave Device: In Vitro Findings and Clinical Assessment in Comparison to a Dry Heat Warming System

Roth-Henschker H, Holzberg E, Oppitz K-H, Lehmann C (Städtisch Krankenhaus München-Neuperlach, West Germany)
Anaesthesist 37:321–330, 1988   13–39

The Fenwal BW-5 dry-heat blood warmer has long been used to warm cold-stored red blood cell concentrates suspended in saline solution in preparation for transfusion. However, the process is time-consuming and complicated. The Infusotherm 407 is a newly developed microwave blood warmer that requires less time for rewarming and is easier to operate. The methods were compared using 211 units containing packed red blood cells diluted in a disposable plastic bag holding 100 ml of saline. The Fenwal BW-5 was used to warm 96 units, and the Infusotherm 407, to warm 115 units.

Both blood warmers caused a slight elevation in hemolysis, but the changes were within the acceptable range for stored packed red blood cells according to the standards set by the European Public Health Committee. Neither the osmotic fragility nor the mean corpuscular volume was affected by either of the warming devices.

Previous studies have shown that erythrocytes in whole blood with a normal hematocrit contained in full-sized blood units are not affected by microwave warming but that small blood units and packed red blood cell units develop considerable hemolysis and distinct changes in mean corpuscular volume and osmotic fragility. The present results demonstrate that it is not the microwave per se that damages red blood cells; rather, local overheating caused by the small volume, insufficient blood mixing, a high hematocrit, and high viscosity are responsible for the development of hemolysis.

Microwave warming using the Infusotherm 407 is a new and rapid method for preparing small and large blood units for transfusion.

▶ Unbelievably, the microwave oven approach to warming blood has reappeared. The units that were used previously intermittently markedly hemolyzed red cells, resulting in some very unfortunate reactions. Is this new microwave oven safe enough that it will not hemolyze packed red cells?—R.D. Miller, M.D.

Use of Rh Positive Blood in Emergency Situations
Schmidt PJ, Leparc GF, Samia CT (Southwest Florida Blood Bank, Tampa; Univ of South Florida)
Surg Gynecol Obstet 167:229–233, September 1987   13–40

Most physicians order units of red blood cells (RBCs) that are both O and Rh negative for emergency transfusions. This precaution, however, proves to be necessary in only a few cases. Furthermore, this practice depletes the supply of O Rh-negative blood for those patients who must have it for routine transfusions. A 2-year study at hospitals supplied by the Southwest Florida Blood Bank evaluated the use of O Rh-positive RBC for emergency situations.

Most of the transfusions were given to trauma victims, and 40% of the 449 patients studied did not survive the emergency episode. Two thirds of the patients were male. Of 418 typed patients, only 20 were Rh-negative females. Half of these, or 2% of all patients, were of childbearing age.

Of 377 transfused patients who did not undergo antibody screening or cross matching, no acute hemolytic reactions occurred. One Rh-negative woman with a ruptured ectopic pregnancy was typed during transfusion, then switched to Rh-negative blood followed by Rh immune globulin.

It is not commonly understood that Rh-positive blood does not cause an immediate transfusion reaction in Rh-negative patients. Nor does O Rh negative imply no donor antigens at all. In this study, only 0.9% of the patients were young Rh-negative women. With this statistic in mind, there seems little reason to require O Rh-negative blood in all emergencies. A national survey of 4,791 delayed hemolytic reactions revealed that only 1.4% were anti-Rh reactions. The routine use of Rh-positive blood in the emergency room can prevent serious shortages of Rh-negative blood.

▶ This article speaks for itself and adds flexibility to blood therapy during emergency surgery and anesthesia.—R.D. Miller, M.D.

Seven Years Experience With Group O Unmatched Packed Red Blood Cells in a Regional Trauma Unit
Lefebre J, McLellan BA, Coovadia AS (Univ of Toronto)
Ann Emerg Med 16:1344–1349, December 1987   13–41

A person with group O blood has long been considered the universal donor. The introduction of blood component systems made group O unmatched packed red blood cells (G O UPRBCs) available for emergency treatment of hypovolemic shock. Seven years' experience with using G O UPRBCs was reviewed to determine the rate of complications.

In the 7 years, 537 units were transfused into 133 trauma patients, for a total of 9.1% of all transfusions in a regional trauma unit during this time period. Ten of the 116 patients who were tested had positive results on direct antiglobulin tests. Seven of 10 received more than 8 units of G O UPRBCs. Among the 89 patients who survived longer than 24 hours after the trauma, 5 had positive results for direct antiglobulin tests (table). Three of the 5 received more than 8 units of G O UPRBCs. There were no clinical complications in this series of patients.

Group O unmatched packed red blood cells are safe and effective in the treatment of hemodynamically unstable trauma patients. They should

---

Patients Who Survived More Than 24 Hours After Trauma and Had Positive Direct Antiglobulin Tests

Patient	Age	Sex	Blood Group	Units of G O UPRBCs	Units Packed Cells (in first 24 hours)	Class of Blood Pressure on Arrival	Direct Antiglobulin Test Results
1	21	F	B-pos	13	13	3	DAT positive (1½) at 7 hr DAT negative at 48 hr
2	23	M	A-pos	6	14	3	DAT positive (½) at 1½ hr DAT negative at 48 hr
3	65	M	AB-pos	9	13	2	DAT positive (½) at 48 hr DAT negative 5 days later
4	33	M	A-neg	17	17	3	DAT positive (½) at 18 hr DAT negative at 48 hr
5	31	M	A-pos	4	13	3	DAT positive (½) at 10 hr DAT negative at 72 hr

(Courtesy of Lefebre J, McLellan BA, Coovadia AS: *Ann Emerg Med* 16:1344–1349, December 1987.)

be used when a patient is in hypovolemic shock and grouping and typing the patient is too time-consuming and carries too high a risk of clerical error.

▶ Whether this approach is better than using typed-specific blood can only be determined with long-term immunologic studies.—R.D. Miller, M.D.

A Clinical Experience With Adsol Preserved Erythrocytes
Valeri CR, Pivacek LE, Palter M, Dennis RC, Yeston N, Emerson CP, Altschule MD (Boston Univ)
Surg Gynecol Obstet 166:33–46, January 1988   13–42

The 24-hour posttransfusion survival rate of human erythrocytes preserved in adenine, glucose, mannitol, and sodium chloride (ADSOL) and stored at 4 C for 35, 42, and 49 days was determined.

Samples of ADSOL-preserved blood were used for in vitro studies for as long as 49 days. Blood was examined periodically throughout the storage period. Volunteers also received autologous and homologous transfusions with ADSOL-preserved erythrocytes stored for the same period. Other volunteers received transfusions with compatible but identifiable

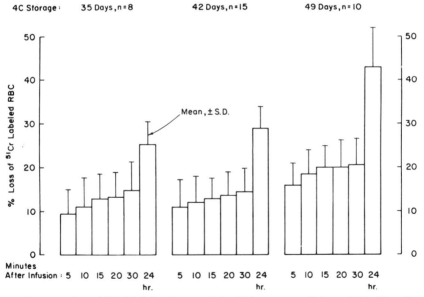

Fig 3–11.—Loss of ^{51}Cr-labeled erythrocytes during 24-hour posttransfusion period in 33 studies. These autologous ADSOL-preserved erythrocytes were stored at 4 C for as long as 49 days. Survival value of 100% was estimated from radioactivity associated with ^{51}Cr-labeled erythrocytes *(RBC)* and erythrocyte volume of volunteers measured from ^{125}I-labeled albumin plasma volume and total body hematocrit value. ADSOL solution was added to erythrocyte concentrate within 4 hours of blood collection and storage at room temperature; ADSOL-resuspended erythrocytes were stored at 4 C for as long as 49 days. (Courtesy of Valeri CR, Pivacek LE, Palter M, et al: *Surg Gynecol Obstet* 166:33–46, January 1988.)

erythrocytes stored under the same protocol. Three methods were used to estimate the 100% survival rate used in the calculation of the 24-hour posttransfusion survival time.

In all of the autologous and homologous transfusions, ADSOL-preserved erythrocyte 24-hour posttransfusion survival values were only 75% after 35 days (Fig 3–11). The nonviable erythrocytes were removed by an extravascular procedure. Plasma hemoglobin levels did not increase, nor was there any decrease in haptoglobin value. Oxygen-transport function was less than 10% of normal 2,3 diphosphoglycerate levels after 2 weeks' storage.

The rate of restoration of 2,3 diphosphoglycerate in ADSOL-preserved erythrocytes may be impaired by prolonged storage. This finding is particularly important in light of other risks currently associated with blood transfusion. Patients should receive preserved erythrocytes of the highest quality.

▶ This study emphasizes the problems of clinicians evaluating various preservatives of red blood cells. The national standard is simply to define the 24-hour survival rate of red blood cells without regard to their overall function. This article indicates that, while it is legal to store red cells for 49 days, perhaps their overall function is hampered sufficiently that perhaps that time should be reduced. In any event the pursuit for long-term storage persists.—R.D. Miller, M.D.

Further Evidence Supporting a Cause and Effect Relationship Between Blood Transfusion and Earlier Cancer Recurrence

Blumberg N, Heal J, Chuang C, Murphy P, Agarwal M (Univ of Rochester; American Red Cross Blood Services, Rochester Region, Rochester, NY; Upjohn Co, Kalamazoo, Mich)
Ann Surg 207:410–415, April 1988   13–43

Studies on the relationship between perioperative blood transfusions and later recurrence of solid tumors have yielded conflicting results, partly because of differing patterns of blood component usage. A previous analysis of data on patients given transfusions suggested that tumor recurrence was associated with transfusion of whole blood as opposed to red blood cell concentrates. Additional analyses of 216 transfused patients with cancers of the colon, rectum, cervix, and prostate were undertaken to determine whether those receiving whole blood, red blood cells only, or no transfusions had differing outcomes. A total of 354 nontransfused patients with cancer served as control.

Patients given at least 1 unit of whole blood had significantly uniform poor outcomes compared with nontranfused patients. In contrast, patients receiving only red blood cells had progressively worse recurrence and death rates with increasing number of transfusions, suggesting a dose-effect relationship. Multivariate analysis showed that blood transfusions of 3 or fewer units of blood, including at least 1 unit of whole blood, were significantly and independently associated with earlier recurrences and death caused by cancer. In contrast, transfusions of 3 or fewer units of red blood cell concentrates only were associated with no greater risk of recurrence than that in nontransfused patients.

Blood transfusion with plasma-rich components (e.g., whole blood) appears to increase the risk of solid tumor recurrence. Strategies for reducing this risk include avoidance of whole blood transfusions when only 1– 3 units are required, more conservative transfusion practices, use of autologous blood transfusions, and, perhaps, use of red blood cells washed free of plasma and white blood cell debris.

▶ The immunodepressant effects of homologous blood transfusions are well documented. Many reports are now appearing that blood transfusions have an influence on the development of cancer and other immunodepressive diseases such as AIDS.— R.D. Miller, M.D.

Autologous Blood Transfusion in a Pediatric Population: Safety and Efficacy
Novak RW (Children's Hosp Med Ctr, Akron, Ohio)
Clin Pediatr (Phila) 27:184–187, April 1988   13–44

The potential for transmission of viral infections via blood transfusions has increased the popularity of autologous blood transfusion in adults. An autologous transfusion program was established specifically for pediatric patients.

During a 2-year period, 82 patients aged 8–16 years, who underwent 82 surgical procedures, participated in a blood transfusion program for the preoperative collection and intraoperative salvage of autologous blood. To donate at least 200 ml of blood safely at a time, children had to weigh more than 45 kg, be able to cooperate with the donation procedure, and be free of medical conditions that would contraindicate blood donation.

Of 34 patients who had blood collected before operation, 22 also participated in the intraoperative blood salvage program. The other 48 patients participated only in the intraoperative salvage program because they did not meet the requirements for preoperative blood collection. The surgical procedures included 76 (93%) spinal fusions for scoliosis, 3 other orthopedic procedures, and 3 plastic surgical procedures.

For the 48 patients in the blood salvage only program, volumes of blood salvaged and reinfused ranged from 100 ml to 1,490 ml, constituting a salvage of 9% to 53% of the patient's calculated blood volume, with a median of 18% of blood volume being salvaged. Autologous blood obtained by salvage accounted for an average of 48% of the blood used in surgery. Five patients (10%) had all of their blood needs met by salvaged blood. For the 12 patients in the blood-donation-only program, preoperatively collected blood met an average of 74% of blood needs when used alone, and in 6 (50%) patients it was the only blood required.

For the 22 patients in the combined program, autologous blood accounted for an average of 94% of the blood used, and 17 patients (77%) required only autologous blood for their surgery. No intraoperative or postoperative complications could be attributed to either the salvage of blood or its reinfusion.

The results demonstrate that programs of elective preoperative autologous blood collection and intraoperative salvage of autologous blood in a pediatric population are safe.

▶ It is encouraging to know that this very useful form of blood transfusion can be applied to the pediatric population.—R.D. Miller, M.D.

An Automatic Autotransfusion System With a Centrifugal Pump: A Hematologic Evaluation in Dogs
ten Duis HJ, Harder MP, Wabeke E, Elstrodt J, Wildevuur CRH (Univ Hosp Groningen, the Netherlands)
Surgery 103:74–78, January 1988   13–45

An on-line autotransfusion system (ATS) must have sufficient capacity for reinfusing shed blood, optimal hemocompatibility, ability to prevent reinfusion of aspirated air, and ease of operation. Previously, a diaphragm pump was tested in a pneumatically driven ATS that met these requirements. In a further study, a centrifugal pump was tested as an outflow pump in the same system.

The conventional ATS was driven by 2 roller pumps. One was used to aspirate blood into a cardiotomy reservoir, and the other, to reinfuse the blood from the reservoir into the systemic circulation. Anesthetized mongrel dogs were treated with either a centrifugal pump or a diaphragm pump. Platelet numbers in both groups decreased to about 25% of initial values within the first few minutes of autotransfusion. Platelet numbers gradually recovered, the centrifugal pump group's at a lower level. Platelet function was well preserved during autotransfusion in both groups. Plasma hemoglobin concentrations steadily increased during autotransfusion. Concentrations in the centrifugal pump group increased at lower values.

The newly developed ATS combined with a centrifugal pump met the requirements for an on-line system. The ATS caused little damage to the blood elements. It can process a sufficient amount of blood and can be used easily and safely be inexperienced operators.

▶ In the continuing evolution of autotransfusion systems, this article presents the success of the centrifugal pump that is on-line and can meet the requirements of being easy to set up and operate by nonspecialized personnel and be relatively inexpensive. Unfortunately, a complete description of this system is not provided. One of the key parts that seems to be advanced in this system is that an aspiration of air along with blood was prevented by an electronically regulated suction system with 2 electrodes mounted on the sucker tip, which measured blood level and regulated the vacuum by activating a tubing clamp that compressed the suction line over a distance of 3 mm. In this way, the blood level was kept constant above the opening in the tip, preventing air from entering the suction line. Whether this system would be useful where the surgeon has to see the field at all times is not clear in my mind, and I wait for further trials of this system.—M.F. Roizen, M.D.

Synthetic Blood Products

Deleterious Effects of Stroma-Free Hemoglobin Used as Resuscitative Fluid for Rats With Ischemic Intestinal Shock

Dawidson I, Drukker S, Hedlund B, Marks DH, Reisch J (Univ of Texas, Dallas; Univ of Minnesota; Letterman Army Inst of Research, Presidio of San Francisco)
Crit Care Med 16:606–609, June 1988   13–46

There has long been considerable interest in developing a stroma-free hemoglobin solution (SFHS) as a resuscitative fluid for use in the treatment of shock. Whereas other resuscitative fluids (e.g., lactated Ringer's solution, albumin, and dextran) provide adequate volume expansion and oncotic pressure, they lack oxygen-carrying capacity. The effect of an SFHS containing Ringer's lactate and 3% human serum albumin on recovery from ischemic intestinal shock was evaluated in 4 groups of 8 Wistar rats subjected to shock and catheter placement.

After the induction of shock, resuscitative fluid was administered intravenously for a 6-hour period. Eight rats were treated Ringer's lactate alone; 8 rats, with 3% albumin alone; and 8 rats, with SFHS; 8 rats served as controls. The hematocrit was used to estimate changes in intravascular volume.

All 8 control animals died within 24 hours. All 8 given Ringer's lactate and 7 of the 8 albumin-treated animals survived for the 7-day study period. Only 2 of the 8 SFHS-treated animals survived for 7 days; the other 6 animals died within the first 24 hours. The difference between the control group and the SFHS group was not statistically significant.

Hemoconcentration developed in the 8 control animals, and all had a 50% loss in plasma volume. Stroma-free hemoglobin solution only partially expanded the intravascular volume. This finding was surprising, as identical volumes of albumin-containing solution were administered to the albumin-treated animals and to the SFHS-treated animals. Several mechanisms could be responsible for the failure of hemoglobin to afford protection during the postshock period, including the intrinsic nephrotoxicity of the hemoglobin solution, or the interference of hemoglobin with the repair process. Further studies to examine these mechanisms are in progress.

▶ Stroma-free hemoglobin has long been thought to be a possibility for developing a synthetic hemoglobin-carrying solution. Unfortunately, it looks as if the toxicity will prevent its usefulness.—R.D. Miller, M.D.

Protection Against Myocardial Ischaemia by Prior Haemodilution With Fluorocarbon Emulsions

Faithfull NS, Fennema M, Erdmann W (Hope Hosp, Salford, England; Erasmus Univ, Rotterdam, the Netherlands)
Br J Anaesth 60:773–778, 1988   13–47

Fluorocarbons have a high solubility for respiratory and other gases. Fluosol-DA 20% (FDA) is a plasma substitute consisting of emulsified fluorocarbons with an oxygen solubility about 2.5 times that of plasma. When used for hemodilution in experimental animals, FDA decreases myocardial infarction by improving intramyocardial oxygen tension. Whether hemodilution with FDA could be used prophylactically to protect against subsequent myocardial ischemia was investigated.

Precalibrated oxygen microelectrodes were inserted into the myocardium of the left ventricle in 2 groups of anesthetized immature pigs. One group of pigs were hemodiluted by removal of blood and immediate volume replacement with FDA. The other group of animals served as controls. Both groups received 100% oxygen plus halothane for at least 30 minutes before the lower third of the left anterior descending coronary artery (LAD) was occluded by tightening the perivascular ligature. The experiments were concluded 3 hours after occlusion by ventilating the animals' lung with 100% nitrous oxide.

Before LAD occlusion, cardiac output in the FDA-treated animals was significantly greater, and systemic vascular resistance was significantly less than in the controls, but there were no significant differences in whole body oxygen consumption or flux (table). There were no significant changes in cardiovascular variables or indices of oxygenation immediately after occlusion of the LAD in either group. However, at 1, 2, and 3 hours after LAD occlusion, whole body oxygen delivery and consumption values in the FDA-treated group were significantly higher than those in the control group (Figs 13–12 and 13–13), suggesting greater hyperemic compensatory response in ischemic border areas in FDA-treated animals.

Changes in Mean Whole Body Oxygen Delivery and Consumption After Terminal Left Anterior Coronary Artery (LAD) Occlusion in Pigs in Control or Fluosol-DA 20% Diluted Animals (FDA)

	Before LAD occlusion		1 h		2 h		3 h	
	Control	FDA	Control	FDA	Control	FDA	Control	FDA
Whole body oxygen	14.3	20.1	13.4	16.6	14.1	18.1	15.9	17.1
delivery (ml min^{-1} kg^{-1})	±2.69	±1.92	±2.57	±0.96	±2.45	±1.05	±1.67	±2.01
n	4	5	4	5	4	5	4	5
Whole body oxygen	6.2	8.9	5.5	8.9*	6.2	9.3*	6.8	8.7*
consumption (ml min^{-1} kg^{-1})	±0.75	±0.86	±0.88	±0.57	±0.97	±0.46	±0.38	±0.67
n	4	5	4	5	4	5	4	5

n, number of observations.
*Significant difference from control group.
(Courtesy of Faithful NS, Fennema M, Erdmann W: Br J Anaesth 60:773–778, 1988.)

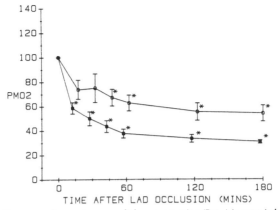

Fig 13–12.—Percentage changes in myocardial oxygen tension (Pmo₂) in most ischemic area of myocardial infarction in pigs. *Shaded squares,* control group. *Open squares,* group receiving prior hemodilution with Fluosol-DA 20%. *Significant decrease in Pmo₂. (Courtesy of Faithfull NS, Fennema N, Erdmann W: *Br J Anaesth* 60:773–778, 1988.)

Although prior hemodilution with FDA did not completely prevent decreases in myocardial oxygen tension in ischemic areas in this pig model of myocardial infarction, FDA reduced the changes in myocardial oxygen tension substantially, and delayed the onset of ischemia.

► For some reason that currently defies logic, the fluorocarbon emulsion Fluosol-DA 20% provides protection against CNS ischemia and has been reported to protect during balloon angioplasty of the coronary arteries when perfused through the open end of the angioplasty catheter. In this study, the hypothesis was advanced that hemodilution used with fluorocarbon emulsion as a diluent would in fact provide protection against an experimental myocardial ischemic episode induced in a pig. Pigs were used because their circulation re-

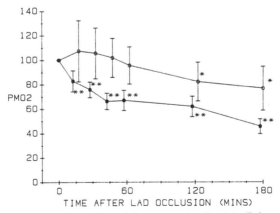

Fig 13–13.—Percentage changes in myocardial oxygen tension (Pmo₂) in all electrodes during myocardial infarction in pigs. *Shaded squares,* control group. *Open squares,* group receiving prior hemodilution with Fluosol-DA 20%. *Significant decrease in Pmo₂. (Courtesy of Faithfull NS, Fennema N, Erdmann W: *Br J Anaesth* 60:773–778, 1988.)

sembles that of the human being, as do their responses to ischemia. Interestingly enough, and again defying logic, the emulsion was protective. Possible reasons why the emulsion was protective involve the fact that hemodilution alone would be protective, and that's a deficit of this study: there was no control group of hemodilution alone. A second reason that could be advanced is that the emulsions have lower viscosity, and thus the viscosity characteristics of blood improve. Fluosol-DA by itself shouldn't deliver more O_2, but somehow it seems to do so. Nevertheless, it seems that this Fluosol-DA 20% has a role in protecting against ischemia. Were this to be its initial indication instead of as a blood substitute, it probably would already be available to use. It looks like there is a use for this, but exactly where it will fit clinically remains to be determined.—M.F. Roizen, M.D.

Sociology

Ventilator Use in Progressive Neuromuscular Disease: Impact on Patients and Their Families
Miller JR, Colbert AP, Schock NC (Tufts Univ; Lexington, Mass)
Dev Med Child Neurol 30:200–207, April 1988   13–48

Patients with progressive neuromuscular disease experience respiratory failure in the final stages of the disease. The use of ventilators to extend their lives is controversial. A number of practical and ethical questions are relevant to the decision to request or refuse mechanical assistance. Quality of life, individual and family stress, and financial factors all must be considered. For the first phase of a 4-part project, 15 individuals— patients and family members—who had chosen ventilator assistance were interviewed.

The study involved 8 patients with Duchenne muscular dystrophy (DMD), 1 with myotubular myopathy, and 1 with type II spinal atrophy. Daily time required on the ventilator ranged from 2 to 24 hours. The patient interviewees were aged between 16 and 31 years.

Although the progress of the disease was predictable, most believed that the decision to ventilate was made at a time of crisis; the onset of respiratory failure. Most saw the ventilator as a way to increase patient comfort, not as a life-extending device. Family members felt the burden of being continuously tied to machine monitoring. The possibility of respiratory infection and equipment breakdown were constant worries. Patients had similar concerns, as well as feelings of inadequacy and loneliness. Almost all of those with DMD felt physically better as a result of ventilator use.

Families agreed on the need for increased community resources, counseling, and financial assistance. A discussion of problems and options before ventilator use is necessary would allow patients and their families to make a well-informed choice. Many may decide not to extend life, and that choice should be supported.

▶ There is, of course, no right answer to the question of ventilator support in fatal illness. When I read this article, I was reminded of similar studies concerning mechanical ventilation of AIDS patients. The medical, ethical, and sometimes legal questions are among the most difficult to answer for critical care practitioners. They obviously are even more difficult for patients and their families.—R.R. Kirby, M.D.

Electroencephalographic Activity After Brain Death
Grigg MM, Kelly MA, Celesia GG, Ghobrial MW, Ross ER (Loyola Univ, Maywood, Ill)
Arch Neurol 44:948–954, September 1987   13–49

The reliability of the EEG to confirm brain death continues to be controversial. A study was done to determine how often EEG activity persists in patients who fulfill all clinical criteria for brain death.

From January 1984 through May 1986, 56 patients at 1 institution were clinically diagnosed as brain dead. Every patient had at least 1 EEG recording after this diagnosis. Eleven (19.6%) exhibited EEG activity after the diagnosis of brain death. The duration of the observed EEG activity was 2–168 hours, with a mean of 36.6 hours. Three patterns of EEG activity were noted. The first was low-voltage, 4–20 μV, theta or beta activity, recorded for 9 patients (16.1%) for as long as 72 hours after brain death. In 1 of these patients, neuropathologic studies revealed hypoxic-ischemic neuronal changes involving all cell layers of the cerebral cortex, basal ganglia, brain stem, and cerebellum.

The second pattern noted was a sleep-like activity: a mixture of synchronous 30–40 μV theta and delta activity and 60–80 μV, 10–12 Hz spindle-like potentials. This was observed in 2 patients (3.6%) for as long as 168 hours after brain death. Pathologic studies in both patients demonstrated ischemic necrosis of the brain stem with relative preservation of the cerebral cortex. The third pattern was an alpha-like activity—monotonous, unreactive, anteriorly predominant, 25–40 μV, 9–12 Hz activity—noted in 1 patient (1.8%) 3 hours after brain death. No patients recovered irrespective of EEG activity.

Using EEG activity after brain death as a confirmatory test of brain death appears to be of questionable value.

▶ I don't like to quibble with a choice of words, but "dead is dead." These patients may have been persistently vegetative and irreversibly comatose, but their brains were not dead. Maybe this distinction makes no clinical difference (a point that has been debated vigorously for the past 15–20 years), but the finding of some electrical activity in patients who are declared brain dead on clinical grounds is commonplace. One of the reasons the original Harvard criteria for brain death were challenged was that they were so rigid; they allowed no possibility to apply clinical judgment to an obviously hopeless but possibly long-term unconscious existence. In view of the fact that none of the patients in Grigg's series survived, the abnormal EEG activity they noted certainly was predictable of a bad outcome, even if it did not equate with cerebral electrical silence.—R.R. Kirby, M.D.

Risk Preference and Decision Making in Critical Care Situations
Nightingale SD, Grant M (Cook County Hosp, Chicago)
Chest 93:684–687, April 1988   13–50

Risk and uncertainty are common elements of critical care situations. The physicians' attitudes toward risk may influence their behavior in these situations. To determine whether this risk preference is associated with the attitudes and practices of physicians in instituting and terminating maximal efforts to prolong life, physicians' responses to a questionnaire about risk were compared with their preferences for "intubation" or "current therapy without intubation" for a hypothetical patient with end-stage lung disease whose condition deteriorated despite appropriate medical therapy. The duration of cardiopulmonary resuscitation before they declared their efforts unsuccessful was also assessed.

In the face of loss, the choice of risky alternative was significantly associated with greater preference for "intubation" and with longer duration of resuscitation efforts. The physicians' risk preferences in the face of gain was not associated with the use of critical care resources.

These results indicate that at least part of the variation in physician attitudes and practices in the care of critically or terminally ill patients reflects measurable psychological differences among individual physicians.

▶ Obviously, physician attitudes play a role in their decision making. Whether these attitudes can be ascertained correctly with a questionnaire in the controlled setting of a quiet office is open to question. Having participated in similar surveys in the past, I am aware of the difficulty in differentiating my actual preference for a given course of action from what I thought was the "correct" answer. Nevertheless, studies such as these are important as a means to understanding our motives and responses.— R.R. Kirby, M.D.

Interpreting Survival Rates for the Treatment of Decompensated Diabetes: Are We Saving Too Many Lives?
Yudkin JS, Doyal LT, Hurwitz BS (Whittington Hosp, London; Middlesex Polytechnic, London)
Lancet 2:1192–1195, Nov 21, 1987   13–51

As many as 25% of elderly patients with decompensated diabetes die. The recent admission of such a patient raised ethical concerns on the part of the medical staff. Two-hundred diabetologists and an equal number of cardiologists were surveyed as to their management of diabetes and their therapeutic approaches to cardiac arrest in 3 elderly patients admitted with severe decompensated diabetes. The response rate was only 27%.

The patients were more likely to be treated for decompensated diabetes than for cardiac arrest. In some circumstances, however, the respondents would not treat the diabetes. In the most problematic patients, the acute event might be a terminal manifestations of irreversible underlying disease; in other patients, the quality of life might be so low that treatment would merely prolong suffering. Cardiac arrest often is a euphemism for death. Even when it is not, the risks are greater than in other patients with decompensated diabetes. However, treatment of decompensated diabetes often is merely symptomatic, and it is more difficult to define decompensated diabetes than cardiac arrest.

If a clinical ethics committee is formed, resuscitation policies can be explicitly drawn up. Discussions of specific cases are a logical part of this approach.

▶ This article looked at the decision to resuscitate from decompensated diabetes. In this case, decompensated diabetes was described as diabetic ketoacidosis with a bicarbonate of less than 14 mmole/L and hyperosmolar state. "Resuscitated from cardiac arrest" was descriptive of a patient who had to have full resuscitative measures. The authors then surveyed the physicians in their hospital to see who would propose resuscitation of patients from these situations.

I think the usefulness of the article is its confirmation of most of the thought patterns I have seen practiced. As the authors state, many decisions about resuscitation in life-threatening medical emergencies need to be made without delay and with little background information. In those circumstances, the patient is usually given full resuscitation. In other circumstances, when more time is available and more information is known about the patient, a consistent ethical approach would be to provide care as vigorously as necessary at all times to produce an improvement in the quality of life of the patient, a state of enjoying life at the present moment despite any physical or mental limitations and with a pleasurable anticipation for the future. However, this quality-of-life judgment has usually been left up to the physician.

The physicians in this study almost universally resuscitated patients from diabetic decompensation, even though treatment of severe decompensated diabetes often does no more than provide symptom relief. Of the diabetic patients decompensated, between 50% and 80% of them survived the acute hospitalization. On the other hand, cardiac arrest patients have a much lower in-hospital survival rate. As it turned out, most physicians would provide total resuscitation from dysrhythmia-induced cardiac arrest, and many fewer would provide full resuscitation from mechanically induced cardiac arrest.

In addition, the article points out that studies have shown poor agreement between patients' stated views about their wishes to be resuscitated and those of their doctors. This finding suggests that the concordance between a proxy decision by doctors about the patient's quality of life and the patient's decision would be low. In the absence of a living will, much of the decision making about resuscitation is ad hoc and informal, and it seems incongruous that the person upon whom the decision is going to have the most effect is the one least likely to be consulted or to have known about it.

It seems likely to conclude that, in Great Britain and probably in the United States, patients should assume that they will receive emergency resuscitation treatment unless they have specifically and in writing requested otherwise. We are being told that we have to be especially concerned about spending so much money for so little gain in the quality of life in the last year of life. Perhaps we should be educating patients more about their ability to control their desire for their own resuscitation because clearly, if they don't make a decision, the survey indicates that they will be resuscitated.—M.F. Roizen, M.D.

Mortality and Quality of Life After Intensive Care for Critical Illness
Jacobs CJ, van der Vliet JA, van Roozendaal MT, van der Linden CJ (Univ Hosp, Maastricht, the Netherlands)
Intensive Care Med 14:217–220, 1988   13–52

Treating critically ill patients in high-technology intensive care units (ICUs) is complex and expensive. Reproducible cost-benefit data are needed urgently to assess the efficacy of intensive care for the various types of critical illness. The long-term quality of life and early and late mortality were investigated in ICU survivors.

Of 313 ICU patients studied, 118 were long-term survivors. The survival rate at discharge from the ICU was 76%, dropping to 61% at 6 months and to 58% at 1 year. A simplified acute physiology score was determined at admission to the ICU. Also recorded were age, length of stay in the ICU, and number of complications during intensive care. Information on housing, drug use, hospital admissions, physical condition, and functional status 2 years after ICU discharge was elicited from long-term survivors by means of a questionnaire. No significant changes in housing were reported, but drug use and the number of hospital admissions were significantly increased. Twenty-one percent of the patients had a deteriorating condition, 77% remained unchanged, and 2% were improved, compared with their condition before their acute illness (Table

TABLE 1.—Physical Complaints 2 Years After Intensive Care

		Minor complaints	Major complaints	
Age	<53 y ($n = 35$)	26 (74.3%)	9 (25.7%)	$p<0.001$ [a]
Age	>53 y ($n = 55$)	25 (45.5%)	30 (54.5%)	
SAPS	<10.7 ($n = 42$)	33 (78.6%)	9 (21.4%)	$p<0.001$ [a]
SAPS	>10.7 ($n = 48$)	18 (37.5%)	30 (62.5%)	
ICU-stay				
	<4 days ($n = 66$)	41 (62.1%)	25 (37.9%)	NS
ICU-stay				
	>4 days ($n = 24$)	10 (41.7%)	14 (58.3%)	
No				
Complications ($n = 74$)		43 (58.1%)	31 (41.9%)	NS
Complications ($n = 16$)		8 (50.0%)	8 (50.0%)	

[a]Chi-square test.
(Courtesy of Jacobs CJ, van der Vliet JA, van Roozendaal MT, et al: *Intensive Care Med* 14:217–220, 1988.)

TABLE 2.—Functional Status 2 Years After Intensive Care

		No to mild restriction	Severe to total restriction	
Age	<53 y (n = 35)	27 (77.1%)	8 (22.9%)	$p < 0.025$[a]
Age	>53 y (n = 55)	29 (52.7%)	26 (47.3%)	
SAPS	<10.7 (n = 42)	34 (81.0%)	8 (19.0%)	$p > 0.005$[a]
SAPS	>10.7 (n = 48)	22 (45.8%)	26 (54.2%)	
ICU-stay				
	<4 days (n = 66)	43 (65.2%)	23 (34.8%)	NS
ICU-stay				
	>4 days (n = 24)	13 (54.2%)	11 (45.8%)	
No				
Complications (n = 74)		46 (62.2%)	28 (37.8%)	NS
Complications (n = 16)		10 (62.5%)	6 (37.5%)	

[a]Chi-square test.
(Courtesy of Jacobs CJ, van der Vliet JA, van Roozendaal MT, et al: *Intensive Care Med* 14:217–220, 1988.)

1). Thirty-eight percent of the patients had major functional impairment (Table 2). The long-term physical condition and functional status were correlated with simplified acute physiology score and age on ICU admission, but the best indicator of quality of life after intensive care proved to be health status before acute illness.

Previous health status strongly influences the long-term outcome and simplified acute physiology score is a good indicator of the risk of death from critical illness. Most of the patients in this series did not suffer from major physical complaints and functioned without assistance after 2 years. Compared with functional status before ICU admission, 21% worsened to a state of dependency.

▶ This study is important because it says that the quality of life after a stay in the intensive care unit is more dependent on the patient's health status before illness than on the acute nature of the illness. This conclusion is controversial in that most people and most logic would dictate that the acute illness would have a major role on the quality of life after ICU care. But apparently the people who were severely ill died. Of the 313 intensive care unit patients admitted to the ICU, 58% of those survived 1 year. Of those who were able to be assessed (and those who were admitted to the intensive care unit because of drug intoxications were not), 38% of the patients were found to have major functional impairments. Thus, of 313 patients admitted, approximately 56 had excellent functional status 2 years after discharge from the intensive care unit.

In this day when we are trying to look at benefit-risk analysis and cost-benefit analysis so that we can more appropriately deploy medical resources, studies like this are important preliminary steps in determining what the medical profession's position should be on where to devote resources for medical care.

This study clearly implied that health status before illness was an important gauge of how vigorously one should pursue and treat. Unfortunately, health status measures for perioperative care in the nonintensive care unit patient are not well established and are expensive to obtain. I believe this article points out the need to get better measures of health status and then to study how valuable those are in predicting outcome and benefits of care.—M.F. Roizen, M.D.

14 Management of Cardiac Pain

Concerning the Management of Pain Associated With Herpes Zoster and of Postherpetic Neuralgia
King RB (State Univ of New York, Syracuse)
Pain 33:73–78, April 1988   14–1

Pain relief for patients with acute shingles or chronic postherpetic neuralgia is difficult to achieve because the available therapeutic regimens are usually only marginally effective. A simple method was developed for controlling the severe pain of acute shingles. Findings for 12 recently treated patients were reviewed.

Method.—The method involves crushing 2 aspirin tablets to a fine powder, after which 15–30 ml of chloroform is added and stirred to uniform cloudiness. A sterile cotton ball is saturated with the suspension and daubed onto the painful hyperpathic area in such a manner that the skin is uniformly covered with powdered aspirin after the chloroform has evaporated. Pain relief is evaluated after 30 minutes.

Three males and 3 females aged 13–84 years with moderate to severe pain from acute herpes zoster, and 3 men and 3 women aged 58–84 years with moderate to severe pain from postherpetic neuralgia, were treated with the aspirin-chloroform suspension. Seven patients experienced pain relief within 10 minutes of application. After 30 minutes, all patients reported significant pain relief. Patients with moderate pain usually reported less dramatic relief. Pain relief generally lasted for 4–6 hours and then gradually returned, but some patients experienced relief for 10–12 hours after only 1 application. Patients usually had to apply the suspension 2–3 times per day to maintain adequate pain relief, with the third application scheduled to coincide with bedtime.

Chloroform alone, applied in 3 patients, cooled the skin but gave no lasting relief. Similarly, a solution of crushed aspirin suspended in water was ineffective. Aspirin in acetone, applied in 2 patients, was useful but not as effective as aspirin in chloroform. It is thought that the chloroform functions as a solvent, cleansing the skin of fats, waxes, and oils and leaving the aspirin in the interstices of the abnormal skin surface in close proximity to cutaneous nociceptors at the site of the herpetic inflammatory process.

▶ This is an unbelievable combination in which the number of patients studied is too small to provide any convincing results. However, this is such a horrible disease, with the results of various treatments largely ineffective, that this suggestion deserves serious consideration.— R.D. Miller, M.D.

Factors Influencing the Duration of Treatment of Acute Herpetic Pain With Sympathetic Nerve Block: Importance of Severity of Herpes Zoster Assessed by Maximum Antibody Titers to Varicella-Zoster Virus in Otherwise Healthy Patients
Higa K, Dan K, Manabe H, Noda B (Fukuoka Univ, Fukuoka, Japan)
Pain 32:147–157, February 1988   14–2

It is generally accepted that aging is the most important risk factor in prolonged treatment of acute herpetic pain and in the possible progression to postherpetic neuralgia. Most studies, however, have not taken into account the severity of herpes zoster. To determine whether there are mutual relationships among severities of skin lesions of herpes zoster, maximum antibody titers to varicella-zoster virus (VZV), and duration of treatment for acute hepatic pain, antibody responses to VZV were serially investigated by the complement fixation test in 72 Japanese individuals with herpes zoster but otherwise healthy. Based on severity of skin lesions, the patients were subdivided into mild (26 patients), moderate (26), and severe (20) groups. All were treated with regional sympathetic nerve blocks until pain relief was achieved.

Irrespective of age, the maximum antibody titers to VZV closely paralleled the severities of the skin lesions of herpes zoster. The duration of treatment for acute herpetic pain became significantly longer as herpes zoster increased in severity. In the entire group of patients, a highly significant positive linear correlation was demonstrated between maximum antibody titers and duration of treatment.

These findings show that, irrespective of age, the severity of herpes zoster in otherwise healthy patients can be defined objectively and quantitatively by the maximum antibody titers to VZV, and that the severity of herpes zoster itself rather than age greatly influences the duration of treatment of acute herpetic pain with intensive sympathetic nerve blocks. Reports concerning the treatment of acute herpetic pain should include data on the severity of herpes zoster, and the results should be analyzed according to this severity, defined preferably by the maximum antibody titers to VZV in otherwise healthy patients.

▶ A devastating disease; this study is encouraging in that we can provide better predictive data as to how effective we will be in treating it.— R.D. Miller, M.D.

The Effects of Myofascial Trigger Point Injections Are Naloxone Reversible
Fine PG, Milano R, Hare BD (Univ of Utah)
Pain 32:15–20, January 1988   14–3

A myofascial trigger point is a hyperirritable spot within a band of skeletal muscle or its fascia, which is painful when compressed. Injection of such a point with local anesthetic is a safe and effective treatment. In a double-blind crossover study, a 1-ml dose of 0.25% bupivacaine was injected into adults having acute or long-standing muscle pain when a trigger point was identified. Naloxone, 10 mg, or a saline placebo was then administered intravenously.

Trigger point injection of local anesthetic consistently relieved pain in the 10 patients who completed crossover trials. In addition, range of motion increased and palpable bands disappeared. All these effects were reversed by intravenously administered naloxone, compared with placebo.

Much of the improvement that follows injection of a trigger point with local anesthetic is reversed by naloxone, which implies that an endogenous opioid system mediates the lessening of pain seen with trigger point injection. The trigger point may represent sensitization of spinal wide-dynamic-range neurons by a peripheral nociceptive stimulus. These neurons then respond to otherwise subthreshold mechanical afferent volleys such as those produced by pressure, stretch, and tonic posture.

▶ This is a fascinating observation. However, the "cause and effect" relationship is unclear. Is naloxone a more complicated drug than we had once thought? In other words, does it have more activity than simply being a narcotic antagonist? It is not surprising that relief of pain is involved with the endogenous opioid system. However, it is difficult to imagine that the simple injection of a local anesthetic would result in an increase in opioids. What would happen if the trigger points were simply penetrated with needles without local anesthetic, i.e., acupuncture? Independent of the mechanism, this is a fascinating article.— R.D. Miller, M.D.

A Retrospective Analysis of the Efficacy of Epidural Steroid Injections
Rosen CD, Kahanovitz N, Bernstein R, Viola K (Hosp for Joint Diseases Orthopaedic Inst, New York)
Clin Orthop 228:270–272, March 1988   14–4

Epidural steroid injection in the management of low back pain and sciatica from spinal stenosis or a herniated lumbar disk is considered a more aggressive form of treatment than standard conservative therapy but less aggressive than surgery. Because few studies have systematically and accurately assessed the efficacy of epidural steroid injections, the records of 40 patients who had received this form of treatment were reviewed retrospectively.

All 40 patients had symptoms and findings consistent with a herniated lumbar disk or spinal stenosis; 39 had symptoms of sciatica in addition to low back pain. The patients ranged in age from 26 to 79 years and were treated on an inpatient basis. Each patient received 1–5 epidural injections with 2 cc of Depomedrol–40. All patients were injected by the same anesthesiologist. Limited ambulation was allowed on the night of the injection. Each patient was asked to rate the pain in the legs and back on a 10-point rating scale immediately after injection and at the time of follow-up examination. Follow-up ranged from 3 to 24 months (average, 8 months).

Thirty-six patients (90%) received either 1, 2, or 3 injections; the other 4 patients received 4 or 5 injections. Sixteen patients (40%) claimed no relief at all in the immediate postinjection period, whereas the other 24 (60%) reported relief of leg and back pain. At follow-up evaluation only 10 (25%) patients remained asymptomatic; 13 (32%) reported varying degrees of improvement, and 17 (43%) claimed no relief by preinjection pain. Further, 53% of the patients had been unable to return to normal activities at the time of follow-up, and 12% eventually had to undergo operation. Half of the patients stated that they were dissatisfied with epidural injection as a form of treatment.

Because epidural steroid injections yielded a positive clinical response in only half of the treated patients, this form of therapy should be considered of questionable clinical value and should not be used in the long-term management of spinal stenosis or nerve root compression.

▶ Even if the epidural steroid yields improvement in only half of the treated patients, doesn't this justify its continued use.—R.D. Miller, M.D.

Regional Sympathetic Blockade in Primary Fibromyalgia
Bengtsson A, Bengtsson M (Univ Hosp, Linköping, Sweden)
Pain 33:161–167, May 1988   14–5

Primary fibromyalgia is characterized by chronic pain, stiffness, muscle fatigue, and the presence of trigger points or tender points. The condition occurs predominantly in women. Recent studies have shown that these patients have disturbances of the microcirculation. An attempt was made to determine whether sympathetic blockade, which is known to improve the microcirculation, would reduce the rest pain and the number of trigger points in patients with primary fibromyalgia.

The study population consisted of 27 women and 1 man with primary fibromyalgia. Eight patients received regional sympathetic blockade initially with bupivacaine and 14 days later with guanethidine intravenously; 10 patients received placebo blockade using saline solution; and 10 others were given intramuscular bupivacaine injections. After treatment, each patient underwent repeated pin-prick testing. Skin blood flow was recorded with a laser Doppler flowmeter and skin temperature with a fast responding thermistor-thermometer; the trigger points of the arm, shoulder, and neck on the side of blockade were counted by digital pressure provocation. Rest pain was evaluated on a linear visual analog pain scale.

Analysis of the data shows that complete sympathetic blockade produced by a stellate ganglion blockade markedly reduced the number of trigger points and markedly decreased rest pain. Although guanethidine blockade reduced the number of trigger points, it had no effect on rest pain. Sham stellate ganglion blockade with saline and bupivacaine injections intramuscularly did not significantly affect either rest pain or the number of trigger points in any of the control patients.

Complete sympathetic blockade produced by stellate ganglion blockade using a local anesthetic markedly reduces the rest pain and the number of trigger points in patients with primary fibromyalgia.

▶ This looks to be another pain syndrome of which anesthesiologists should be familiar.— R.D. Miller, M.D.

Subject Index

A

Accidents
  hypothermia after, severe, prognostic
    factors in, 303
  motor vehicle, advanced life support
    after, 297
  during surgery, 80
Acebutolol
  to control cardiovascular response to
    endotracheal intubation, 88
Acid base
  changes, umbilical cord, and perinatal
    cardiac failure, 191
Acidosis
  Carbicarb for hypoxia in, 310
  Carbicarb as substitute for $NaHCO_3$ in,
    309
  metabolic, predictive value in perinatal
    brain damage, 188
Acquired immunodeficiency syndrome (see
    AIDS)
ADSOL
  preserved red blood cells, 323
Age
  morphine dose after abdominal
    hysterectomy and, 243
Aged
  hip fracture, mortality after anesthesia
    for, 141
AIDS
  confidentiality, legal limits of, 7
  directed blood donations and, as
    dilemma, 9
  HIV infection, health care workers
    exposed to blood from, 83
  HIV transmission by transfusion
    screened as negative for HIV
    antibody, 10
  risk for recipients of blood components
    from donors with later AIDS, 9
  virus infection, documentation of, 8
Air (see Embolism, air)
Airway
  management of supraglottitis in
    children, 295
  upper airway obstruction after adult
    respiratory distress syndrome, 282
Alarms
  auditory, during anesthesia monitoring,
    208
Albumin
  lymphatic, effects of Hespan on, 315
Alcohol
  as analgesic, 23
Alcoholic
  liver disease, vecuronium in, 41

Alfentanil
  binding to extracorporeal circuit, 117
  enflurane-sparing effect of (in dog),
    19
Allergy
  to suxamethonium, 55
Alveolar
  capillary perfusion and PEEP, 270
Ambulatory (see Surgery, ambulatory)
Amnesia
  relation to midazolam in surgical
    patients, 28
Analgesia
  catheter, interpleural, for pancreatic
    pain, 239
  epidural
    continuous vs. intermittent, for labor
      and delivery, 173
    implying high forceps rate, 172
    for labor (see Labor, epidural
      analgesia for)
    postoperative, and postoperative
      pulmonary complications, 245
  fentanyl, continuous epidural, in blunt
    chest injury, 307
  opioid, at peripheral sites, 22
  patient-controlled
    for cesarean section pain, epidural vs.
      intramuscular narcotics for, 235
    for children, 233
    after colon surgery, 232
    with narcotics for post-cesarean
      section pain, 235
    for pain management, acute, 234
    after thoracotomy with bupivacaine via
      intrapleural catheter in children,
      238
Analgesic
  alcohol as, 23
Anaphylactic reactions
  to suxamethonium, 54
Anaphylaxis
  to furosemide, IV, 55
Anastomotic
  disruption, colonic, in myasthenia
    gravis, 38
Angiography
  fluorescein, for retinal microvascular
    studies, 107
Anesthesia
  balanced, vecuronium by bolus and
    infusion during, 36
  brachial plexus, bupivacaine in, 103
  for cesarean delivery and neonatal
    status, 194
  contribution to operative mortality, 1
  critical incidents detected by pulse
    oximetry during, 209

343

Author Index

A

Abbott, D., 168
Abboud, T.K., 198
Abouleish, E., 204
Abrouk, F., 265
Acharya, P.A., 105
Acker, D., 192
Adams, S., 114
Adler, S., 115
Admed, S., 162
Agarwal, M., 324
Aguilar, C., 225
Ahlen, K., 105
Ahmed, S.W., 256
Alarcon, J., 245
Alazia, M., 54
Albert, J.M., 232
Albritton, W.L., 165
Aldridge, L.M., 16
Alexander, C.M., 21, 28
Alexander, J.C., 252
Alexander, S.S., 8
Alford, F.P., 111
Ali, H.H., 50, 53
Alila, A., 42
Allan, L.G., 16
Allen, J.R., 9, 10
Alpert, J.S., 211
Altschule, M.D., 323
Amar, R., 24
Anand, K.J.S., 156
Andersen, H.F., 194
Anderson, C.M., 165
Angel, J.J., 166
Ansley, D.M., 212
Antrobus, J.H.L., 62
Aps, C., 110
Arden, J.R., 41
Argov, Z., 226
Arieff, A.I., 310
Arnaud, A., 54
Arnold, J.V., 107
Aromaa, U., 90
Aronson, S., 114
Arthur, G.R., 104
Artru, A.A., 34
Ashton, J., 307
Askanazi, J., 285, 289
Auster, G.H., 194
Avram, M.J., 36, 40
Aynsley-Green, A., 156

B

Bader, A.M., 104, 178
Baguneid, S., 105
Baker, M.D., 244
Banner, M.J., 271
Barach, P.G., 269

Bardgett, D.M., 279
Barnette, R.E., 251
Barnhart, G.R., 300
Baron, L., 260
Barone, D.L., 124
Barrett, J., 301
Barrie, W.W., 81
Barry, M.J., 132, 134, 136
Bartle, E.J., 13, 309
Bartlett, R.L., 297
Basta, S.J., 50, 53
Baumgarten, R.K., 32
Bayer, A.J., 230
Becker, G.L., 200
Beckett, G.J., 16
Bedder, M.D., 103
Beemer, G.H., 48
Benedetti, C., 237
Bengtsson, A., 340
Bengtsson, M., 340
Benotti, P.N., 285
Bent, J.M., 212
Bentley, M.W., 162
Benzarti, M., 54, 55
Berg, A., 152
Bergqvist, D., 262
Bernstein, R., 339
Berrier, J., 69
Berry, W.R., 253
Bersin, R.M., 310
Best, J.D., 111
Bevan, D.R., 44
Bierkamper, G.G., 39
Biondi, J.W., 269
Biscoping, J., 37
Bistrian, B.R., 285
Bizousky, F.P., 290
Bjornson, K.M., 109
Black, J.W., 274
Blackburn, G.L., 285
Blair, E., 189
Blancato, L.S., 186
Blauth, C.I., 107
Blery, C., 72
Blom-Muilwijk, M.C., 281
Blumberg, N., 324
Bodner, D., 137
Boeke, S., 79
Bond-Taylor, W., 97
Bone, M.E., 112
Bonke, B., 79
Bonn, G.G., 159
Bonsu, A.K., 46
Borron, S.W., 49
Bourgain, J.L., 245
Bouwhuis-Hoogerwerf, M.L., 79
Bovill, J.G., 79
Bowen, K.A., 15
Bowie, E.J.W., 261
Bowman, R.J., 11
Boys, R.J., 170
Boysen, P.G., 271

Brand-Elnaggar, J., 83
Brandom, B.W., 51, 52
Brar, H.S., 191
Braunstein, L.T., 49
Bredenberg, C.E., 270
Brett, C.M., 158
Britten, J.S., 296
Brizgys, R.V., 201
Brodsky, D.A., 158
Brook, R.H., 120
Brough, S.J., 81
Brousseau, C., 150
Brown, C.G., 307
Brown, C.K., 171
Brown, D.A.J., 192
Brown, D.E., 195
Brown, J.L., 32
Browner, W., 215
Bubolz, T., 132
Burke, T.J., 176
Burns, H.J.G., 2
Burris, J.F., 221
Burrows, R.F., 167
Busch, E.H., 256
Butler, B.D., 35, 131

C

Cahalan, M.K., 219
Cahalan, M.T., 219
Caldwell, F.T., Jr., 303
Calvey, T.N., 33
Campbell, E.J., 244
Campbell, W.A., 187
Camu, F., 27
Canfell, P.C., 41
Cannon, J.C., 41
Caplan, R.A., 93
Caplan, R.C., 237
Caprini, J.A., 252
Carlon, G.C., 286
Carpenter, R.J., Jr., 43
Carrico, C.J., 260
Carter, C.E., 32
Carter, D.C., 2
Carvalho, J.C.A., 197
Cason, B.A., 218
Caspi, J., 24
Cassisi, N.J., 140
Castagnoli, K.P., 41
Castro, J.L., 186
Celesia, G.G., 331
Chadwick, H.S., 237, 243
Chalmers, T.C., 69
Chance, B., 226
Channa, A.B., 305
Chant, A.D.B., 248
Chaplin, D.D., 55
Charlton, A.J., 151
Charlton, J.E., 113

363